International

REVIEW OF

Neurobiology

Volume 97

International
REVIEW OF
Neurobiology

Volume 97

Translating Mechanisms of Orofacial Neurological Disorder

EDITED BY

MASAYUKI KOBAYASHI

Nihon University School of Dentistry, Tokyo, Japan

NORIAKI KOSHIKAWA

Nihon University School of Dentistry,Tokyo, Japan

KOICHI IWATA

Nihon University School of Dentistry,Tokyo, Japan

JOHN L. WADDINGTON

Molecular & Cellular Therapeutics,
Royal College of Surgeons in Ireland, Dublin, Ireland

ELSEVIER

AMSTERDAM • BOSTON • HEIDELBERG • LONDON
NEW YORK • OXFORD • PARIS • SAN DIEGO
SAN FRANCISCO • SINGAPORE • SYDNEY • TOKYO
Academic Press is an imprint of Elsevier

Academic Press is an imprint of Elsevier
32 Jamestown Road, London, NW1 7BY, UK
Radarweg 29, PO Box 211, 1000 AE Amsterdam, The Netherlands
225 Wyman Street, Waltham, MA 02451, USA
525 B Street, Suite 1900, San Diego, CA 92101-4495, USA

This book is printed on acid-free paper.

For information on all Elsevier publications
visit our website at elsevierdirect.com

ISBN: 978-0-12-385198-7

Printed and bound by CPI Group (UK) Ltd, Croydon, CR0 4YY

Transferred to Digital Print 2011

CONTENTS

Regulation of Orofacial Movement: Amino Acid Mechanisms and Mutant Models

KATSUNORI TOMIYAMA, COLM M.P. O'TUATHAIGH AND JOHN L. WADDINGTON

The Trigeminal Circuits Responsible for Chewing

KARL-GUNNAR WESTBERG AND ARLETTE KOLTA

Ultrastructural Basis for Craniofacial Sensory Processing in the Brainstem

YONG CHUL BAE AND ATSUSHI YOSHIDA

Mechanisms of Nociceptive Transduction and Transmission: A Machinery for Pain Sensation and Tools for Selective Analgesia

Alexander M. Binshtok

Peripheral and Central Mechanisms of Orofacial Inflammatory Pain

Barry J. Sessle

The Role of Trigeminal Interpolaris-Caudalis Transition Zone in Persistent Orofacial Pain

Ke Ren and Ronald Dubner

Physiological Mechanisms of Neuropathic Pain: the Orofacial Region

Koichi Iwata, Yoshiki Imamura, Kuniya Honda and Masamichi Shinoda

Neurobiology of Estrogen Status in Deep Craniofacial Pain

DAVID A BEREITER AND KEIICHIRO OKAMOTO

Macroscopic Connection of Rat Insular Cortex: Anatomical Bases Underlying its Physiological Functions

MASAYUKI KOBAYASHI

The Balance Between Excitation And Inhibition And Functional Sensory Processing in the Somatosensory Cortex

ZHI ZHANG AND QIAN-QUAN SUN

CONTRIBUTORS

Numbers in parentheses indicate the pages on which the authors contributions begin.

Noriaki Koshikawa (1), Department of Pharmacology, Nihon University School of Dentistry, 1-8-13 Kanda-Surugadai, Chiyoda-ku, Tokyo 101-8310, Japan; Division of Oral and Craniomaxillofacial Research, Dental Research Centre, Nihon University School of Dentistry, 1-8-13 Kanda-Surugadai, Chiyoda-ku, Tokyo 101-8310, Japan

Satoshi Fujita (1), Department of Pharmacology, Nihon University School of Dentistry, 1-8-13 Kanda-Surugadai, Chiyoda-ku, Tokyo 101-8310, Japan; Division of Oral and Craniomaxillofacial Research, Dental Research Centre, Nihon University School of Dentistry, 1-8-13 Kanda-Surugadai, Chiyoda-ku, Tokyo 101-8310, Japan

Kazunori Adachi (1), Department of Diagnostic and Therapeutic Sciences, Meikai University School of Dentistry, 1-1 Keyaki-dai, Sakado, 350-0283, Japan

John L. Waddington (39, 61), Molecular and Cellular Therapeutics, Royal College of Surgeons in Ireland, Dublin 2, Ireland

Gerard J. O'Sullivan (39), Molecular and Cellular Therapeutics, Royal College of Surgeons in Ireland, Dublin 2, Ireland

Katsunori Tomiyama (39, 61), Advanced Research Institute for the Sciences and Humanities, Nihon University, Tokyo 102, Japan; Department of Pharmacology, Nihon University School of Dentistry, Tokyo 101, Japan

Colm M.P. O'Tuathaigh (61), Molecular and Cellular Therapeutics, Royal College of Surgeons in Ireland, Dublin 2, Ireland; School of Medicine, University College Cork, Cork, Ireland

Karl-Gunnar Westberg (77), Department of Integrative Medical Biology, Section for Physiology, Umeå University, SE-901 87 Umeå, Sweden

Arlette Kolta (77), Faculté de Médecine Dentaire, Université de Montréal, and Groupe de Recherches sur le Système Nerveux Central du FRSQ, Université de Montréal

Yong Chul Bae (99), Department of Oral Anatomy, Neurobiology, School of Dentistry, Kyungpook National University, Daegu 700-412, Korea

Atsushi Yoshida (99), Department of Oral Anatomy, Neurobiology, Graduate School of Dentistry, Osaka University, Suita, Osaka 565-0871, Japan

Alexander M. Binshtok (143), Department of Medical Neurobiology, Institute for Medical Research Israel Canada and Center for Research on Pain, The Hebrew University Medical School, Jerusalem, Israel

Barry J. Sessle (179), Faculty of Dentistry, University of Toronto, 124 Edward Street, Toronto, ON M5G 1G6

Ke Ren (207), Department of Neural and Pain Sciences, Dental School; & Program in Neuroscience, University of Maryland, Baltimore, MD 21201-1586, USA

Ronald Dubner (207), Department of Neural and Pain Sciences, Dental School; & Program in Neuroscience, University of Maryland, Baltimore, MD 21201-1586, USA

Koichi Iwata (227), Department of Physiology, Nihon University School of Dentistry, 1-8-13 Kanda-Surugadai, Chiyoda-ku Tokyo, 101-8310, Japan

Yoshiki Imamura (227), Department of Oral Diagnosis, Nihon University School of Dentistry, 1-8-13 Kanda-Surugadai, Chiyoda-ku Tokyo, 101-8310, Japan

Kuniya Honda (227), Department of Physiology, Nihon University School of Dentistry, 1-8-13 Kanda-Surugadai, Chiyoda-ku Tokyo, 101-8310, Japan; Department of Physiology and Oral and Maxillofacial Surgery, Nihon University School of Dentistry, 1-8-13 Kanda-Surugadai, Chiyoda-ku Tokyo, 101-8310, Japan

Masamichi Shinoda (227), Department of Physiology, Nihon University School of Dentistry, 1-8-13 Kanda-Surugadai, Chiyoda-ku Tokyo, 101-8310, Japan

David A. Bereiter (251) Department of Diagnostic and Biological Sciences, University of Minnesota School of Dentistry, Minneapolis, MN 55455 USA

Keiichiro Okamoto (251) Department of Diagnostic and Biological Sciences, University of Minnesota School of Dentistry, Minneapolis, MN 55455 USA

Masayuki Kobayashi (285), Department of Pharmacology, Nihon University School of Dentistry, 1-8-13 Kanda-Surugadai, Chiyoda-ku, Tokyo 101-8310, Japan; Division of Oral and Craniomaxillofacial Research, Dental Research Center, Nihon University School of Dentistry, 1-8-13 Kanda-Surugadai, Chiyoda-ku, Tokyo 101-8310, Japan; Functional Probe Research Laboratory, Molecular Imaging Research Program, RIKEN, 6-7-3 Minatojima-minamimachi, Chuo-ku, Kobe 650-0047, Japan

Zhi Zhang (305), Department of Zoology and Physiology, University of Wyoming, Laramie, WY 82071

Qian-Quan Sun (305), Department of Zoology and Physiology, University of Wyoming, Laramie, WY 82071

PREFACE

Orofacial movements constitute fundamental motor patterns with essential roles in consummatory behavior, self-care, defensive and attack behaviors, vocalization, and, in higher mammals, verbal as well as nonverbal communication. Clinically, dysfunction in orofacial movement is evident in numerous dental, craniomaxillofacial, and neuropsychiatric disorders, including dysphagia, Huntington's disease, Parkinson's disease, and schizophrenia. These fundamental motor patterns are regulated, often as programmed sequences of coordinated movements, by complex neuronal networks that involve diverse brain regions, particularly the basal ganglia and cerebral cortex. Among these, one of the most important features of orofacial function is the recruitment of multimodal sensory information, which is integrated in the brainstem and higher brain regions that also involve the basal ganglia and cerebral cortex. Sensation in the orofacial regions consists of not only somatoform tactile/pressure/thermal/deep sensation but also unique sensations, including periodontal mechanoreception, tooth pain, and chemical senses of gustation and olfaction. These sensory stimuli play important roles in regulating oromaxillofacial motor functions, including mastication, swallowing, and vocalization, that require complex and precise temporal and spatial muscle movements. For example, during mastication, gustation and olfaction play a role in detecting what kind of food is present in the mouth; mechanoreception of the periodontal ligaments and deep sensation of muscle spindles monitor masticatory force; somatosensation perceives the texture of food, and thermal sensation contributes to judgment as to whether food is of adequate hotness to consume. These highly coordinated interactions between motor and sensory processes are considered to be mechanistically distinct from those regulating other body regions such as the limbs and trunk. When these regulatory processes are disrupted, a variety of functional impairments can emerge, for example neuropathic pain in dental and craniomaxillofacial disorders, the dysphagia of Parkinson's disease, and the involuntary orofacial movements of Huntington's disease. In this volume, members of the International Translational Research Network on Orofacial Neurological Disorders and invited experts provide authoritative overviews of new aspects of motor function and sensation relating to neurological disorders in orofacial regions.

BEHAVIORAL PHARMACOLOGY OF OROFACIAL MOVEMENT DISORDERS

Noriaki Koshikawa[1,2], Satoshi Fujita[1,2] and Kazunori Adachi[3]

[1]Department of Pharmacology, Nihon University School of Dentistry, 1-8-13 Kanda-Surugadai, Chiyoda-ku, Tokyo 101-8310, Japan
[2]Division of Oral and Craniomaxillofacial Research, Dental Research Center, Nihon University School of Dentistry, 1-8-13 Kanda-Surugadai, Chiyoda-ku, Tokyo 101-8310, Japan
[3]Department of Diagnostic and Therapeutic Sciences, Meikai University School of Dentistry, 1-1 Keyaki-dai, Sakado, 350-0283, Japan

I. Introduction

Within mammalian behavior, orofacial movements constitute fundamental motor patterns with essential roles in consummatory behavior, self-care, defensive and attack behaviors, vocalization and, in higher mammals, verbal as well as non-verbal communication. Clinically, dysfunction in orofacial movement is evident in numerous dental, craniomaxillofacial and neurological disorders, including dysphagia, Parkinson's disease [L-3, 4-dihydroxy phenylalanine (L-DOPA)-induced dyskinesia], Huntington's disease, and schizophrenia [tardive dyskinesia].

There is a considerable body of evidence indicating the important role of the basal ganglia and associated dopaminergic (DAergic) mechanisms in the regulation of orofacial movements (Adachi *et al.*, 2002; Delfs and Kelley, 1990; Koshikawa

INTERNATIONAL REVIEW OF NEUROBIOLOGY, VOL. 97
DOI: 10.1016/B978-0-12-385198-7.00001-1

et al., 1989). The effects of dopamine (DA) are attributed to activation of two receptor subtypes, namely D1 and D2 receptors (Kebabian and Calne, 1979). In the early 1990s, DNA cloning techniques led to previously uncharacterized DA receptors such as D3 (Sokoloff *et al.*, 1990), D4 (Van Tol *et al.*, 1991) and D5 (Tiberi *et al.*, 1991; Sunahara *et al.*, 1991) receptors. However, due to similarities in structure and intracellular signaling systems, together with limitations of the available selective ligands to pharmacologically distinguish these receptor subtypes, DA receptors are still classified as D1-like (D1 and D5) and D2-like (D2, D3, and D4) receptor subfamilies. D1 and D5 receptors are thought to be closely related in terms of pharmacological binding profiles (Gingrich and Caron, 1993), and activation of these receptors stimulates a Gs protein that then stimulates adenylyl cyclase (Stoof and Kebabian, 1981; Zhou *et al.*, 1990). The highest densities of D1 receptors are found in the projection areas of the substantia nigra pars compacta and the ventral tegmental area, namely in the caudate-putamen (striatum), the nucleus accumbens and the olfactory tubercle; significant amounts are also present in the neocortex, the globus pallidus and the amygdala (Boyson, McGonigle, and Molinoff, 1986; Richfield, Penney, and Young, 1989; Mansour *et al.*, 1990). D5 receptors are less abundantly present in the brain; however, relatively high densities are found in the hippocampus, the hypothalamus and the parafascicular nucleus of the thalamus (Tiberi *et al.*, 1991; Meador-Woodruff *et al.*, 1992; Bergson *et al.*, 1995). D2, D3, and D4 receptors have more diversity in binding characteristics (Gingrich and Caron, 1993), and activation of these receptors inhibits a Gi protein that then inhibits adenylyl cyclase (Stoof and Kebabian, 1981). Short and long isoforms of the D2 receptor, produced by alternative splicing of the same gene, exist (Dal Toso *et al.*, 1989; Giros *et al.* 1989). Highest densities of D2 receptors are present in the caudate putamen, the nucleus accumbens, the olfactory tubercle, and the substantia nigra pars compacta, while intermediate densities are found in the central nucleus of amygdala, the lateral septum, the entorhinal cortex, the superior colliculus and the hippocampus (Boyson *et al.*, 1986; Richfield *et al.*, 1989; Mansour *et al.*, 1990). D3 receptors are predominantly found in the olfactory tubercle and the shell of the nucleus accumbens (Sokoloff *et al.*, 1990). The density of D4 receptors is very low; however, moderate levels are found in the frontal cortex, the amygdala and, to a lesser extent, the striatum (Defagot and Antonelli, 1997).

Elucidating the relative involvement of individual DA receptor subtypes in the processes and the identification of DA-mediated behaviors has been impeded by incompatibility at the behavioral pharmacology-molecular biology interface (Waddington *et al.*, 2001, 2005). Specifically, the extent to which gene cloning has revealed greater diversity in DA receptor typology beyond the original D1/D2 classification, has not been matched by similar progress in developing selective agonists and antagonists for these receptors (O'Sullivan *et al.*, 2010).

It is well recognized that DA receptor subtypes, particularly those of the D1-like family and involving interactions with their D2-like counterparts, exert a critical role in the regulation of orofacial movements (Delfs and Kelley, 1990; O'Sullivan *et al.*, 2010; Rosengarten and Friedhoff, 1998; Waddington *et al.*, 1995, 2005). As an important example, bilateral co-stimulation of both D1-like and D2-like receptors, particularly in the ventrolateral part of the striatum, readily elicits repetitive jaw movements in rats (Adachi *et al.*, 2002; Delfs and Kelley, 1990; Koshikawa *et al.*, 1989; Uchida *et al.*, 2005a).

Dysfunction in orofacial movement is evident in the clinic particularly in schizophrenia, Parkinson's disease, and Huntington's disease. Treatment of schizophrenia with antipsychotics, having a property of D2-like receptor antagonism, often results in serious side effects. Most prominent are the so-called extrapyramidal side effects and tardive orofacial dyskinesia, one of the most serious extrapyramidal side effects; in contrast with other extrapyramidal symptoms, tardive dyskinesia occurs only after prolonged treatment with most typical antipsychotic drugs. Although chronic antipsychotic treatment was thought to be the principal cause for inducing tardive orofacial dyskinesia, recent studies suggest that it may be more complicated (Whitty et al., 2009) In addition, the prototypic atypical antipsychotic, clozapine, appears to have a better clinical profile. It ameliorates symptoms in some patients that are unresponsive to other antipsychotics, and it induces hardly any extrapyramidal side effects. Therefore, studies on antipsychotic-induced tardive orofacial dyskinesia should consider the vulnerability of an individual and the differences between the typical and atypical antipsychotics. In addition, tardive dyskinesia and Parkinson-like symptoms can often coexist in the same patient. This phenomenon might be explained by the hypothesis that orofacial dyskinesia is a disturbance in the mesolimbic DAergic systems rather than that of the nigrostriatal system (Cools, 1983).

Treatment of Parkinson's disease with L-DOPA, which is converted to DA and then stimulates both D1-like and D2-like receptors, also often results in orofacial dyskinesia. It is well recognized that the L-DOPA-induced orofacial dyskinesia and typical Parkinson symptoms can co-occur in the same Parkinson's disease patient (Jankovic and Casabona, 1987). There is circumstantial evidence that L-DOPA-induced orofacial dyskinesia in humans might be the consequence of a hyperfunctioning mesolimbic-pallidal circuitry, in which the mesolimbic region occupies a central role, in contrast to the typical Parkinson symptoms which are inherent to hypofunction in nigrostriato-nigral circuitry. Thus, orofacial dyskinesias are considered to arise when hierarchically lower order output stations of the mesolimbic region become dysfunctional as a consequence of the arrival of distorted information sent by the mesolimbic region. This hypothesis fits in with the idea postulated in the early 1970s that changes in GABAergic activity of striatal efferents, rather than changes in DAergic activity within the striatum that would underlie the appearance of orofacial dyskinesia in humans (Pakkenberg *et al.*, 1973).

In animal studies on orofacial dyskinesia, the above-mentioned neurological disorders, e.g. schizophrenia (tardive orofacial dyskinesia) and Parkinson's disease

(L-DOPA-induced dyskinesia), have been considered as starting points to elucidate the underlying mechanisms. Such studies in rats involve complexities in the assessment of orofacial behaviors (Waddington, 1990). As a result of the great variety of methods used, it is difficult to assess the orofacial movements quantitatively, or even qualitatively. There are some experimental designs providing more objective and detailed measures, such as those in which variations in the distance between points on the maxilla and mandible of rat by using fluorescence dye, light-emitting diode or magnet are quantified (Ellison *et al.*, 1987; Koshikawa *et al.*, 1989; Lee *et al.*, 2003). These designs provide detailed information on the amplitude and the frequency of the jaw movements. By using these methods, involvements of neurotransmitter systems and functional neural connections within the basal ganglia have been studied in rat rhythmical jaw movements. Regarding the neurotransmitter systems, DAergic (Koshikawa *et al.*, 1989, 1990a, 1990b, 1991a), cholinergic (Adachi *et al.*, 2002; Kikuchi de Bertrán *et al.*, 1992), γ-aminobutyric acid (GABA) ergic (Adachi *et al.*, 2002; Uchida *et al.*, 2005b) and glutamatergic (Fujita *et al.*, 2010b) systems have been shown to be involved in the display of rat rhythmical jaw movements. The involved neural connections have also been investigated, and research has focused on the differential role between (1) The dorsal and ventral part of the striatum (Koshikawa *et al.*, 1989; 1990a), (2) The shell and core of the nucleus accumbens (Cools *et al.*, 1995) and (3) The output pathways from the striatum and the nucleus accumbens (Adachi *et al.*, 2002; Uchida *et al.*, 2005b).

This chapter seeks to provide an overview of findings across several orofacial movement disorders and interpret new insights in the context of the limitations of techniques in behavioral pharmacology and prior knowledge of the regulation of behavior by DA receptors. Particularly, this chapter focuses on pharmacological approaches that have been instrumental in defining DA-, GABA-, and glutamate-dependent mechanisms in the regulation of orofacial behaviors; it is complemented by the following chapters that focus on mutant ["knockout"] mouse models (Waddington *et al.*, 2011, this volume; Tomiyama *et al.*, 2011, this volume). The purpose here is to review how studies in rats have helped to elucidate the relative involvement of such neuronal systems in spontaneous and drug-induced unconditioned orofacial behavior.

II. Orofacial Movement Disorders in Schizophrenia

A. Clinical Description

The syndrome of abnormal involuntary orofacial movements gained special attention following the introduction of antipsychotic drugs in the early 1950s. It was initially referred to as "persistent involuntary syndrome", or "terminal extrapyramidal insufficiency syndrome", and the term "tardive dyskinesia", introduced by Faurbye *et al.*, (1964) was derived from the Latin word "tardus (= late)" which refers generally to late onset of the syndrome after continuous use of antipsychotics. Until now the exact mechanisms underlying this syndrome are unknown and there is no successful treatment available.

Tardive orofacial dyskinesia is characterized by repetitive, involuntary, purposeless movements of oral-lingual-buccal region that usually resemble continual chewing motions with intermittent tongue protrusion and abnormal movements of the lips. The abnormal involuntary movements, as described for tardive orofacial dyskinesia, occur in a variety of medicated and non-medicated people. Although epidemiological data point to neuroleptic exposure as being the most significant etiologic factor in the development, some authors have questioned this relationship. Movements quite similar to tardive orofacial dyskinesia are also described in different neurological/psychiatric disorders, including untreated schizophrenia; long before the introduction of antipsychotic drugs, spontaneous hyperkinetic dyskinesias of "grimacing" and "irregular movements of tongue and lips" were described in psychotic patients (Owens *et al.*, 1982; Casey, 1985; Waddington, 1989; see Whitty *et al.*, 2009). Stereotypies (purposeless, meaningless actions) and mannerisms (peculiar ways of carrying out normal actions) of psychosis are part of a differential diagnosis of tardive orofacial dyskinesia. However, it is not known whether these movements are behavioral indications of a comparable pathogenesis in these different disorders. Nevertheless, it has been hypothesized that the invariable association of antipsychotic drugs with tardive orofacial dyskinesia has impaired the search for its neurobiological substrate.

Although chronic antipsychotic treatment was thought to be the principal cause of tardive orofacial dyskinesia, many studies suggest that it may be more complicated. A large number of factors determine the vulnerability of an individual to develop tardive orofacial dyskinesia: there is a correlation between tardive orofacial dyskinesia and patients with negative symptoms and cognitive impairment (Waddington, 1989; Whitty *et al.*, 2009). Moreover, tardive orofacial dyskinesia is influenced by gender and, particularly, by age. It can be concluded that antipsychotics induce tardive orofacial dyskinesia in vulnerable individuals. However, it also has a high incidence in patients with organic brain diseases, like dementia (Waddington, 1989; Whitty *et al.*, 2009).

The prototypic atypical antipsychotic, clozapine, appears to have a better clinical profile. It ameliorates many symptoms and is therapeutically effective in some of the patients that are unresponsive to other antipsychotics (Leppig *et al.*, 1989). Although it has weak DA receptor antagonistic activity, it has more potent antagonistic activity at several other neurotransmitter sites, i.e. serotonergic, cholinergic, histaminergic, and α-adrenergic. Clozapine induces exceptionally low rates of acute extrapyramidal syndromes and there are no well-documented cases of tardive dyskinesia from extended clozapine use; the effect of clozapine on tardive dyskinesia is highly variable, as in some patients the drug suppresses the syndrome while in others it does not (Casey, 1989; Margolese *et al.*, 2005a, b). Since experience with clozapine is limited due to the risk of agranulocytosis (1–2%), it is unwise to draw firm conclusions about the liability of clozapine to produce tardive dyskinesia. The prevalence of tardive dyskinesia steadily increases with age (Smith and Baldessarini, 1980; Margolese *et al.*, 2005a, b). Most, but not all, studies show that tardive dyskinesia occurs more often in women (Yassa and Jeste, 1992; Margolese *et al.*, 2005a, b).

Treating tardive dyskinesia is a clinical challenge. Unfortunately, almost no drugs are uniformly safe and effective over extended treatment periods. Apart from a recent case report showing efficacy of atypical antipsychotics (Peritogiannis and Tsouli, 2010) and clinical reports investigating the effects of calcium-channel blocker drugs on treating tardive dyskinesia (e.g. Soares-Weiser and Rathbone, 2004), the long list of the many drugs used to study these symptoms attests to their general lack of therapeutic benefits (Casey, 1990; Margolese *et al.*, 2005a, b). Without following up the symptoms over time, one may misunderstand the course of tardive dyskinesia. For example, the disorder may emerge or worsen when the drug dosage is decreased because symptoms are unmasked. This unmasking could also occur when anticholinergic agents are added. Similarly, tardive dyskinesia symptoms may lessen when the dose of antipsychotic is increased or when anticholinergic agents are decreased because symptoms are masked.

B. Pathophysiology of Tardive Orofacial Dyskinesia

Despite decades of clinical and animal research, the neurological substrate of tardive dyskinesia has remained unknown. However, several hypotheses have been postulated on various grounds as outlined below.

The DA receptor supersensitivity hypothesis is based on striatal (caudate-putamen) DAergic hyperfunctioning and has long been the leading hypothesis for tardive dyskinesia. The basic idea is that DA or some other DA-related factor in the basal ganglia and limbic forebrain may be overactive. Such a state of relative excess of DAergic activity may be ascribed to increased number or effectiveness of postsynaptic DA receptors (Tarsy and Baldessarini, 1977; Margolese *et al.*, 2005a, b), and this aspect has played a central role in the DA hypothesis. This originates from animal research showing that, following the withdrawal from subchronic antipsychotic treatment, rodents are sensitive to the development of perioral stereotyped behaviors when challenged with a DA receptor agonist. The mechanism underlying this effect is thought to be an adaptive response consisting of an increase in the number of DA receptors after prolonged blockade of DA receptors by neuroleptics (Tarsy and Baldessarini, 1977; Margolese *et al.*, 2005a, b). Such receptor supersensitivity was directly demonstrated in the striatum of neuroleptic-treated animals using radioligand binding (Muller and Seeman, 1978; Margolese *et al.*, 2005a, b).

Although this hypothesis has been widely accepted, a major shortcoming of the hypothesis is the temporal discrepancy between the change in DA receptors and occurrence of tardive dyskinesia. In addition, the DA receptor hypothesis cannot explain why tardive dyskinesia and Parkinson-like symptom can coexist in the same patient at the same time (Richardson and Craig, 1982; Wolf *et al.*, 1983; Jankovic and Casabona, 1987; Margolese *et al.*, 2005a, b). Finally, there is little or no direct evidence for DAergic hyperfunctioning in patients with tardive dyskinesia, as assessed either in vivo, using positron emission tomography (PET) or singe photon emission computed tomography (SPECT) imaging, or in postmortem brain tissue (Margolese *et al.*, 2005a, b). Parkinson-like symptoms are presumed to reflect DAergic hypofunction, which would appear to be pathophysiologically incompatible with DAergic hyperfunction. In view of these objections, several other hypotheses have been postulated for tardive orofacial dyskinesia.

Cools (1983) postulated that orofacial dyskinesia is a disturbance in mesolimbic DAergic systems. This hypothesis may explain why tardive dyskinesia and Parkinson-like symptoms can coexist in the same patient. Other hypotheses are related to structural damage induced by antipsychotics. Thus, the GABA hypothesis is based on an decrease in the number of striatal neurons by chronic treatment with antipsychotics which would result in a decrease in the output region of the striatum (Pakkenberg *et al.*, 1973; Margolese *et al.*, 2005a, b), and similar neuron damage by free radicals, which are known to be formed as metabolic products of antipsychotics, may also contribute to the pathogenesis of tardive orofacial dyskinesia (Rollema *et al.*, 1994; Margolese *et al.*, 2005a, b). These different hypotheses are quite diverse, which may be due to the fact that tardive orofacial dyskinesia is not a unitary syndrome and multiple causes may be involved. Therefore, a multidisciplinary investigation of the neuronal substrate involved in tardive orofacial dyskinesia may provide new insights into this syndrome.

III. Orofacial Movement Disorders in Parkinson's Disease and Huntington's Disease

A. Clinical Description

Hypokinesia of the muscles of facial expression and orofacial motor abnormalities have long been recognized in Parkinson's disease (Hunker *et al.*, 1982; Schneider *et al.*, 1986). In fact, patients with Parkinson's disease often complain of difficulties in chewing and swallowing (Leopold and Kagel, 1996). These disturbances are thought to depend on hypokinesia of the muscles in the orofacial region but little is known of the mechanism behind the movement disturbances and their pathophysiology. The primary pathology of Parkinson's disease is the selective degeneration of DAergic neurons in the substantia nigra pars compacta and the ensuing loss of caudate-putamen DA content is held responsible for the onset of motor symptoms. Although peripheral structures are involved in various oral motor acts, such as chewing, swallowing, and speaking, distinct basal ganglia circuits may be used to generate the various motor patterns (Hoover and Strick, 1993). Indeed, a circuit that may influence rhythmic jaw movements is a projection from the caudate-putamen to the substantia nigra pars reticulata and then to neurons in the reticular formations of brainstem, the area has connections with the trigeminal and facial motor complex (Adachi *et al.*, 2002; Iwata *et al.*, 1996; Mogoseanu *et al.*, 1993, 1994; von Krosigk and Smith 1991). Until now, little information has been available on how Parkinson's disease affects motor control of the orofacial area. Patients suffering from Parkinson's disease, for the first few years, experience a satisfactory response to L-DOPA, which is converted to DA in the brain and then stimulates both D1-like and D2-like receptors. Thereafter, the majority eventually develop motor response complications such as dyskinesia, on-off fluctuations and wearing-off effects (Marsden and Parkes 1976; Chase *et al.* 1993; Calabresi *et al.*, 2010).

In contrast, orofacial dyskinesia is an intrinsic feature of Huntington's disease. While Huntington's disease is historically conceptualized as a disorder of chore-iform *hyper*kinesias, particularly of the orofacial region, the clinical trajectory of motor dysfunction over the course of illness is characterized by transitions from dyskinesia to rigidity and other *hypo*kinetic features; indeed, that *hypo*kinesias as well as *hyper*kinesias can be present, especially in the early onset of variants and late in the course following more a typical onset, is one of the reasons underpinning contemporary preference for the term Huntington's disease rather than Huntington's chorea (Walker, 2007; Ross and Tabrizi, 2011).

B. Pathophysiology of Orofacial Dyskinesia in Parkinson's Disease and Huntington's Disease

Concerning the hypothesis that L-DOPA-induced orofacial dyskinesia in humans is the consequence of hyperfunction in the mesolimbic region, though no direct proof is currently present, there are clinical data which are in line with this hypothesis. The hypothesis predicts that compounds that enhance DAergic activity within the mesolimbic region worsen orofacial dyskinesia. Given the fact that monoamine oxidase B (MAO-B) is especially active in mesolimbic regions in animals, it could be predicted that selegiline, which selectively inhibits MAO-B, would worsen orofacial dyskinesia; this is indeed the case for Parkinson's disease patients receiving both L-DOPA and selegiline (Yahr, 1978; Youdim, 1978;

Garrick and Murphy, 1980; Calabresi *et al.*, 2010). This hypothesis also predicts that agents which attenuate DAergic activity within the mesolimbic region will ameliorate orofacial dyskinesia. Given the fact that D1 receptors are present in regions innervated by mesolimbic fibres, it can be predicted that compounds inhibiting D1 receptors ameliorate orofacial dyskinesia (Offermeier and van Rooyen, 1983). In this context it is relevant to mention that ceruletide, an analogue of cholecystokinin octapeptide (CCK-8), is known to prevent the development of hypersensitive DA receptors in mesolimbic regions (Fuxe *et al.*, 1981), and that CCK-8 is known to occur primarily in mesolimbic regions (Hökfelt *et al.*, 1980). The finding that ceruletide ameliorates orofacial dyskinesia in humans (Nishikawa *et al.*, 1985, 1986) underlines again the importance of the mesolimbic region in the control of orofacial dyskinesia in humans. In addition, inhibition of GABA receptors within the subcommissural part of the globus pallidus, a primary output station of the mesolimbic region, elicits intense, and vigorous orofcial dyskinesias in cats (Cools *et al.*, 1989). This may imply that GABA agonist may also be effective in attenuating orofacial dyskinesia in humans, though studies to date have been less than successful.

In Huntington's disease, progressive cell loss occurs primarily in the striatum, cerebral cortex, thalamus, and subthalamic nucleus, involving loss of GABAergic and glutamatergic neurons. Medium spiny neurons of the caudate nucleus and putamen are preferentially affected, with loss not only of GABAergic and glutamatergic elements but also of D1 and D2 receptors (Walker, 2007; Ross and Tabrizi, 2011). However, little is known on the relative roles of loss of D1 vs. D2 receptors in the motor features of Huntington's disease.

In summary, there is circumstantial evidence that L-DOPA-induced orofacial dyskinesia in man might be the consequence of a hyperfunctioning mesolimbic-pallidal circuitry, in which the mesolimbic region occupies a central role. Orofacial dyskinesia is thought to arise when output stations of the mesolimbic region start to dysfunction as a consequence of the arrival of distorted information sent by the mesolimbic region. This hypothesis fits in with the earlier reported hypothesis that changes in GABAergic activity of striatal efferents, rather than changes in DAergic activity within the striatum, and would underlie the appearance of orofacial dyskinesia in humans (Pakkenberg *et al.*, 1973; Calabresi *et al.*, 2010). Recent evidence supports the involvement not only of GABAergic but also glutamatergic dysfunction in L-DOPA-induced dyskinesias (Samadi *et al.*, 2008a, b). Orofacial dyskinesia, involving hyperfunction in mesolimbic-pallidal circuity, and typical Parkinsonian symptoms, involving hypofunction in nigrostriato-nigral circuity, can co-occur in the same Parkinson's disease patient (Jankovic and Casabona, 1987; Calabresi et al., 2010). Huntington's disease can involve not only *hyper*kinesia but also transitions from dyskinesia to rigidity and other *hypo*kinetic features, in the face of a distinct neurodegenerative process involving primarily GABAergic and glutamatergic processes, with secondary loss of D1-like and D2-like receptors (Walker, 2007; Ross and Tabrizi, 2011).

This attests the difficulty in resolving the diversity of mechanisms involved in regulating orofacial movements and orofacial movement disorder. Such problems emphasize the need for more appropriate animal models for the study of orofacial function and dysfunction, particularly in rodents, to delineate the differential involvement of DAergic, GABAergic, glutamatergic and other neuronal processes.

IV. Orofacial Movement Disorders: Studies in Rats

A. Experimental Approaches to Studying Orofacial Movement Disorders

1. *Methods to Assess Orofacial Behavior*

Animal studies on orofacial behavior in rats are beset by methodological difficulties in assessment. As a result of the great variety of methods used, it is difficult to quantitatively, or even qualitatively, compare the outcome of the available studies. There are some experimental designs providing more objective and detailed measures, such as designs in which variations in the distance between points on the maxilla and mandibe of rats, by using fluorescence dye, light-emitting diode or magnet, are quantified (Adachi *et al.*, 2002; Ellison *et al.*, 1987; Koshikawa *et al.*, 1989; Lee *et al.*, 2003). Inspection of the perioral region while the animal is lightly anesthetized or confined in a tube can involve direct observation, video recording or automated videotracking of any markers or transducers applied to the jaw (Koshikawa *et al.*, 1989; Levy and Ellison, 1987; Rosengarten and Friedhoff, 1998; Waddington, 1990). However, quantitative advantages are compromized by their invasive nature and/or resolution of only a single topography of orofacial movement; this severely limits investigation of relationships to other behavioral sequences and, critically, generalization to physiologically relevant conditions. In fact, in the so-called tube test, jaw movement are measured in animals that are placed in a tube (Ellison *et al.*, 1987) which restricts the animals and accordingly creates a stressful situation. In other experimental designs, the animals are lightly anesthetized to fix their head to frames, inhibiting thereby the display of any non-oral behavior (Koshikawa *et al.*, 1989). Apart from these attempts to quantify oral behavior in restricted rats, there are studies in freely moving rats (Collins *et al.*, 1991, 1993; Lee *et al.*, 2003).

Traditionally, oral behaviors of rats were analyzed by visual observation. The display of spontaneous oral movements such as vacuous chewing is often considered as a valid animal model of tardive orofacial dyskinesia occurring in schizophrenia patients treated chronically with antipsychotics. The behavior is characterized by vertical jaw movements in the absence of any chewable material in the mouth. The number of episodes of vacuous chewing movements, each consists of distinct bursts of three to five jaw movements (Diana *et al.*, 1992), was visually counted. Its predictive validity is illustrated by the fact that long-term treatment (>4 months) with the typical antipsychotic haloperidol, but not atypical antipsychotic clozapine increased spontaneous vacuous jaw movements (Gunne *et al.*, 1986; Rupniak *et al.*, 1983). Face validity of the model is underlined by the observation that both the morphology and the onset of the oral movements elicited in rats bear a certain resemblance to those seen in humans (Waddington, 1990). Attempts have been made to improve the efficiency of this model by reducing the duration of the treatment, but the results of these studies are inconsistent. Some studies (Ikeda *et al.*, 1999; See and Ellison, 1990) do not show an effect after 4 weeks, whereas others demonstrate an increase of vacuous jaw movements with 1–4 weeks haloperidol treatment (Diana *et al.*, 1992; Egan *et al.*, 1996; Rupniak *et al.*, 1985), casting some doubt on the predictive validity of this relatively simple animal model of tardive dyskinesia. Using the above-mentioned technique, in which jaw movements are recorded by means of a light-emitting diode attached to the mandible of rats anesthetized lightly so as to fix their head to frames, both apomorphine and a mixture of D1-like and D2-like receptor agonists (SKF 38393 and quinpirole) have been found to increase jaw movements in haloperidol-treated, but not clozapine-treated rats (Ikeda *et al.*, 1999); the study presents an animal model of tardive dyskinesia with predictive validity, reliability, and efficiency.

2. *Magnetic Sensor Technology in Freely Moving Rats*

The preferred approach would be a technique that could provide both quantitative resolution of orofacial movements in freely moving animals and allow these to be related to other behavioral sequences in the natural repertoire. A magnetic sensor system has been described, with concurrent electromyography, for quantifying vertical jaw movements in freely moving rats (Lee *et al.*, 2003) and this was applied to study jaw movements induced by the non-selective DA receptor agonist apomorphine (Lee *et al.*, 2004). Recently, this technology was extended to study distinct topographies of orofacial movements and their relationship to other behaviors in the rodent repertoire under challenge with two distinct D1-like agonists that have been reported to exert differing effects on orofacial movements using observational or non-naturalistic paradigms (Fujita *et al.*, 2010a). The study tested a system for monitoring jaw movements in freely moving rats. A Hall-effect transducer was fixed to the skull in order to sense voltage changes induced by variations in the position of a magnet fixed to the mandible. By measuring DA receptor-mediated jaw movements, this system produces data comparable to that obtained using a light-sensitive transducer system in anesthetized rats, while also measuring the vertical component of jaw movements in freely moving rats (Fig. 1). In combination with conventional visual observation, this system may provide a useful tool for assessing movements of the orofacial region during spontaneous and drug-induced behavior.

These above-mentioned methods are believed to lay a firm foundation for studies on the nature and occurrence of orofacial movements in the animal models of orofacial dyskinesia.

B. Brain Structures Involved in Orofacial Movement Disorders

1. *Basal Ganglia Anatomy*

The majority of DA-containing nerve cells are found in the midbrain. Several different forebrain projections from the midbrain DAergic cell groups are distinguished, including the mesostriatal, mesocortical, and mesolimbic projections (Loughlin and Fallon, 1984). There are minor species differences in the anatomical organization of the striatum and associated structures in rodents and primates (Wu and Parent, 2000). The primate striatum contains structurally distinct caudate nucleus and putamen, whereas these structures are not differentiated in the rodent brain and are collectively referred to as the caudate-putamen or neostriatum. The striatum of both primates and rodents contains a rostroventral extension which is referred to as the nucleus accumbens. The nigrostriatal projection comprises the dorsal component of the mesostriatal system, which originates primarily from DA cells of the substantia nigra pars compacta and, to a lesser extent, from DA cells of the retrorubral field and the ventral tegmental area (Gerfen *et al.*, 1987a, b). These areas are believed to have a predominant role in motor control. The basal ganglia consist of five closely interlinked structures, i.e. the caudate-putamen, the internal and external segment of the globus pallidus, the subthalamic nucleus and the substantia nigra pars reticulata. The GABAergic medium spiny neurons of the striatum are projected by the DAergic neurons from the substantia nigra pars compacta. These neurons also receive massive glutamatergic input from the neocortex via the cortico-striatal pathway, and from the cerebellum via the intralaminar nuclei of the thalamus. Within the basal ganglia, information is processed via pathways from the medium spiny neurons of the striatum to the output structures of the basal ganglia, the substantia nigra pars reticulata and the internal segment of the globus pallidus (entopeduncular nucleus). When movements are absent, the neurons in the substantia nigra pars reticulata and the entopeduncular nucleus are tonically active, and their constant release of GABA produces a powerful inhibition of target cells in the ventral thalamic nuclei, superior colliculus, pedunculo pontine nucleus, and reticular formation of brainstem. The medium spiny neurons affect the activity of the substantia nigra pars reticulata and

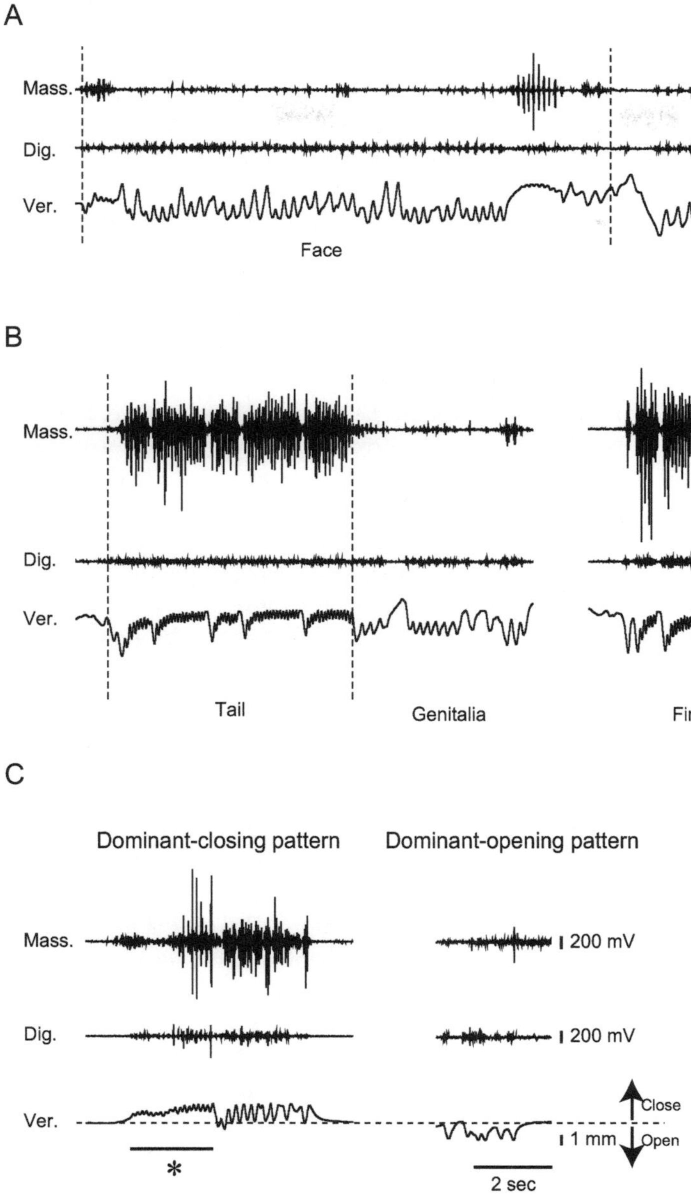

FIG. 1. Magnetic sensor recordings of vertical jaw movements (Ver) and electromyographic recordings from masseter (Mass) and digastric (Dig) muscles during (A) Syntactic grooming of the face and trunk, (B) Non-syntactic grooming of the tail, genitalia and fingers and (C) Vacuous chewing of dominant-closing and dominant-opening patterns; * indicates high frequency, small amplitude, bruxism-like movements that frequently preceded the dominant-closing pattern (For experimental details, see Fujita *et al.*, 2010a).

entopeduncular nucleus neurons through two pathways: a subclass of medium spiny neurons projects directly to the substantia nigra pars reticulata and the entopeduncular nucleus, whereas another subgroup projects to the output nuclei through an indirect route that includes the external segment of the globus pallidus, which in turn project to the subthalamic nucleus. All medium spiny neurons release GABA.

Medium spiny neurons which contribute to the direct and indirect pathways express markedly different DA receptor subtypes. Striatoentopeduncular neurons of direct pathway principally express D1 receptors whereas striatopallidal neurons of indirect pathway preferentially express D2 receptors (Gerfen, 1992a, b). Through molecular biological studies it is now recognized that there are families of D1-like and D2-like receptors (Missale *et al.*, 1998; O'Sullivan *et al.*, 2010), which show specific regional distributions, within the striatum. For example, D3 receptors are not expressed by medium spiny neurons of either type in the neostriatum but they are found within the nucleus accumbens (Kawaguchi, 1997). D1 receptor stimulation of medium spiny neurons leads to a rapid silencing of inhibitory entopeduncular nucleus and substantia nigra pars reticulata neurons through the direct pathway. Consequently, thalamic, collicular pontine and brainstem neurons exhibit a burst of activity. In the indirect pathway, D2 receptor stimulation of striatal GABAergic neurons to the external segment of the globus pallidus suppresses the activity of the neurons which release GABAergic neurons in the external segment of the globus pallidus from inhibition, and in turn produce tonic inhibition on the gultamatergic subthalamic nucleus neurons, which results in reduction in activity of the entopeduncular nucleus and substantia nigra pars reticulata. As a result, the innervation of medium spiny neurons by nigral DAergic fibres releases the thalamic and brainstem nuclei from the tonic suppressing effects of the external segment of the globus pallidus and substantia nigra pars reticulata. Increased activity of brainstem nuclei increases their glutamatergic output to the various areas involved in motor control. Thus, it is suggested that the basal ganglia influence the output to the lower brainstem areas, including the superior colliculus (Hikosaka and Wurtz, 1985) and the pedunculo-pontine nucleus (Spann and Grofova, 1991), to exert direct effects on motor control (Jaspers *et al.*, 1989).

The major cortical inputs to the caudate-putamen arise from the neocortex, whereas the nucleus accumbens receives inputs from the limbic cortex, in particular the hippocampus and the cingulate cortex (Groenewegen *et al.*, 1980; McGeorge and Faull, 1989). It is generally assumed that the nucleus accumbens, in keeping with these strong limbic connections, plays a critical role in the control of motivated behaviors (Mogenson *et al.*, 1980). Thus, manipulations of the nucleus accumbens in experimental animals tend to result in changes in motivated behaviors such as locomotion and exploratory behaviors. Whilst the strict functional dissociation of the caudate-putamen and nucleus accumbens in terms of motor control versus control of motivated behaviors is no longer tenable, it is now clear that the nucleus accumbens is involved in control of orofacial motor behaviors (Koshikawa *et al.*, 1990b; Cools *et al.*, 1995).

C. Functional Dorsal and Ventral Division Within the Striatum

Stereotyped movements induced by apomorphine are largely due to an action on DAergic mechanisms within the striatum. However, the action of apomorphine is not simple, since its effects may be blocked by the injection of the D2-like receptor antagonist, sulpiride, into the ventral region of the striatum but potentiated by injection of sulpiride into the dorsal region of the striatum (Arnt, 1985; Koshikawa *et al.*, 1987). These results suggest that the striatum is a heterogeneous structure and this is further supported by studies examining stereotyped jaw movements in ketamine-anesthetized rats. Thus, repetitive jaw movements induced by apomorphine are prevented by injections of either sulpiride or SCH 23390, a D1-like receptor antagonist, into the ventral part of the striatum and are mimicked by co-injection of the D1-like and D2-like receptor agonists, SKF 38393 and quinpirole, into sites in the selected ventral part of the striatum from which repeated jaw movements could also be obtained by electrical stimulation (Koshikawa *et al.*, 1989). The combined effect of these two selective agonists is considerably greater than the additive effects of each drug given alone, i.e. they show synergism. The fact that the ventral, particularly ventrolateral, part of the striatum plays an important role in eliciting repetitive jaw movement has also been confirmed by stimulation of not only DAergic (Delfs and Kelley, 1990) but also cholinergic receptors (Kelley *et al.*, 1989) in these structures. Since injection of these two agonists together into the dorsal part of the striatum failed to evoke rhythmical jaw movements, this synergism may also be due to ventrolateral striatal mechanisms. In contrast, injection of sulpiride into the dorsal part of the striatum markedly potentiates the effects of apomorphine, an action that is prevented by administering sulpiride with SCH 23390. In order to generalize this finding made with sulpiride (Koshikawa *et al.*, 1989), another D2-like antagonist YM-09151-2 (Terai *et al.*, 1983), has been tested. YM-09151-2 injected into the ventrolateral striatum blocked apomorphine-induced jaw movements but potentiated this behavior when injected into the dorsal part of the striatum (Koshikawa *et al.*, 1990a). Similarly, co-administration of SCH 23390 with YM-09151-2 into the dorsal striatum prevents the potentiating effects of the latter compound on apomorphine-induced jaw movements (Koshikawa *et al.*, 1990a). In addition, local application of the D1-like receptor agonists, SKF 38393 and SKF 75670, into the dorsal part of the striatum potentiates apomorphine-induced jaw movements, while a D2-like receptor agonist, quinpirole, injected into the same site attenuates these movements (Koshikawa *et al.*, 1990a).

Although the reason why injection of D2-like receptor antagonists into the dorsal part of the striatum potentiates apomorphine-induced jaw movements is not well understood, it can be proposed that increased DAergic activity induced by blockade of presynaptic D2-like receptors (Westerink and De Vries, 1989) in the dorsal striatum is responsible for the facilitation, via postsynaptic D1-like receptors, of apomorphine-induced jaw movements (Koshikawa *et al.*, 1989; 1990a). Another way to interpret these results is that postsynaptic D2-like receptors have an opposite function in different areas of the striatum.

Dorsal/ventrolateral differential control is also present in cholinergic mechanisms in the striatum. Orofacial movements induced by apomorphine are potentiated by carbachol injected into the dorsal striatum, while these movements are inhibited by carbachol injected into the ventrolateral striatum (Kikuchi de Beltrán *et al.*, 1992).

1. *Functional Shell and Core Division Within the Nucleus Accumbens*

In animal studies on orofacial dyskinesia, neurological disorders have been considered as a starting point. It is well recognized that both the tardive dyskinesia in schizophrenia and L-DOPA-induced orofacial dyskinesia in Parkinson's disease can co-occur with Parkinsonian symptoms in the same patient. There is circumstantial evidence that orofacial dyskinesias in humans might be the consequence of a hyperfunctioning mesolimbic-pallidal circuitry, in which the mesolimbic region occupies a central role, in contrast to typical Parkinsonian symptoms, which involve hypofunction in nigrostriato-nigral circuity. In this context, attempts have been made to clarify the extent to which the nucleus accumbens plays a crucial role in the elicitation of involuntary repetitive jaw movements. It was found that both D1-like and D2-like receptors in the nucleus accumbens are involved in the manifestation of apomorphine-induced jaw movements (Koshikawa *et al.*, 1990b), in a way similar to that demonstrated in the ventrolateral part of the striatum (Koshikawa *et al.*, 1989), and that the expression of these movements requires concurrent activation of D1-like and D2-like receptors (Koshikawa *et al.*, 1990b).

The nucleus accumbens is known as a heterogeneous structure and differences have been found between the core and shell with respect to anatomy (Heimer *et al.*, 1991; Jongen-Rêlo *et al.*, 1994; Zahm and Brog, 1992), receptor density (Deutch and Cameron, 1992) and electrophysiology (Pennartz *et al.*, 1992). In line with a report emphasizing the importance of the shell in oral behavior of freely moving rats (Prinssen *et al.*, 1994), D1-like and D2-like receptors in the shell, but not the core, of the nucleus accumbens are found to be critically involved in the control of jaw movements of the rat, providing the evidence that D1-like and D2-like receptors in the shell of the nucleus accumbens mediate a particular behavior (Cools *et al.*, 1995; Koshikawa *et al.*, 1996), while mesolimbic D3 receptors play almost no role in DA-dependent and shell-specific jaw movements (Koshikawa *et al.*, 1996).

2. *Output Pathways from the Ventrolateral Striatum: Involvement in Rat Jaw Movements*

One of the central tenets of the basal ganglia model is segregation of striatal output pathways. Early retrograde cell labeling studies have supported the idea of distinct striatofugal projections arising from separate neuronal populations in the striatum (Beckstead and Cruz, 1986; Loopuijt and van der Kooy, 1985; Parent *et al.*, 1984). In the most widely accepted scheme of basal ganglia organization, the striatum is thought to exert its function via direct and/or indirect pathways (Albin *et al.*, 1989; DeLong, 1990; Smith *et al.*, 1998; Wichmann and DeLong, 1996). As mentioned in the above section, the direct pathway originates from GABAergic neurons projecting monosynaptically on neurons of the entopeduncular nucleus and substantia nigra pars reticulata, while the indirect pathway arises from GABAergic neurons projecting polysynaptically to entopeduncular nucleus/ substantia nigra pars reticulata via relays in the globus pallidus and the subthalamic nucleus. Each of the pathways is thought to serve a particular function. However, a single-cell labeling study in rats revealed the existence of striatal projection neurons with collateralized axons that provide branches to several striatal recipient structures. For example, Wu *et al.* (2000) provided evidence that there are three types of neurons in the striatum, i.e. (a) Neurons projecting to the globus pallidus, entopeduncular nucleus and substantia nigra pars reticulata, (b) Neurons projecting to the globus pallidus and substantia nigra pars reticulata, and (c) Neurons projecting only to the globus pallidus. This finding suggests that each of these may serve a separate function.

Activation of DA or acetylcholine receptors in the ventrolateral part of the striatum has been found to elicit repetitive jaw movements in rats (Delfs and Kelley, 1990; Kelley *et al.*, 1989; Koshikawa *et al.*, 1989), each of these marked by its own movement profile (Kikuchi de Beltrán *et al.*, 1992). GABAergic neurons arising from the ventrolateral striatum primarily converge onto neurons in the dorsolateral part of the substantia nigra pars reticulata (Iwata *et al.*, 1996; von Krosigk *et al.*, 1992) and in the entopeduncular nucleus (Parent, 1990; Takada *et al.*, 1994), which in turn project directly, or indirectly via the superior colliculus, to the parvicellular reticular formation (Takada *et al.*, 1994; Yasui *et al.*, 1992, 1994, 1995). This area is connected directly with the orofacial motor nuclei and gives rise to neurons that converge onto neurones in the trigeminal motor nucleus (Fort *et al.*, 1990; Travers and Norgren, 1983). The ventral pallidum, a ventral portion of the globus pallidus, is also known to receive GABAergic input from the striatum, especially the ventral striatum encompassing the nucleus accumbens (Groenewegen and Russschen, 1984; Zahm and Brog, 1992). It has been reported, using electromyography and a phototransduction system, that, two distinct types of jaw movements can be elicited by bilateral injections of DA and acetylcholine receptor agonists into the ventrolateral striatum (Kikuchi de Beltrán *et al.*, 1992). Regarding the hypothesis that DA receptor-mediated and acetylcholine receptor-mediated jaw movements are funnelled via distinct GABAergic output channels, the agonist and antagonist of $GABA_A$ receptors, muscimol, and bicuculline, were injected bilaterally into the ventral pallidum, entopeduncular nucleus or dorsolateral part of the substantia nigra pars reticulata of rats treated with bilateral injections into the ventrolateral striatum of the D1-like and D2-like receptor agonists mixture, SKF 82958 and quinpirole, or the acetylcholine receptor agonist carbachol (Adachi *et al.*, 2002). The study shows that bilateral injections of both muscimol and bicuculline into the ventral pallidum, entopeduncular nucleus or dorsolateral part of the substantia nigra pars reticulata essentially inhibit DA receptor-mediated jaw movements to varying degrees. In contrast, acetylcholine receptor-mediated jaw movements are inhibited by muscimol given into the entopeduncular nucleus and dorsolateral part of the substantia nigra pars reticulata, whereas these movements are enhanced by bicuculline. These acetylcholine receptor-mediated jaw movements are not affected by muscimol injections into the ventral pallidum, but are inhibited by bicuculline injections (Table 1). These data allow the conclusion that DA receptor-mediated and acetylcholine receptor-mediated jaw movements are two distinct types of jaw movements that are funnelled via separate GABAergic output channels (Adachi *et al.*, 2002).

It was suggested by Adachi *et al.* (2002) that the three different profiles of responses to GABAergic drugs in animals showing either DA receptor-mediated or acetylcholine receptor-mediated jaw movements reflect the involvement of three distinct types of output neurons of the striatum (Wu *et al.*, 2000), namely: Type I: Neurons with collateralized axons to the ventral pallidum, entopeduncular nucleus, and dorsolateral part of the substantia nigra pars reticulata, mediating the DAreceptor-mediated jaw movements; Type II: Neurons with collateralized axons to the globus pallidus that, in turn, project to the entopeduncular nucleus and the dorsolateral part of the substantia nigra pars reticulata, mediating directly the acetylcholine receptor-mediated jaw movements; and Type III: Neurons with a single axon to the ventral pallidum, mediating indirectly the acetylcholine receptor-mediated movements.

The superior colliculus is known to receive tonic GABAergic inhibitory inputs from the dorsolateral part of the substantia nigra pars reticulata and the entopeduncular nucleus (Redgrave *et al.*, 1992; Takada *et al.*, 1994; Yasui *et al.*, 1995), and the superior colliculus in turn sends an excitatory output to the parvicellular reticular formation, predominantly at the contralateral side (Redgrave *et al.*, 1990; Yasui *et al.*, 1994). Both the substantia nigra pars reticulata and the entopeduncular nucleus are also connected with the ventrolateral striatum, where stimulation of either DA or acetylcholine receptors has been found to elicit distinct types of jaw movements in rats (Kikuchi de Beltrán *et al.*, 1992). It has long been

Table 1
Summary of Overall Effects of Local Injections of Muscimol and Bicuculline Into the Ventral Pallidum (VP), Entopeduncular Nucleus (EP) and Dorsolateral Part of the Substantia Nigra Pars Reticulata (DlSNR) on Ventrolateral Striatal Dopamine and Acetylcholine Receptor-mediated Jaw Movements (for Experimental Details, See Adachi *et al.*, 2002).

Stimulation	Areas	Muscimol	Bicuculline
Dopamine receptor	VP	⬇	↓
	EP	⬇	⬇
	dlSNR	↓	⬇
Acetylcholine receptor	VP	0	⬇
	EP	↓	↑
	dlSNR	↓	↑

known that the superior colliculus is involved in the control of DA-dependent oral stereotypy (Dean *et al.*, 1982; Redgrave *et al.*, 1980) and other oral behaviors in rats (Redgrave *et al.*, 1981; Scheel-Krüger, 1986; Taha *et al.*, 1982). Subsequently, the role of $GABA_A$ receptors in the superior colliculus in the production of rat repetitive jaw movements was examined by Adachi *et al.*, (2003). They found that bicuculline dose-dependently produces repetitive jaw movements only when injected bilaterally into a circumscribed region of the lateral deeper layers of the superior colliculus; this region is known to receive input predominantly from the dorsolateral part of the substantia nigra pars reticulata. The effects of bicuculline are $GABA_A$ receptor specific because the effects are abolished by muscimol given into the same site. The bicuculline-induced jaw movements differ qualitatively from those elicited by D1-like/D2-like (Koshikawa *et al.*, 1989; Kikuchi de Beltrán *et al.*, 1992; Adachi *et al.*, 2002) or acetylcholine receptor stimulation (Kikuchi de Beltrán *et al.*, 1992) in the ventrolateral striatum. Nevertheless, injection of muscimol into the lateral deeper layers of the superior colliculus inhibited jaw movements evoked by the D1-like/D2-like receptor stimulation. Conversely, the jaw movements evoked by acetylcholine receptor stimulation are enhanced by injection of muscimol into the superior colliculus. It was suggested by Adachi *et al.* (2003) that $GABA_A$ receptor blockade in a circumscribed region of the lateral deeper layers of the superior colliculus elicits characteristic repetitive jaw movements, and the $GABA_A$ receptors in that region modulate the D1-like/D2-like receptor-mediated and acetylcholine receptor-mediated jaw movements in an opposite manner.

3. *Output Pathways from the Nucleus Accumbens Shell: Involvement in Rat Jaw Movements*

The ventral pallidum is known to receive GABAergic input from the nucleus accumbens (Groenewegen and Russschen, 1984; Zahm and Brog, 1992). The retrorubral field is also known to receive GABAergic input from the nucleus accumbens (Zahm and Heimer, 1993). Although GABAergic manipulation of the ventral pallidum does not elicit repetitive jaw movements (Adachi *et al.*, 2002), it has been found to modulate the jaw movements induced by bilateral injections of a mixture of SKF 82958 and quinpirole into the ventrolateral striatum (Adachi *et al.*, 2002). It is well known that DAergic neurons in the retrorubral field project primarily to the striatum (Gerfen *et al.*, 1987a, b). This region also contains a neural population that projects to the parvicellular reticular formation, a region that contains orofacial premotor nuclei and gives rise to neurons that converge onto neurons in the trigeminal motor nucleus (Fort *et al.*, 1990; Travers and Norgren, 1983). For that reason, it became of interest to compare the role of the retrorubral field with that of the ventral pallidum. Activation of DA receptors in the nucleus accumbens has been found to elicit repetitive jaw movements in rats (Koshikawa *et al.*, 1990b). Subsequently, it has been found that these DA receptor-mediated jaw movements are elicited predominantly by co-activation of D1-like and D2-like receptors in the shell, but not the core, of the nucleus accumbens (Cools *et al.*, 1995; Koshikawa *et al.*, 1996).

The retrorubral field is reported to be involved in the control of oral behaviors in cats (Arts *et al.*, 1998) and the area contains DAergic neurons projecting to the region of the striatum that encompasses its ventrolateral part (Gerfen *et al.*, 1987a, b), where repetitive jaw movements can be elicited by D1-like/D2-like receptor stimulation (Adachi *et al.*, 2002, 2003; Delfs and Kelley, 1990; Koshikawa *et al.*, 1989). The retrorubral field also receives a GABAergic inhibitory input from the nucleus accumbens and is connected with the parvicellular reticular formation, a region that is directly connected with the orofacial motor nuclei. Uchida *et al.* (2005b) examined the role of $GABA_A$ receptors in the retrorubral field in the production of rat repetitive jaw movements using electromyography and a phototransduction system, and found that the $GABA_A$ receptor antagonist bicuculline produces repetitive jaw movements when injected bilaterally into the retrorubral field, but not the ventral pallidum. The effects of bicuculline are $GABA_A$ receptor specific, because they are abolished by muscimol given into the same site. When focusing on the characteristics of jaw movement patterns, bicuculline-induced jaw movements differ qualitatively from those elicited by D1-like/D2-like receptor stimulation in the nucleus accumbens shell. Nevertheless, injections of muscimol into the retrorubral field significantly inhibit jaw movements evoked by the D1-like/D2-like receptor stimulation in the nucleus accumbens shell; injections of bicuculline also reduce the D1-like/D2-like receptor-mediated jaw movements. Essentially similar effects are obtained when muscimol and bicuculline are given into the ventral pallidum, a region that is also known to receive GABAergic inhibitory inputs from the nucleus accumbens. Thus, the study by Uchida *et al.* (2005b) demonstrates that $GABA_A$ receptor blockade in the retrorubral field elicits a characteristic type of repetitive jaw movements that fully differs from those elicited by stimulation of D1-like/D2-like receptors in the nucleus accumbens shell. Furthermore, evidence is provided that $GABA_A$ receptors in the retrorubral field control accumbens shell-specific D1-like/D2-like receptor-mediated jaw movements in a manner essentially similar to that of the $GABA_A$ receptors in the ventral pallidum.

D. Receptors Involved In Orofacial Movement Disorders

1. *D1-like/D2-like Receptor Interaction*

It is well recognized that DA receptor subtypes, particularly those of the D1-like and D2-like families interact to exert a critical role in the regulation of orofacial movements, with which cooperative/synergistic and oppositional interactions are documented (Delfs and Kelley, 1990; O'Sullivan *et al.*, 2010; Rosengarten and Friedhoff, 1998; Waddington *et al.*, 1995, 2001, 2005). As an important example, bilateral co-stimulation of both D1-like and D2-like receptors, particularly in the ventrolateral part of the striatum (Delfs and Kelley, 1990; Koshikawa *et al.*, 1989; Lee *et al.*, 2003) and the nucleus accumbens shell (Cools *et al.*, 1995; Koshikawa *et al.*, 1996), readily elicits repetitive jaw movements in rats. Specifically, in studies using a light-emitting diode attached to the mandible that permits a detailed qualitative and quantitative analysis of jaw movements in rats, D1-like receptor stimulation with systemically administered SKF 38393 produces frequent bursts of teeth chattering. D2-like receptor stimulation by quinpirole produces infrequent bursts of jaw movements, which were characterized by low frequency jaw opening and closure movements from the rest position of the jaw and absence of tongue protrusions; an additional stimulation of D1-like receptors by giving SKF 38393 produces an almost continuous pattern of jaw openings but less closure movements from the rest position, and the openings were accompanied by frequent tongue protrusions, demonstrating that the type of oral behavior produced by stimulation of D1-like and D2-like receptors together is qualitatively different from that produced by stimulation of either D1-like or D2-like receptors alone (Koshikawa *et al.*, 1991a). As mentioned above, such functional interaction between D1-like and D2-like receptors occurs also when both receptor agonists are focally injected into the ventrolateral part of the striatum (Delfs and Kelley, 1990; Koshikawa *et al.*, 1989; Lee *et al.*, 2003) or the nucleus accumbens shell (Cools *et al.*, 1995; Koshikawa *et al.*, 1996); in the latter case, though D3 receptor specificity of the employed compound 7-OH-DPAT is required, mesolimbic D3 receptors may not play any role in D1-like/D2-like receptor-dependent and shell-specific jaw movements (Koshikawa *et al.*, 1996). Simultaneous electromyographic recording of masseter (jaw closing) muscle and digastric (jaw opening) muscle reveals that DA receptor-mediated jaw movements are marked by a dominant digastric muscle activity during jaw opening and a dominant masseter activity during jaw closing (digastric/masseter type), whereas the acetylcholine receptor-mediated jaw movements were marked by a dominant digastric activity during jaw opening without any significant change in the masseter activity during jaw closing (digastric type) (see Fig. 2). These jaw movements induced by D1-like/D2-like receptor stimulation appear to be affected by central neuromodulatory systems, including acetylcholine (Kikuchi de Beltrán *et al.*, 1992), serotonin (Fujita *et al.*, 2008) and adenosine (Lee *et al.*, 2004).

These behavioral findings have led to the hypothesis that DA receptor-mediated jaw movements are mediated via mechanisms that differ from those involved in the acetylcholine receptor-mediated jaw movements.

2. *D1-like Receptors Coupled to Adenylyl Cyclase vs Phosphoinositide Hydrolysis*

While D1-like receptors have been defined conventionally in terms of their linkage to the stimulation of adenylyl cyclase, neurochemical, neurophysiological and behavioral evidence indicates also the existence of a D1-like receptor coupled to a transduction system additional to adenylyl cyclase, with phosphoinositide hydrolysis being the most widely studied candidate (Mahan *et al.*, 1990; Undie and Friedman, 1994; Undie *et al.*, 1994, 2000; Waddington *et al.*, 1995). However, any role for such a site at other levels of function is poorly understood. There are two relatively specific compounds available for studying functional role of these D1-like receptors: SKF 83822, which stimulates D1-like receptors coupled to adenylate cyclase (Andersen and Jansen, 1990; O'Sullivan *et al.*, 2004; Undie *et al.*, 1994) and SKF 83959, which stimulates D1-like receptors coupled to phosphoinositide hydrolysis (Deveney and Waddington, 1995; Jin *et al.*, 2003; Panchalingam and Undie, 2001; Undie *et al.*, 1994).

In a study examining the effects on orofacial movement topography of SKF 83822 in comparison with SKF 83959 in rats, SKF 83822 alone induces chattering, while SKF 83959 alone exerted little effect. SKF 83822 and SKF 83959 each in combination with the D2-like agonist quinpirole results in synergistic induction of non-chattering movements with tongue protrusions (Adachi *et al.*, 1999, 2003; Hasegawa *et al.*, 2001; Fujita *et al.*, 2006). These effects are blocked by the D1-like receptor antagonist SCH 23390 (Adachi *et al.*, 1999; Fujita *et al.*, 2006). However, the D2-like receptor antagonist YM-09151-2 exerts a biphasic effect on synergism with SKF 83822: chattering is initially released but antagonized thereafter (Fujita *et al.*, 2006). While both adenylyl cyclase- and phosphoinositide-coupled D1-like receptors participate in synergistic D1-like/D2-like receptor interactions, topographically specific synergistic and oppositional D1-like/D2-like interactions evident with SKF 83822 reflect the involvement primarily of D1-like receptors coupled to adenylyl cyclase rather than phosphoinositide hydrolysis. Thus, distinct topographies of jaw movement appear to be regulated differentially by adenylyl cyclase- vs. phosphoinositide hydrolysis-coupled D1-like receptor mechanisms and their interactions with D2-like receptors. These findings may be relevant for the pathogenesis and treatment of conditions characterized by orofacial movement disorder, such as tardive dyskinesia, where inter alia abnormalities of DAergic function are implicated.

Another study has applied new magnetic sensor-electromyographic technology to record jaw movements in freely moving rats so as to analyze topographies of orofacial movements that occur in association with individual elements of behavior under challenge with two D1-like receptor agonists, SKF 83822 and SKF 83959 (Fujita *et al.*, 2010a). As can be seen in Fig. 1, grooming of the snout/face involves primarily dominant-mouth opening jaw movements with small activation of digastric muscles; subsequent grooming of the flank/trunk is characterized by repetitive, uniform jaw movements with small activation of digastric and masseter muscles. In contrast, grooming of the fingers and tail typically involves high-frequency jaw movements with variable vertical jaw movements and/or strong activation of masseter muscles. Vacuous chewing involves two distinct patterns of jaw movements: a dominant-closing pattern, with strong activation of masseter muscles, and a dominant-opening pattern, with slight activation of masseter muscles. Thus, these agonists exert differential effects on jaw movements, as SKF 83959 induces more jaw movements per episode of syntactic grooming than SKF 83822, while SKF 83822 induces more jaw movements during non-syntactic grooming than SKF 83959 (Fujita *et al.*, 2010a). Magnetic sensor technology in freely moving animals resolved distinct topographies of orofacial movement and informs on their relationship to other behaviors in the rodent repertoire and to D1-like receptor function.

3. *Cholinergic Receptors*

In studies on cholinergic involvement in the regulation of orofacial behavior in rats, acetylcholine receptor agonists given either systemically or into the

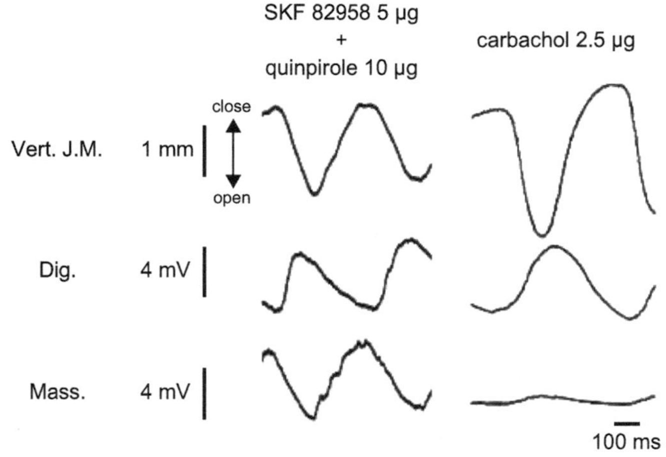

FIG. 2. Difference in pattern of jaw movements elicited by dopamine D1-like/D2-like receptor and acetylcholine receptor stimulation in the ventrolateral striatum. For D1-like/D2-like receptor stimulation, injection of a mixture of SKF 82958 (5 μg) and quinpirole (10 μg) was used; acetylcholine receptor stimulation was with the injection of carbachol (2.5 μg). Averaged values of 10 consecutive vertical component of jaw movements (Vert. J.M.) and associated electromyographic (EMG) activity recorded from digastric (Dig.) and masseter (Mass.) muscles are shown (For experimental details, see Adachi *et al.*, 2002).

ventrolateral striatum induce repetitive oral movements (Kikuchi de Beltrán *et al.*, 1992; Adachi *et al.*, 2002). These acetylcholine receptor-mediated jaw movements are marked by a dominant digastric activity during jaw opening, without any significant change in masseter activity during jaw closing (digastric type), whereas, as mentioned in the above section, DA receptor-mediated jaw movements are marked by a dominant digastric activity during jaw opening and a dominant masseter activity during jaw closing (digastric/masseter type) (see Fig. 2). These acetylcholine receptor-mediated jaw movements are inhibited by the $GABA_A$ receptor agonist muscimol given into the entopeduncular nucleus and dorsolateral part of the substantia nigra pars reticulata, whereas these movements are enhanced by the $GABA_A$ receptor antagonist bicuculline. In contrast, acetylcholine receptor-mediated jaw movements are not affected by muscimol injections into the ventral pallidum, but are inhibited by bicuculline (Adachi *et al.*, 2002) (Table 1).

Striatal DArgic/cholinergic interactions in the regulation of oral behavior in rats were also studied (Kikuchi de Beltrán *et al.*, 1992). Orofacial movements induced by apomorphine are potentiated by carbachol injected into the dorsal striatum, while inhibition is found following carbachol injections into the ventrolateral striatum. Orofacial movements induced by injection of carbachol into the ventral striatum are enhanced by injection of a combination of D1-like/D2-like receptor agonists (SKF 38393 and quinpirole) into the same site and are inhibited by the DA receptor antagonist (*cis*)-flupentixol. These behavioral findings have led to the hypothesis that acetylcholine receptor-mediated jaw movements are mediated via mechanisms that differ from those involved in DA receptor-mediated jaw movements, and that the striatal DA/acetylcholine interaction in their regulation is neither simply antagonistic or synergistic, nor reciprocal.

Cholinergic stimulation is also known to elicit tremulous jaw movements in rats. The movements share some characteristics with Parkinsonian tremor (Mayorga *et al.*, 1997, 1999; Salamone *et al.*, 1998), and are dependent on ventrolateral striatal mechanisms (Cousins *et al.*, 1999) as well as the related GABAergic output pathways (Finn *et al.*, 1997). The tremulous jaw movements induced by cholinomimetics appear to be affected by central neuromodulatory systems including DA (Salamone *et al.*, 2005), serotonin (Carlson *et al.*, 2003) and adenosine (Collins *et al.*, 2010).

4. *Thyrotropin-releasing Hormone*

Thyrotropin-releasing hormone (TRH) has been shown to elicit a variety of biological activities (Ikegami *et al.*, 1989; Yamamoto *et al.*, 1990; Matsui *et al.*, 1994). Some of these effects appear to share a DAergic mechanism; for example, inhibition of D1-like/D2-like receptors attenuates TRH effects (Popoli *et al.*, 1991). DAergic terminal areas, such as the nucleus accumbens, receive a dense innervation of TRH-containing fibres (Hökfelt *et al.*, 1975) and contain a high concentration of TRH receptors (Taylor and Butt, 1982). The TRH has the ability to enhance the release of DA (Méndez *et al.*, 1993; Ogata *et al.*, 1998), while it is also able to inhibit the uptake of DA (Ikegami *et al.*, 1989). YM-14673, a TRH analogue, is known to elicit sniffing and hyperlocomotion, behaviors generally thought to be mediated by DAergic mechanisms (Yamamoto *et al.*, 1990). When injected into the nucleus accumbens, the ventrolateral striatum and the dorsal striatum, YM-14673 produces repetitive jaw movements in a dose-dependent manner. These effects are greatest in the nucleus accumbens and smallest in the ventrolateral striatum and are blocked by non-selective DA receptor antagonist, (*cis*)-flupentixol. The pattern of these movements differs from that produced by injections of a mixture of SKF 38393 and quinpirole; frequent tongue protrusions are evident in rats treated with the mixture but those are not seen in YM-14673-treated rats (Miwa *et al.*, 1995). Since TRH does not evoke jaw movements from any of these sites, the mechanisms giving rise to the display of jaw movements after intrastriatal injections of YM-14673 remain unknown. Nevertheless, stimulation of D1-like/D2-like receptors may at least partly contribute to these effects (Miwa *et al.*, 1995). These findings, together with other reports (Kawada *et al.*, 1995), suggest that neuropeptides in the basal ganglia play important roles in the manifestation of orofacial dyskinetic symptoms.

5. *Cholecystokinin*

The CCK-8 is known to coexist with DA in some mesolimbic DAergic neurons, for example in the medial region of the nucleus accumbens but not in the lateral region, which appears to be devoid of CCK (Hökfelt *et al.*, 1980). These two regions are considered to be almost equivalent to the widely accepted subdivisions characterized in later studies, i.e. shell and core of the nucleus accumbens, respectively (Heimer *et al.*, 1991; Zahm and Brog, 1992; Jongen-Rêlo *et al.*, 1994). Both antagonistic effects of CCK-8 towards DA (Stoessl *et al.*, 1989; Zetler, 1985) and facilitatory effects (Stittsworth and Mueller, 1990; Weiss *et al.*, 1988) have been reported. It is possible that these differences may relate to anatomical and functional heterogeneity within the nucleus accumbens. CCK-8 and its analogue caerulein injected into the dorsomedial nucleus accumbens increase the frequency of apomorphine-induced jaw movements (Koshikawa *et al.*, 1991b). The potentiation is prevented by administration of the CCK-A (CCK_1) receptor antagonist lorglumide together with CCK-8 or caerulein; injection of lorglumide alone does not alter apomorphine-induced jaw movements. Moreover, injections of CCK-8 and caerulein into adjacent sites (the ventrolateral nucleus accumbens, the dorsal striatum, and the ventrolateral striatum) do not affect the responses elicited by apomorphine (Koshikawa *et al.*, 1991b). These results demonstrate that CCK-8 modulates responses elicited by the DA receptor agonist apomorphine in a region of the brain where CCK-8 is known to coexist with DA.

These findings, together with other reports (Kawada *et al.*, 1995; Miwa *et al.*, 1995), suggest that neuropeptides in the basal ganglia play important roles in the manifestation of orofacial dyskinetic symptoms.

6. *NMDA Receptors*

Although D1-like/D2-like receptors in ventrolateral striatum play a critical role in the regulation of orofacial movements (Delfs and Kelley, 1990; Koshikawa *et al.*, 1989), there are important interactions with other neurotransmitters in this region. The striatum receives glutamatergic projections from the cerebral cortex; this information is then modified in the striatum and transmitted downstream via GABAergic medium spiny neurons. Medium spiny neurons receive dense DAergic projections from the substantia nigra pars compacta (Hallett and Standaert, 2004) and contain high levels of NMDA receptors (Albin *et al.*, 1992; Standaert *et al.*, 1999). As mentioned above, the striatum is thought to exert its function via a direct and an indirect pathway. In the ventrolateral part of the striatum, the direct pathway originates from GABAergic neurons that project monosynaptically upon neurons of the substantia nigra pars reticulata, and the indirect pathway arises from GABAergic neurons that project polysynaptically upon the substantia nigra pars reticulata via relays in the globus pallidus and the subthalamic nucleus (Gerfen, 1992a, b; Smith *et al.*, 1998). In contrast to the well-documented role of the GABAergic direct pathway in rat jaw movements evoked by D1-like/D2-like receptor stimulation in the ventrolateral striatum (Adachi *et al.*, 2002), the role of the indirect pathway remains unclear. The neurons in the subthalamic nucleus that project to the substantia nigra pars reticulata are known to be glutamatergic (Delong, 1990; Parent and Hazrati, 1995). Regarding the functional role of the indirect pathway, the glutamate NMDA receptor subtype antagonists, AP-5 and MK-801, have been shown to enhance locomotor activity at a level of the substantia nigra pars reticulata (Murer *et al.*, 1996; St-Pierre and Bédard, 1994). For orofacial movements evoked by D1-like/D2-like receptor stimulation in the ventrolateral striatum, bilateral injections of NMDA or MK-801 into the substantia nigra pars reticulata, which alone do not produce jaw movements, reduce DAergic repetitive jaw movements (Uchida *et al.*, 2005a). Moreover, other behaviors such as grooming, rearing, yawning, vacuous chewing, and locomotor activity that occur after D1-like/D2-like receptor stimulation are not significantly altered by bilateral injections of NMDA or MK-801 into the substantia nigra pars reticulate (Uchida *et al.*, 2005a). Given the previous results showing that both an agonist and an antagonist of $GABA_A$ receptors injected into the substantia nigra pars reticulata inhibit jaw movements elicited by D1-like/D2-like receptor stimulation in the ventrolateral striatum (Adachi *et al.*, 2002), these results suggest that there are complex functional interactions between NMDA and $GABA_A$ receptors within the substantia nigra pars reticulata that may be responsible for the common orofacial profiles in the effects of NMDA and $GABA_A$ receptor agents.

In studies on the role of NMDA receptors at the level of the ventrolateral striatum (Kelley and Delfs, 1994; Fujita *et al.*, 2010b), apomorphine-induced repetitive jaw movements are reduced by bilateral microinjections of the NMDA into the ventrolateral striatum. Apomorphine-induced repetitive jaw movements are also reduced by bilateral microinjections of the NMDA receptor antagonists AP-5 or MK-801. The inhibitory effect of NMDA is reduced by co-administration of MK-801. Microinjections of drugs into the ventrolateral striatum in the absence of apomorphine do not affect jaw movements (Fujita *et al.*, 2010b). These results suggest that NMDA receptors in the ventrolateral striatum play an important modulatory role in the expression of D1-like/D2-like receptor-mediated jaw movements. However, similar effects of NMDA and NMDA receptor antagonists echo previous paradoxical findings and indicate that interactions between DA and NMDA receptors are complex and multifaceted.

7. *Overview*

Studies on the roles of different anatomical regions and distinct receptor systems in the regulation of orofacial movements indicate complex interactions between D1-like/D2-like receptors, GABA receptors, glutamate receptors, and other neurotransmitter and neuropeptide receptors. These interactions take place not only within the basal ganglia, nucleus accumbens and their efferent systems, but involve also their connections with cortical, other subcortical, and brainstem regions. Additionally, there is the challenge of how these mechanisms subserve not only the orofacial movements in general but, rather, the numerous individual patterns and topographies of orofacial behavior that constitute the mammalian repertoire.

Acknowledgments

This work was funded by a grant for promotion of multidisciplinary research projects entitled "Translational Research Network on Orofacial Neurological Disorders," from the Ministry of Education, Culture, Sports, Science and Technology, Japan.

References

Adachi, K., Ikeda, H., Hasegawa, M., Nakamura, S., Waddington, J.L., and Koshikawa, N. (1999). SK&F 83959 and non-cyclase-coupled dopamine D1-like receptors in jaw movements via dopamine D1-like/D2-like receptor synergism. *Eur. J. Pharmacol.* **367**, 143–149.

Adachi, K., Hasegawa, M., Fujita, S., Sato, M., Miwa, Y., Ikeda, H., Koshikawa, N., and Cools, A.R. (2002). Dopaminergic and cholinergic stimulation of the ventrolateral striatum elicit rat jaw movements that are funnelled via distinct efferents. *Eur. J. Pharmacol.* **442**, 81–92.

Adachi, K., Hasegawa, M., Ikeda, H., Sato, M., Koshikawa, N., and Cools, A.R. (2003). The superior colliculus contains a discrete region involved in the control of jaw movements: role of $GABA_A$ receptors. *Eur. J. Pharmacol.* **464**, 147–154.

Albin, R.L., Makowiec, R.L., Hollingsworth, Z.R., Dure, L.S.,4th, 4th Penney, J.B., and Young, A.B. (1992). Excitatory amino acid binding sites in the basal ganglia of the rat: a quantitative autoradiographic study. Neuroscience ***46***, 35–48

Andersen, P.H., and Jansen, J.A. (1990). Dopamine receptor agonists: selectivity and dopamine D1 receptor efficacy. *Eur. J. Pharmacol.* **188**, 335–347.

Arnt, J. (1985). Antistereotypic effects of dopamine D-1 and D-2 antagonists after intrastriatal injection in rats. Pharmacological and regional specificity. *Naunyn Schmiedebergs Arch. Pharmacol.* **330**, 97–104.

Arts, M.P., Bemelmans, F.F., and Cools, A.R. (1998). Role of the retrorubral nucleus in striatally elicited orofacial dyskinesia in cats: effects of muscimol and bicuculline. Psychopharmacology (Berl.) **140**, 150–156.

Beckstead, R.M., and Cruz, C.J. (1986). Striatal axons to the globus pallidus, entopeduncular nucleus and substantia nigra come mainly from separate cell populations in cat. *Neuroscience* **19**(1); 147–158.

Bergson, C., Mrzljak, L., Smiley, J.F., Pappy, M., Levenson, R., and Goldman-Rakic, P.S. (1995). Regional, cellular, and subcellular variations in the distribution of D1 and D5 dopamine receptors in primate brain. *J. Neurosci.* **15**, 7821–7836.

Boyson, S.J., McGonigle, P., and Molinoff, P.B. (1986). Quantitative autoradiographic localization of the D1 and D2 subtypes of dopamine receptors in rat brain. *J. Neurosci.* **6**, 3177–3188.

Calabresi, P., Di Filippo, M., Ghiglieri, V., Tambasco, N., and Picconi, B. (2010). Levodopa-induced dyskinesias in patients with Parkinson's disease: filling the bench-to-bedside gap. *Lancet Neurol.* **9**, 1106–1117.

Carlson, B.B., Wisniecki, A., and Salamone, J.D. (2003). Local injections of the 5-hydroxytryptamine antagonist mianserin into substantia nigra pars reticulate block tremulous jaw movements in rats: studies with a putative model of Parkinsonian tremor. *Psychopharmacology (Berl.)* **165**, 229–237.

Casey, D.E. (1985). Spontaneous and tardive dyskinesia: Clinical and laboratory studies. *J. Clin. Psychiatry* **46**, 42–47.

Casey, D.E. (1989). Clozapine: neuroleptic-induced EPS and tardive dyskinesia. *Psychopharmacology (Berl.)* **99**(Suppl); S47–S53.

Casey, D.E. (1990). Tardive dyskinesia. *West. J. Med.* **153**, 535–541.

Chase, T.N., Mouradian, M.M., and Engber, T.M. (1993). Motor response complications and the function of striatal efferent systems. *Neurology* **43**(12 Suppl 6); S23–S27.

Collins, L.E., Galtieri, D.J., Brennum, L.T., Sager, T.N., Hockemeyer, J., Müller, C.E., Hinman, J.R., Chrobak, J.J., and Salamone, J.D. (2010). Oral tremor induced by the muscarinic agonist pilocarpine is suppressed by the adenosine A2A antagonists MSX-3 and SCH58261, but not the adenosine A1 antagonist DPCPX. *Pharmacol Biochem Behav.* **94**, 561–569.

Collins, P., Broekkamp, C.L., Jenner, P., and Marsden, C.D. (1991). Drugs acting at D-1 and D-2 dopamine receptors induce identical purposeless chewing in rats which can be differentiated by cholinergic manipulation. *Psychopharmacology (Berl.)* **103**, 503–512.

Collins, P., Broekkamp, C.L., Jenner, P., and Marsden, C.D. (1993). Electromyographical differentiation of the components of perioral movements induced by SKF 38393 and physostigmine in the rat. *Psychopharmacology (Berl.)* **112**, 428–436.

Cools, A.R. (1983). Mesolimbic system and tardive dyskinesia: new perspectives for therapy. *Mod. Probl. Pharmacopsychiatry* **21**, 111–123.

Cools, A.R., Spooren, W., Bezemer, R., Cuypers, E., Jaspers, R., and Groenewegen, H. (1989). Anatomically distinct output channels of the caudate nucleus and orofacial dyskinesia: critical role of the subcommissural part of the globus pallidus in oral dyskinesia. *Neuroscience* **33**, 535–542.

Cools, A.R., Miwa, Y., and Koshikawa, N. (1995). Role of dopamine D1 and D2 receptors in the nucleus accumbens in jaw movements of rats: a critical role of the shell. *Eur. J. Pharmacol.* **286**, 41–47.

Cousins, M.S., Finn, M., Trevitt, J., Carriero, D.L., Conlan, A., and Salamone, J.D. (1999). The role of ventrolateral striatal acetylcholine in the production of tacrine-induced jaw movements. *Pharmacol. Biochem. Behav.* **62**, 439–447.

Dal Toso, R., Sommer, B., Ewert, M., Herb, A., Pritchett, D.B., Bach, A., Shivers, B.D., and Seeburg, P.H. (1989). The dopamine D2 receptor: two molecular forms generated by alternative splicing. *EMBO J.* **8**, 4025–4034.

Dean, P., Redgrave, P., and Eastwood, L. (1982). Suppression of apomorphine-induced oral stereotypy in rats by microinjection of muscimol into midbrain. *Life Sci.* **30**, 2171–2179.

Defagot, M.C., and Antonelli, M.C. (1997). Autoradiographic localization of the putative D4 dopamine receptor in rat brain. *Neurochem. Res.* **22**, 401–407.

Delfs, J.M., and Kelley, A.E. (1990). The role of D1 and D2 dopamine receptors in oral stereotypy induced by dopaminergic stimulation of the ventrolateral striatum. *Neuroscience* **39**, 59–67.

DeLong, M.R. (1990). Primate models of movement disorders of basal ganglia origin. *Trends Neurosci.* **13**, 281–285.

Deutch, A.Y., and Cameron, D.S. (1992). Pharmacological characterization of dopamine systems in the nucleus accumbens core and shell. *Neuroscience* **46**, 49–56.

Deveney, A.M., and Waddington, J.L. (1995). Pharmacological characterization of behavioural responses to SK&F 83959 in relation to 'D1-like' dopamine receptors not linked to adenylyl cyclase. *Br. J. Pharmacol.* **116**, 2120–2126.

Diana, M., Collu, M., Mura, A., and Gessa, G.L. (1992). Haloperidol-induced vacuous chewing in rats: suppression by alpha-methyl-tyrosine. *Eur. J. Pharmacol.* **211**, 415–419.

Egan, M.F., Hurd, Y., Ferguson, J., Bachus, S.E., Hamid, E.H., and Hyde, T.M. (1996). Pharmacological and neurochemical differences between acute and tardive vacuous chewing movements induced by haloperidol. *Psychopharmacology (Berl.)* **127**, 337–345.

Ellison, G., See, R., Levin, E., and Kinney, J. (1987). Tremorous mouth movements in rats administered chronic neuroleptics. *Psychopharmacology (Berl.)* **92**, 122–126.

Faurbye, A., Rasch, P.J., Petersen, P.B., Brandborg, G., and Pakkenberg, H. (1964). Neurological symptoms in pharmacotherapy of psychoses. *Acta. Psychiatr. Scand.* **40**, 10–27.

Finn, M., Mayorga, A.J., Conlan, A., and Salamone, J.D. (1997). Involvement of pallidal and nigral GABA mechanisms in the generation of tremulous jaw movements in rats. *Neuroscience* **80**, 535–544.

Fort, P., Luppi, P.H., Sakai, K., Salvert, D., and Jouvet, M. (1990). Nuclei of origin of monoaminergic, peptidergic, and cholinergic afferents to the cat trigeminal motor nucleus: a double-labeling study with cholera-toxin as a retrograde tracer. *J. Comp. Neurol.* **301**, 262–275.

Fujita, S., Lee, J., Kiguchi, M., Uchida, T., Cools, A.R., Waddington, J.L., and Koshikawa, N. (2006). Topographical resolution of jaw movements mediated by cyclase- vs. non-cyclase-coupled dopamine D_1-like receptors: studies with SK&F 83822. *Eur. J. Pharmacol.* **538**, 94–100.

Fujita, S., Kiguchi, M., Lee, J., Terakado, M., Suga, K., Hatanaka, H., and Koshikawa, N. (2008). 5-HT_{1A} and 5-HT_{1B} receptors in the ventrolateral striatum differentially modulate apomorphine-induced jaw movements in rats. *J. Oral Sci.* **50**, 387–395.

Fujita, S., Kiguchi, M., Kobayashi, M., Kinsella, A., Koshikawa, N., and Waddington, J.L. (2010 a) Assessment of jaw movements by magnetic sensor in relation to topographies of orofacial behaviour in freely moving rats: Studies with the dopamine D1-like receptor agonists SKF 83822 vs SKF 83959. *Eur. J. Pharmacol.* **632**(1–3); 39–44.

Fujita, S., Kiguchi, M., Kobayashi, M., Koshikawa, N., and Waddington, J.L. (2010 b) Involvement of NMDA receptors in the ventrolateral striatum of rats in apomorphine-induced jaw movements. *Brain Res.* **1322**, 30–37.

Fuxe, K., Agnati, L.F., Köhler, C., Kuonen, D., Ogren, S.O., Andersson, K., and Hökfelt, T. (1981). Characterization of normal and supersensitive dopamine receptors: effects of ergot drugs and neuropeptides. *J. Neural Transm.* **51**, 3–37.

Garrick, N.A., and Murphy, D.L. (1980). Species differences in the deamination of dopamine and other substrates for monoamine oxidase in brain. Psychopharmacology (Berl) **72**, 27–33.

Gerfen, C.R. (1992 a) The neostriatal mosaic: multiple levels of compartmental organization. *Trends Neurosci.* **15**, 133–139.

Gerfen, C.R. (1992 b) The neostriatal mosaic: multiple levels of compartmental organization in the basal ganglia. *Annu. Rev. Neurosci.* **15**, 285–320.

Gerfen, C.R., Herkenham, M., and Thibault, J. (1987 a) The neostriatal mosaic: II. *Patch- and matrix-directed mesostriatal dopaminergic and non-dopaminergic systems. J. Neurosci.* **7**, 3915–3934.

Gerfen, C.R., Baimbridge, K.G., and Thibault, J. (1987 b) The neostriatal mosaic: III. *Biochemical and developmental dissociation of patch-matrix mesostriatal systems. J. Neurosci.* **7**, 3935–3944.

Gingrich, J.A., and Caron, M.G. (1993). Recent advances in the molecular biology of dopamine receptors. *Annu. Rev. Neurosci.* **16**, 299–321.

Giros, B., Sokoloff, P., Martres, M.P., Riou, J.F., Emorine, L.J., and Schwartz, J.C. (1989). Alternative splicing directs the expression of two D2 dopamine receptor isoforms. *Nature* **342**, 923–926.

Groenewegen, H.J., Becker, N.E., and Lohman, A.H. (1980). Subcortical afferents of the nucleus accumbens septi in the cat, studied with retrograde axonal transport of horseradish peroxidase and bisbenzimid. *Neuroscience* **5**, 1903–1916.

Groenewegen, H.J., and Russchen, F.T. (1984). Organization of the efferent projections of the nucleus accumbens to pallidal, hypothalamic, and mesencephalic structures: a tracing and immunohistochemical study in the cat. *J. Comp. Neurol.* **223**, 347–367.

Gunne, L.M., Andersson, U., Bondesson, U., and Johansson, P. (1986). Spontaneous chewing movements in rats during acute and chronic antipsychotic drug administration. *Pharmacol. Biochem. Behav.* **25**, 897–901.

Hallett, P.J., and Standaert, D.G. (2004). Rationale for and use of NMDA receptor antagonists in Parkinson's disease. *Pharmacol. Ther.* **102**, 155–174.

Hasegawa, M., Adachi, K., Nakamura, S., Sato, M., Waddington, J.L., and Koshikawa, N. (2001). Ventral striatal vs. accumbal (shell) mechanisms and non-cyclase-coupled dopamine D_1-like receptors in jaw movements. *Eur. J. Pharmacol.* **423**, 171–178.

Heimer, L., Zahm, D.S., Churchill, L., Kalivas, P.W., and Wohltmann, C. (1991). Specificity in the projection patterns of accumbal core and shell in the rat. *Neuroscience* **41**, 89–125.

Hikosaka, O., and Wurtz, R.H. (1985). Modification of saccadic eye movements by GABA-related substances. *II. Effects of muscimol in monkey substantia nigra pars reticulata. J. Neurophysiol.* **53**, 292–308.

Hökfelt, T., Fuxe, K., Johansson, O., Jeffcoate, S., and White, N. (1975). Distribution of thyrotropin-releasing hormone (TRH) in the central nervous system as revealed with immunohistochemistry. *Eur. J. Pharmacol.* **34**, 389–392.

Hökfelt, T., Skirboll, L., Rehfeld, J.F., Goldstein, M., Markey, K., and Dann, O. (1980). A subpopulation of mesencephalic dopamine neurons projecting to limbic areas contains a cholecystokinin-like peptide: evidence from immunohistochemistry combined with retrograde tracing. *Neuroscience* **5**, 2093–2124.

Hoover, J.E., and Strick, P.L. (1993). Multiple output channels in the basal ganglia. *Science* **259**, 819–821.

Hunker, C.J., Abbs, J.H., and Barlow, S.M. (1982). The relationship between Parkinsonism rigidity and hypokinesia in the orofacial system: A quantitative analysis. *Neurology* **32**, 755–761.

Ikeda, H., Adachi, K., Hasegawa, M., Sato, M., Hirose, N., Koshikawa, N., and Cools, A.R. (1999). Effects of chronic haloperidol and clozapine on vacuous chewing and dopamine-mediated jaw movements in rats: evaluation of a revised animal model of tardive dyskinesia. *J. Neural Transm.* **106**, 1205–1216.

Ikegami, H., Spahn, S.A., and Prasad, C. (1989). Neuropeptide-dopamine interactions. *IV. Effect of thyrotropin-releasing hormone on striatal dopaminergic neurons. Peptides* **10**, 681–685.

Iwata, K., Yagi, J., Tsuboi, Y., Koshikawa, N., Sumino, R., and Cools, A.R. (1996). Anatomical connections of the ventral, but not the dorsal part of the striatum with the parvicellular reticular formation: implications for the anatomical substrate of oral movements. *Neurosci. Res. Comm.* **18**, 71–77.

Jankovic, J., and Casabona, J. (1987). Coexistent tardive dyskinesia and Parkinsonism. *Clin. Neuropharmacol.* **10**, 511–521.

Jaspers, R.M., Berkelbach van der Sprenkel, J.W., and Cools, A.R. (1989). Progressive pathology of the caudate nucleus, the substantia nigra pars reticulata and the deeper layers of the colliculus superior: acute behavioural and metabolic effects of intrastriatal kainic acid. *Neuroscience* **28**, 159–169.

Jin, L.Q., Goswami, S., Cai, G., Zhen, X., and Friedman, E. (2003). SKF83959 selectively regulates phosphatidylinositol-linked D1 dopamine receptors in rat brain. *J. Neurochem.* **85**, 378–386.

Jongen-Rêlo, A.L., Voorn, P., and Groenewegen, H.J. (1994). Immunohistochemical characterization of the shell and core territories of the nucleus accumbens in the rat. *Eur. J. Neurosci.* **6**, 1255–1264.

Kawada, Y., Ogawa, N., Asanuma, M., and Mori, A. (1995). Neuropeptide levels in discrete brain regions in the iminodipropionitrile-induced persistent dyskinesia rat model. *Regul. Pept.* **55**, 103–110.

Kawaguchi, Y. (1997). Neostriatal cell subtypes and their functional roles. *Neurosci. Res.* **27**, 1–8.

Kebabian, J.W., and Calne, D.B. (1979). Multiple receptors for dopamine. *Nature* **277**, 93–96.

Kelley, A.E., Bakshi, V.P., Delfs, J.M., and Lang, C.G. (1989). Cholinergic stimulation of the ventrolateral striatum elicits mouth movements in rats: pharmacological and regional specificity. *Psychopharmacology (Berl.)* **99**, 542–549.

Kelley, A.E., and Delfs, J.M. (1994). Excitatory amino acid receptors mediate the orofacial stereotypy elicited by dopaminergic stimulation of the ventrolateral striatum. *Neuroscience* **60**, 85–95.

Kikuchi de Beltrán, K., Koshikawa, N., Saigusa, T., Watanabe, K., Koshida, Y., and Kobayashi, M. (1992). Cholinergic/dopaminergic interaction in the rat striatum assessed from drug-induced repetitive oral movements. *Eur. J. Pharmacol.* **214**, 181–189.

Koshikawa, N., Aoki, S., Tomiyama, K., Maruyama, Y., and Kobayashi, M. (1987). Sulpiride injection into the dorsal striatum increases methamphetamine-induced gnawing in rats. *Eur. J. Pharmacol.* **133**, 119–125.

Koshikawa, N., Aoki, S., Hiruta, M., Tomiyama, K., Kobayashi, M., Tsuboi, Y., Iwata, K., Sumino, R., and Stephenson, J.D. (1989). Effects of intrastriatal injections of selective dopamine D-1 and D-2 agonists and antagonists on jaw movements of rats. *Eur. J. Pharmacol.* **163**, 227–236.

Koshikawa, N., Tomiyama, K., Omiya, K., Kikuchi de Beltrán, K., and Kobayashi, M. (1990 a). Dopamine D-1 but not D-2 receptor stimulation of the dorsal striatum potentiates apomorphine-induced jaw movements in rats. *Eur. J. Pharmacol.* **178**, 189–194.

Koshikawa, N., Koshikawa, F., Tomiyama, K., Kikuchi de Beltrán, K., Kamimura, F., and Kobayashi, M. (1990 b) Effects of dopamine D1 and D2 agonists and antagonists injected into the nucleus accumbens and globus pallidus on jaw movements of rats. *Eur. J. Pharmacol.* **182**, 375–380.

Koshikawa, N., Kikuchi de Beltrán, K., Tomiyama, K., Kobayashi, M., and Cools, A.R. (1991a). Functional interaction between dopamine D1 and D2 receptors in rat jaw movements. *Eur. J. Pharmacol.* **201**, 47–51.

Koshikawa, N., Kikuchi de Beltrán, K., Saigusa, T., Kobayashi, M., and Stephenson, J.D. (1991b). Cholecystokinin octapeptide and caerulein injection into the dorsomedial nucleus accumbens potentiate apomorphine-induced jaw movements in rats. *Eur. J. Pharmacol.* **209**, 75–80.

Koshikawa, N., Miwa, Y., Adachi, K., Kobayashi, M., and Cools, A.R. (1996). Behavioural effects of 7-OH-DPAT are solely due to stimulation of dopamine D2 receptors in the shell of the nucleus accumbens; jaw movements. *Eur. J. Pharmacol.* **308**, 227–234.

Lee, J., Adachi, K., Gionhaku, N., Fujita, S., Uchida, T., and Koshikawa, N. (2003). Measurement of dopamine receptor-mediated jaw movements by a magnet-sensing system in freely moving rats. *Methods Find. Exp. Clin. Pharmacol.* **25**, 525–530.

Lee, J., Adachi, K., Gionhaku, N., Fujita, S., Uchida, T., Gerstner, G.E., and Koshikawa, N. (2004). Evidence that angiotensin II enhances apomorphine-induced jaw movements via AT_1 receptors in the ventrolateral striatum: studies by magnet-sensing system in freely moving rats. *Methods Find. Exp. Clin. Pharmacol.* **26**, 195–199.

Leopold, N.A., and Kagel, M.C. (1996). Prepharyngeal dysphagia in Parkinson's disease. *Dysphagia* **11**, 14–22.

Leppig, M., Bosch, B., Naber, D., and Hippius, H. (1989). Clozapine in the treatment of 121 out-patients. *Psychopharmacology (Berl.)* ***99*(Suppl)**S77–S79

Levy, A.D., and Ellison, G.D. (1987). Interaction between chronic amphetamine and neuroleptic treatments on oral behavior in rats. *Psychopharmacology (Berl.)* **93**, 218–222.

Loopuijt, L.D., and van der Kooy, D. (1985). Organization of the striatum: collateralization of its efferent axons. *Brain Res.* **348**, 86–99.

Loughlin, S.E., and Fallon, J.H. (1984). Substantia nigra and ventral tegmental area projections to cortex: topography and collateralization. *Neuroscience* **11**, 425–435.

Mahan, L.C., Burch, R.M., Monsma Jr., F.J., and Sibley, D.R. (1990). Expression of striatal D1 dopamine receptors coupled to inositol phosphate production and Ca^{2+} mobilization in *Xenopus* oocytes. *Proc. Natl. Acad. Sci. USA* **87**, 2196–2200.

Mansour, A., Meador-Woodruff, J.H., Bunzow, J.R., Civelli, O., Akil, H., and Watson, S.J. (1990). Localization of dopamine D2 receptor mRNA and D1 and D2 receptor binding in the rat brain and pituitary: an in situ hybridization-receptor autoradiographic analysis. *J. Neurosci.* **10**, 2587–2600.

Margolese, H.C., Chouinard, G., Kolivakis, T.T., Beauclair, L., and Miller, R. (2005 a) Tardive dyskinesia in the era of typical and atypical antipsychotics. Part 1: pathophysiology and mechanisms of induction. *Can. J. Psychiatry* **50**, 541–547.

Margolese, H.C., Chouinard, G., Kolivakis, T.T., Beauclair, L., Miller, R., and Annable, L. (2005 b) Tardive dyskinesia in the era of typical and atypical antipsychotics. Part 2: incidence and management strategies in patients with schizophrenia. *Can. J. Psychiatry* **50**, 703–714.

Marsden, C.D., and Parkes, J.D. (1976). "On-off" effects in patients with Parkinson's disease on chronic levodopa therapy. *Lancet* **1**, 292–296.

Matsui, K., Wada, K., and Kwak, S. (1994). Ataxia-ameliorating effects of YM-14673, a potent analog of thyrotropin releasing hormone, in ataxic mutant mice. *Eur. J. Pharmacol.* **254**, 295–297.

Mayorga, A.J., Carriero, D.L., Cousins, M.S., Gianutsos, G., and Salamone, J.D. (1997). Tremulous jaw movements produced by acute tacrine administration: possible relation to Parkinsonian side effects. *Pharmacol. Biochem. Behav.* **56**, 273–279.

Mayorga, A.J., Cousins, M.S., Trevitt, J.T., Conlan, A., Gianutsos, G., and Salamone, J.D. (1999). Characterization of the muscarinic receptor subtype mediating pilocarpine-induced tremulous jaw movements in rats. *Eur. J. Pharmacol.* **364**, 7–11.

McGeorge, A.J., and Faull, R.L. (1989). The organization of the projection from the cerebral cortex to the striatum in the rat. *Neuroscience* **29**, 503–537.

Meador-Woodruff, J.H., Mansour, A., Grandy, D.K., Damask, S.P., Civelli, O., and Watson Jr., S.J. (1992). Distribution of D5 dopamine receptor mRNA in rat brain. *Neurosci. Lett.* **145**, 209–212.

Méndez, M., Morán, J., Wilk, S., Joseph-Bravo, P., and Charli, J.L. (1993). Assessment of the role of TRH in the release of [^{3}H]-dopamine from rat nucleus accumbens-lateral septum slices. *Brain Res. Bull* **31**, 621–625.

Missale, C., Nash, S.R., Robinson, S.W., Jaber, M., and Caron, M.G. (1998). Dopamine receptors: from structure to function. *Physiol. Rev.* **78**, 189–225.

Miwa, Y., Koshikawa, N., Miyata, N., Koshida, Y., Kobayashi, M., and Cools, A.R. (1995). YM-14673, a thyrotropin-releasing hormone analogue, injected into the nucleus accumbens and the striatum produces repetitive jaw movements in rats. *Eur. J. Pharmacol.* **77**, 63–69.

Mogenson, G.J., Jones, D.L., and Yim, C.Y. (1980). From motivation to action: functional interface between the limbic system and the motor system. *Prog. Neurobiol.* **14**, 69–97.

Mogoseanu, D., Smith, A.D., and Bolam, J.P. (1993). Monosynaptic innervation of trigeminal motor neurones involved in mastication by neurones of the parvicellular reticular formation. *J. Comp. Neurol.* **336**, 53–65.

Mogoseanu, D., Smith, A.D., and Bolam, J.P. (1994). Monosynaptic innervation of facial motoneurones by neurones of the parvicellular reticular formation. *Exp. Brain Res.* **101**, 427–438.

Muller, P., and Seeman, P. (1978). Dopaminergic supersensitivity after neuroleptics: time-course and specificity. *Psychopharmacology (Berl.)* **60**, 1–11.

Murer, G., Tseng, K., Sinay, V., Penalva, R., Armando, I., and Pazo, J.H. (1996). Turning behavior induced by injections of glutamate receptor antagonists into the substantia nigra of the rat. *Synapse* **24**, 147–155.

Nishikawa, T., Tanaka, M., Koga, I., and Uchida, Y. (1985). Biphasic and long-lasting effect of ceruletide on tardive dyskinesia. *Psychopharmacology (Berl.)* **86**, 43–44.

Nishikawa, T., Tanaka, M., Tsuda, A., Kuwahara, H., Koga, I., and Uchida, Y. (1986). Effect of ceruletide on tardive dyskinesia: a pilot study of quantitative computer analyses on electromyogram and microvibration. *Psychopharmacology (Berl.)* **90**, 5–8.

Offermeier, J., and van Rooyen, J.M. (1983). Dopamine inhibitory and excitatory systems in tardive dyskinesias. *Mod. Probl. Pharmacopsychiatry* **21**, 124–142.

Ogata, A., Nagashima, K., Yasui, K., Matsuura, T., and Tashiro, K. (1998). Sustained release dosage of thyrotropin-releasing hormone improves experimental Japanese encephalitis virus-induced Parkinsonism in rats. *J. Neurol. Sci.* **159**, 135–139.

O'Sullivan, G.J., Roth, B.L., Kinsella, A., and Waddington, J.L. (2004). SK&F 83822 distinguishes adenylyl cyclase from phospholipase C-coupled dopamine D1-like receptors: behavioural topography. *Eur. J. Pharmacol.* **486**, 273–280.

O'Sullivan, G.J., O'Tuathaigh, C., Tomiyama, K., Koshikawa, N., and Waddington, J.L. (2010). Dopamine receptor subtypes and behaviour: from psychopharmacology to mutant models. In: Neve, K. (Ed.), *"The Dopamine Receptors"*. Totowa, NJ, Humana Press, pp. 323–371.

Owens, D.G., Johnstone, E.C., and Frith, C.D. (1982). Spontaneous involuntary disorders of movement: their prevalence, severity, and distribution in chronic schizophrenics with and without treatment with neuroleptics. *Arch. Gen. Psychiatry* **39**, 452–461.

Pakkenberg, H., Fog, R., and Nilakantan, B. (1973). The long-term effect of perphenazine enanthate on the rat brain. *Some metabolic and anatomical observations. Psychopharmacologia* **29**, 329–336.

Panchalingam, S., and Undie, A.S. (2001). SKF83959 exhibits biochemical agonism by stimulating [^{35}S]GTPγS binding and phosphoinositide hydrolysis in rat and monkey brain. *Neuropharmacology* **40**, 826–837.

Parent, A. (1990). Extrinsic connections of the basal ganglia. *Trends Neurosci.* **13**, 254–258.

Parent, A., Bouchard, C., and Smith, Y. (1984). The striatopallidal and striatonigral projections: two distinct fiber systems in primate. *Brain Res.* **303**, 385–390.

Parent, A., and Hazrati, L.N. (1995). Functional anatomy of the basal ganglia. II. The place of subthalamic nucleus and external pallidum in basal ganglia circuitry. *Brain Res. Rev* **20**, 128–154.

Pennartz, C.M., Dolleman-Van der Weel, M.J., Kitai, S.T., and Lopes da Silva, F.H. (1992). Presynaptic dopamine D1 receptors attenuate excitatory and inhibitory limbic inputs to the shell region of the rat nucleus accumbens studied in vitro. *J. Neurophysiol.* **67**, 1325–1334.

Peritogiannis, V., and Tsouli, S. (2010). Can atypical antipsychotics improve tardive dyskinesia associated with other atypical antipsychotics? Case report and brief review of the literature. *J. Psychopharmacol.* **24**, 1121–1125.

Popoli, P., Caporali, M.G., and Scotti de Carolis, A. (1991). Interactions between dopamine D1 and D2 receptors in the model of thyrotropin-releasing hormone (TRH)-induced behaviour in rabbits. *Eur. J. Pharmacol.* **201**, 11–16.

Prinssen, E.P., Balestra, W., Bemelmans, F.F., and Cools, A.R. (1994). Evidence for a role of the shell of the nucleus accumbens in oral behavior of freely moving rats. *J. Neurosci.* **14**, 1555–1562.

Redgrave, P., Dean, P., Donohoe, T.P., and Pope, S.G. (1980). Superior colliculus lesions selectively attenuate apomorphine-induced oral stereotypy: a possible role for the nigrotectal pathway. *Brain Res.* **196**, 541–546.

Redgrave, P., Dean, P., Souki, W., and Lewis, G. (1981). Gnawing and changes in reactivity produced by microinjections of picrotoxin into the superior colliculus of rats. *Psychopharmacology (Berl.)* **75**, 198–203.

Redgrave, P., Dean, P., and Westby, G.W. (1990). Organization of the crossed tecto-reticulo-spinal projection in rat-I. Anatomical evidence for separate output channels to the periabducens area and caudal medulla. *Neuroscience* **37**, 571–584.

Redgrave, P., Marrow, L., and Dean, P. (1992). Topographical organization of the nigrotectal projection in rat: evidence for segregated channels. *Neuroscience* **50**, 571–595.

Richardson, M.A., and Craig, T.J. (1982). The coexistence of Parkinsonism-like symptoms and tardive dyskinesia. *Am. J. Psychiatry* **139**, 341–343.

Richfield, E.K., Penney, J.B., and Young, A.B. (1989). Anatomical and affinity state comparisons between dopamine D1 and D2 receptors in the rat central nervous system. *Neuroscience* **30**, 767–777.

Rollema, H., Skolnik, M., D'Engelbronner, J., Igarashi, K., Usuki, E., and Castagnoli Jr., N. (1994). MPP^+-like neurotoxicity of a pyridinium metabolite derived from haloperidol: in vivo microdialysis and in vitro mitochondrial studies. *J. Pharmacol. Exp. Ther.* **268**, 380–387.

Rosengarten, H., and Friedhoff, A.J. (1998). A phosphoinositide-linked dopamine D1 receptor mediates repetitive jaw movements in rats. *Biol. Psychiatry* **44**, 1178–1184.

Ross, C.A., and Tabrizi, S.J. (2011). Huntington's disease: from molecular pathogenesis to clinical treatment. *Lancet Neurol.* **10**, 83–98.

Rupniak, N.M., Jenner, P., and Marsden, C.D. (1983). Cholinergic manipulation of perioral behaviour induced by chronic neuroleptic administration to rats. *Psychopharmacology (Berl.)* **79**, 226–230.

Rupniak, N.M., Jenner, P., and Marsden, C.D. (1985). Pharmacological characterisation of spontaneous or drug-associated purposeless chewing movements in rats. *Psychopharmacology (Berl.)* **85**, 71–79.

Salamone, J.D., Mayorga, A.J., Trevitt, J.T., Cousins, M.S., Conlan, A., and Nawab, A. (1998). Tremulous jaw movements in rats: a model of Parkinsonian tremor. *Prog Neurobiol.* **56**, 591–611.

Salamone, J.D., Carlson, B.B., Rios, C., Lentini, E., Correa, M., Wisniecki, A., and Betz, A. (2005). Dopamine agonists suppress cholinomimetic-induced tremulous jaw movements in an animal model of Parkinsonism: tremorolytic effects of pergolide, ropinirole and CY 208-243. *Behav. Brain Res.* **156**, 173–179.

Samadi, P., Grégoire, L., Morissette, M., Calon, F., Hadj Tahar, A., Bélanger, N., Dridi, M., Bédard, P. J., and Di Paolo, T. (2008 a) Basal ganglia group II metabotropic glutamate receptors specific binding in non-human primate model of L-Dopa-induced dyskinesias. *Neuropharmacology* **54**, 258–268.

Samadi, P., Morissette, M., Calon, F., Hadj Tahar, A., Dridi, M., Belanger, N., Meltzer, L.T., Bédard, P.J., and Di Paolo, T. (2008 b) Normalization of $GABA_A$ receptor specific binding in the substantia nigra reticulata and the prevention of L-dopa-induced dyskinesias in MPTP Parkinsonian monkeys. *Synapse* **62**, 101–109.

Scheel-Krüger, J. (1986). Dopamine-GABA interactions: evidence that GABA transmits modulates and mediates dopaminergic functions in the basal ganglia and the limbic system. *Acta Neurol. Scand. Suppl.* **107**, 1–54.

Schneider, J.S., Diamond, S.G., and Markham, C.H. (1986). Deficits in orofacial sensorimotor function in Parkinson's disease. *Ann. Neurol.* **19**, 275–282.

See, R.E., and Ellison, G. (1990). Comparison of chronic administration of haloperidol and the atypical neuroleptics, clozapine and raclopride, in an animal model of tardive dyskinesia. *Eur. J. Pharmacol.* **181**, 175–186.

Smith, J.M., and Baldessarini, R.J. (1980). Changes in prevalence, severity and recovery in tardive dyskinesia with age. *Arch. Gen. Psychiatry* **37**, 1368–1373.

Smith, Y., Bevan, M.D., Shink, E., and Bolam, J.P. (1998). Microcircuitry of the direct and indirect pathways of the basal ganglia. *Neuroscience* **86**, 353–387.

Soares-Weiser, K., and Rathbone, J. (2004). Calcium channel blockers for neuroleptic-induced tardive dyskinesia. *Cochrane Database Syst. Rev.* **1**, CD000206.

Sokoloff, P., Giros, B., Martres, M.P., Bouthenet, M.L., and Schwartz, J.C. (1990). Molecular cloning and characterization of a novel dopamine receptor (D3) as a target for neuroleptics. *Nature* **347**, 146–151.

Spann, B.M., and Grofova, I. (1991). Nigropedunculopontine projection in the rat: an anterograde tracing study with phaseolus vulgaris-leucoagglutinin (PHA-L). *J. Comp. Neurol.* **311**, 375–388.

Stittsworth Jr., J.D., and Mueller, A.L. (1990). Cholecystokinin octapeptide potentiates the inhibitory response mediated by D2 dopamine receptors in slices of the ventral tegmental area of the brain in the rat. *Neuropharmacology* **29**, 119–127.

St-Pierre, J.A., and Bédard, P.J. (1994). Intranigral but not intrastriatal microinjection of the NMDA antagonist MK-801 induces contralateral circling in the 6-OHDA rat model. *Brain Res.* **660**, 255–260.

Standaert, D.G., Friberg, I.K., Landwehrmeyer, G.B., Young, A.B., and Penney Jr., J.B. (1999). Expression of NMDA glutamate receptor subunit mRNAs in neurochemically identified projection and interneurons in the striatum of the rat. *Mol. Brain Res.* **64**, 11–23.

Stoessl, A.J., Dourish, C.T., and Iversen, S.D. (1989). Chronic neuroleptic-induced mouth movements in the rat: suppression by CCK and selective dopamine D1 and D2 receptor antagonists. *Psychopharmacology (Berl.)* **98**, 372–379.

Stoof, J.C., and Kebabian, J.W. (1981). Opposing roles for D-1 and D-2 dopamine receptors in efflux of cyclic AMP from rat neostriatum. *Nature* **294**, 366–368.

Sunahara, R.K., Guan, H.C., O'Dowd, B.F., Seeman, P., Laurier, L.G., Ng, G., George, S.R., Torchia, J., Van Tol, H.H., and Niznik, H.B. (1991). Cloning of the gene for a human dopamine D5 receptor with higher affinity for dopamine than D1. *Nature* **350**, 614–619.

Taha, E.B., Dean, P., and Redgrave, P. (1982). Oral behaviour induced by intranigral muscimol is unaffected by haloperidol but abolished by large lesions of superior colliculus. *Psychopharmacology (Berl.)* **77**, 272–278.

Takada, M., Tokuno, H., Ikai, Y., and Mizuno, N. (1994). Direct projections from the entopeduncular nucleus to the lower brainstem in the rat. *J. Comp. Neurol.* **342**, 409–429.

Tarsy, D., and Baldessarini, R.J. (1977). The pathophysiologic basis of tardive dyskinesia. *Biol. Psychiatry.* **12**, 431–450.

Taylor, R.L., and Burt, D.R. (1982). Species differences in the brain regional distribution of receptor binding for thyrotropin-releasing hormone. *J. Neurochem.* **38**, 1649–1656.

Terai, M., Usuda, S., Kuroiwa, I., Noshiro, O., and Maeno, H. (1983). Selective binding of YM-09151-2, a new potent neuroleptic, to D2-dopaminergic receptors. *Jpn. J. Pharmacol.* **33**, 749–755.

Tiberi, M., Jarvie, K.R., Silvia, C., Falardeau, P., Gingrich, J.A., Godinot, N., Bertrand, L., Yang-Feng, T.L., Fremeau Jr., R.T., and Caron, M.G. (1991). Cloning, molecular characterization, and chromosomal assignment of a gene encoding a second D1 dopamine receptor subtype: differential expression pattern in rat brain compared with the D1A receptor. *Proc. Natl. Acad. Sci. USA* **88**, 7491–7945.

Tomiyama, K., O'Tuathaigh, C., and Waddington, J.L. (2011). Regulation of orofacial movements: aminoacid mechanisms and mutant models. *Int. Rev. Neurobiol.* in press

Travers, J.B., and Norgren, R. (1983). Afferent projections to the oral motor nuclei in the rat. *J. Comp. Neurol.* **220**, 280–298.

Uchida, T., Lee, J., Fujita, S., Kiguchi, M., Matsumoto, M., Oi., Y., Gionhaku, N., and Koshikawa, N. (2005 a) Effects of NMDA and MK-801 injected into the substantia nigra pars reticulata on jaw movements evoked by dopamine D1-/D2 receptor stimulation in the ventrolateral striatum: studies in freely moving rats. *Methods Find. Exp. Clin. Pharmacol.* **27**, 31–37.

Uchida, T., Adachi, K., Fujita, S., Lee, J., Gionhaku, N., Cools, A.R., and Koshikawa, N. (2005 b) Role of $GABA_A$ receptors in the retrorubral field and ventral pallidum in rat jaw movements elicited by dopaminergic stimulation of the nucleus accumbens shell. *Eur. J. Pharmacol.* **510**, 39–47.

Undie, A.S., and Friedman, E. (1994). Inhibition of dopamine agonist-induced phosphoinositide hydrolysis by concomitant stimulation of cyclic AMP formation in brain slices. *J. Neurochem.* **63**, 222–230.

Undie, A.S., Weinstock, J., Sarau, H.M., and Friedman, E. (1994). Evidence for a distinct D1-like dopamine receptor that couples to activation of phosphoinositide metabolism in brain. *J. Neurochem.* **62**, 2045–2048.

Undie, A.S., Berki, A.C., and Beardsley, K. (2000). Dopaminergic behaviors and signal transduction mediated through adenylate cyclase and phospholipase C pathways. *Neuropharmacology* **39**, 75–87.

von Krosigk, M., and Smith, A.D. (1991). Descending projection from the substantia nigra and retrorubral field to the medullary and pontomedullary reticular formation. *Eur. J. Neurosci.* **3**, 260–273.

von Krosigk, M., Smith, Y., Bolam, J.P., and Smith, A.D. (1992). Synaptic organization of GABAergic inputs from the striatum and the globus pallidus onto neurons in the substantia nigra and retrorubral field which project to the medullary reticular formation. *Neuroscience* **50**, 531–549.

Van Tol, H.H., Bunzow, J.R., Guan, H.C., Sunahara, R.K., Seeman, P., Niznik, H.B., and Civelli, O. (1991). Cloning of the gene for a human dopamine D4 receptor with high affinity for the antipsychotic clozapine. *Nature* **350**, 610–614.

Waddington, J.L. (1989). Schizophrenia, affective psychoses, and other disorders treated with neuroleptic drugs: the enigma of tardive dyskinesia, its neurobiological determinants, and the conflict of paradigms. *Int. Rev. Neurobiol.* **31**, 297–353.

Waddington, J.L. (1990). Spontaneous orofacial movements induced in rodents by very long-term neuroleptic drug administration: phenomenology, pathophysiology and putative relationship to tardive dyskinesia. *Psychopharmacology (Berl.)* **101**, 431–447.

Waddington, J.L., Daly, S.A., Downes, R.P., Deveney, A.M., McCauley, P.G., and O'Boyle, K.M. (1995). Behavioural pharmacology of 'D-1-like' dopamine receptors: further subtyping, new pharmacological probes and interactions with 'D-2-like' receptors. *Prog. Neuropsychopharmacol. Biol. Psychiatry* **19**, 811–831.

Waddington, J.L., Clifford, J.J., McNamara, F.N., Tomiyama, K., Koshikawa, N., and Croke, D.T. (2001). The psychopharmacology-molecular biology interface: exploring the behavioural roles of dopamine receptor subtypes using targeted gene deletion ('knockout'). *Prog. Neuropsychopharmacol. Biol. Psychiatry* **25**, 925–964.

Waddington, J.L., O'Tuathaigh, C., O'Sullivan, G., Tomiyama, K., Koshikawa, N., and Croke, D.T. (2005). Phenotypic studies on dopamine receptor subtype and associated signal transduction mutants: insights and challenges from 10 years at the psychopharmacology-molecular biology interface. *Psychopharmacology (Berl.)* **18**, 611–638.

Waddington, J.L., O'Sullivan, G.J., and Tomiyama, K. (2011). Regulation of orofacial movement: dopamine receptor mechanisms and mutant models. *Int. Rev. Neurobiol.* in press

Walker, F.O. (2007). Huntington's disease. *Lancet* **369**, 218–228.

Weiss, F., Tanzer, D.J., and Ettenberg, A. (1988). Opposite actions of CCK-8 on amphetamine-induced hyperlocomotion and stereotypy following intracerebroventricular and intra-accumbens injections in rats. *Pharmacol. Biochem. Behav.* **30**, 309–317.

Westerink, B.H., and de Vries, J.B. (1989). On the mechanism of neuroleptic induced increase in striatal dopamine release: brain dialysis provides direct evidence for mediation by autoreceptors localized on nerve terminals. *Neurosci. Lett.* **99**, 197–202.

Whitty, P., Owoeye, O., and Waddington, J.L. (2009). Neurological signs and involuntary movements in schizophrenia: intrinsic to and informative on systems pathobiology. *Schizophr. Bull.* **35**, 415–424.

Wichmann, T., and DeLong, M.R. (1996). Functional and pathophysiological models of the basal ganglia. *Curr. Opin. Neurobiol.* **6**, 751–758.

Wolf, M.E., Chevesich, J., Lehrer, E., and Mosnaim, A.D. (1983). The clinical association of tardive dyskinesia and drug-induced Parkinsonism. *Biol. Psychiatry* **18**, 1181–1188.

Wu, Y., and Parent, A. (2000). Striatal interneurons expressing calretinin, parvalbumin or NADPH-diaphorase: a comparative study in the rat, monkey and human. *Brain Res.* **863**, 182–191.

Wu, Y., Richard, S., and Parent, A. (2000). The organization of the striatal output system: a single-cell juxtacellular labeling study in the rat. *Neurosci. Res.* **38**, 49–62.

Yahr, M.D. (1978). Overview of present day treatment of Parkinson's disease. *J. Neural Transm.* **43**, 227–238.

Yamamoto, M., Ozawa, Y., Sasamata, M., Koshikawa, N., and Kobayashi, M. (1990). Central dopaminergic actions of YM-14673, a new TRH analogue, in rodents. *Eur. J. Pharmacol.* **180**, 319–324.

Yassa, R., and Jeste, D.V. (1992). Gender differences in tardive dyskinesia: a critical review of the literature. *Schizophr. Bull.* **18**, 701–715.

Yasui, Y., Nakano, K., Nakagawa, Y., Kayahara, T., Shiroyama, T., and Mizuno, N. (1992). Non-dopaminergic neurons in the substantia nigra project to the reticular formation around the trigeminal motor nucleus in the rat. *Brain Res.* **585**, 361–366.

Yasui, Y., Tsumori, T., Ando, A., Domoto, T., Kayahara, T., and Nakano, K. (1994). Descending projections from the superior colliculus to the reticular formation around the motor trigeminal nucleus and the parvicellular reticular formation of the medulla oblongata in the rat. *Brain Res.* **656**, 420–426.

Yasui, Y., Tsumori, T., Ando, A., and Domoto, T. (1995). Demonstration of axon collateral projections from the substantia nigra pars reticulata to the superior colliculus and the parvicellular reticular formation in the rat. *Brain Res.* **674**, 122–126.

Youdim, M.B. (1978). The active centers of monoamine oxidase types "A" and "B": binding with (^{14}C)-clorgyline and (^{14}C)-deprenyl. *J. Neural Transm.* **43**, 199–208.

Zahm, D.S., and Brog, J.S. (1992). On the significance of subterritories in the "accumbens" part of the rat ventral striatum. *Neuroscience* **50**, 751–767.

Zahm, D.S., and Heimer, L. (1993). Specificity in the efferent projections of the nucleus accumbens in the rat: comparison of the rostral pole projection patterns with those of the core and shell. *J. Comp. Neurol.* **327**, 220–232.

Zetler, G. (1985). Antistereotypic effects of cholecystokinin octapeptide (CCK-8), ceruletide and related peptides on apomorphine-induced gnawing in sensitized mice. *Neuropharmacology* **24**, 251–259.

Zhou, Q.Y., Grandy, D.K., Thambi, L., Kushner, J.A., Van Tol, H.H., Cone, R., Pribnow, D., Salon, J., Bunzow, J.R., and Civelli, O. (1990). Cloning and expression of human and rat D1 dopamine receptors. *Nature* **347**, 76–80.

REGULATION OF OROFACIAL MOVEMENT: DOPAMINE RECEPTOR MECHANISMS AND MUTANT MODELS

John L. Waddington[1], Gerard J. O'Sullivan[1] and Katsunori Tomiyama[2]

[1]Molecular and Cellular Therapeutics, Royal College of Surgeons in Ireland, Dublin 2, Ireland
[2]Department of Pharmacology, Nihon University School of Dentistry, Tokyo 101, Japan

I. Introduction

A. The Nature of Orofacial Movements

Given the involvement of the orofacial region in so many diverse and essential functions, the underlying regulatory mechanisms must be complex. While there appear to be generators for "core," down-stream patterns of orofacial movement

INTERNATIONAL REVIEW OF NEUROBIOLOGY, VOL. 97
DOI: 10.1016/B978-0-12-385198-7.00002-3

(Lund and Kolta, 2006; Goulding, 2009), these are likely regulated by multiple, upstream mechanisms that are dependent on the circumstances in which given orofacial movement(s) occur and their intended purpose; these include comsummatory behavior, self-care, defensive and attack behaviors, vocalization and, in higher mammals, verbal as well as non-verbal communication (Graziano, 2006; van der Bilt *et al.*, 2006; Sessle *et al.*, 2007; Pong, Horn, and Gibson, 2008). For example, whether opening of the jaw occurs to eat, yawn, shout or attack a conspecific, or is manifested involuntarily in Huntington's disease, some commonality of motor pattern is driven by higher processes related to the prevailing purpose and its physiological and psychosocial milieu.

B. The Role of Dopamine

A primary role for the neurotransmitter dopamine (DA) in regulating orofacial movements derives from early recognition of (i) The ability of direct and indirect dopaminergic (DAergic) agonist drugs to induce stereotyped behaviors that involve the perioral region, (ii) The effect of long-term treatment with the DA precursor L-dopa to induce *inter alia* orofacial dyskinesia as a late-onset adverse effect in the treatment of Parkinson's disease (PD) and (iii) The effect of long-term treatment with DA receptor antagonists to induce *inter alia* tardive orofacial dyskinesia as a late-onset adverse effect in the treatment of psychotic illness such as schizophrenia (Waddington *et al.*, 1995; Di Chiara 2002; Margolese *et al.*, 2005; Jenner, 2008). Multiple studies have now elaborated this role of DAergic mechanisms (O'Sullivan *et al.*, 2010; see also Koshikawa, Fujita, and Adachi, 2011, this volume). Yet, however important these may be, they constitute only one level of explanation within the broader and deeper neuroscience of how orofacial movements are regulated, from molecular mechanisms, through integration of physiological and psychosocial processes, to ultimate manifestation.

Even though DAergic processes constitute one fundamental level of explanation, two particular challenges endure: (i) How might individual elements of often complex orofacial movement patterns, subserving diverse functions, be regulated differentially and coordinated by DAergic mechanisms, and: (ii) What are the roles of individual DA receptor subtypes and their associated transduction mechanisms in these processes; orofacial movement is a broad, generic term that encompasses multiple, coordinated motor sequences, each of which is composed of numerous individual motor topographies that may be mechanistically distinct.

C. Dopamine Receptor Subtypes, Transduction and Behavior

Molecular approaches have been the essential route to broader subtyping of DA receptors beyond the original, pharmacologically based D1/D2 nomenclature

(Kebabian and Calne, 1979) into D1-like [D1 and D5] and D2-like [D2, D3 and D4] families, together with additional D1-like and D2-like entities, deriving from alternative splicing, evolutionary diversity and phylogenetic heterogeneity, that are of uncertain functional significance (Di Chiara, 2002; Neve, 2010). Medicinal chemistry has failed to keep pace with these developments in terms of identifying selective agonists and antagonists acting at each individual member of these molecular biologically defined families. Thus, until this situation is rectified, systematic resolution of their functional roles depends upon mutant mice with targeted gene deletion [knockout (KO)] or gene insertion [transgenic/knock-in], in comparison with wildtype (WT) controls, for such functional parcellation (Waddington *et al.*, 2005; O'Sullivan *et al.*, 2010). In the present context, such mutants can illuminate the functional roles of individual DA receptor subtypes at two phenotypic levels: (i) Spontaneous orofacial movements, and (ii) Orofacial movements, induced by currently available agonists and antagonists that are able to distinguish *between*, but much less so *within*, the D1-like vs D2-like families. Similarly, mutant mice can illuminate the signalling processes and cascades by which DA receptor-mediated events are transduced, via KO of essential components of these cascades, particularly dopamine- and adenosine 3′,5′-monophosphate-regulated phosphoprotein of 32 kilodaltons (DARPP-32; Svenningsson *et al.*, 2004; Waddington *et al.*, 2005; Neve, 2010).

D. Assessment of Orofacial Movements in Mutant Mouse Models

The ability of mutant mice to inform on the functional roles of individual DA receptor subtypes is critically dependent upon a clear concept of the function at issue. While mutants can be applied, at least theoretically, to study orofacial movements occurring in the course of each of comsummatory, self-care, defensive, attack, and vocalization behaviors, the esential precursor is to study mutant phenotype in terms of spontaneous orofacial movements and those induced by selective DA receptor subtype agonists that can distinguish *between*, though not *within*, D1-like vs D2-like receptor families. Methodologically, study of orofacial movements in rats has a long history (Waddington, 1990; Koshikawa *et al.*, 2011, this volume), the complexities of which are magnified by the physical dimensions of mice that render them even less accessible to detailed assessment. For example, much work in rats has centred on assessment of "vacuous chewing", i.e. chewing movements not directed onto any physical material; however, unless prominent, these are substantialy inaccessible in the mouse (Waddington, 1990; Tomiyama *et al.*, 2001).

A critical choice is the observation of orofacial movements in: (i) Freely moving mice, which has the advantage of physiologically relevant conditions but is limited by inability to resolve individual topographies of orofacial movement under such conditions, vs (ii) Assessment under some restriction device that has the advantage of allowing resolution of individual topographies of orofacial movement but is limited by non-physiological conditions (Waddington, 1990; Koshikawa *et al.*, 2011, this volume). To help address this challenge, we have introduced two complementary techniques for the study of KO vs WT mice, though caution must be exercised in comparing directly these two conceptually distinct experimental conditions.

The first (Clifford *et al.*, 1998; Waddington *et al.*, 2005) accesses and quantifies the natural repertoire of behavioral topographies manifested by the mouse as it initially explores, and then subsequently habituates to a novel environment. This approach defines the broad *ethogram* of murine behavior, among which orofacial movements are a small, relatively inaccessible component; within the *ethogram*, these can be captured reliably only in terms of more general behaviors that involve orofacial movements, such as "sniffing" [i.e. movements of the vibrissae and flaring of the nostrils], "grooming" [whether of any form (i.e. total grooming), or intense, sequential grooming of the snout and then face with the forepaws, followed by vigorous grooming of the flank/anogenital region with the snout (i.e. syntactic grooming)], and as "chewing" [i.e. chewing movements are directed onto any physical material, without consumption; note that food is not usually available during such assessments, unless feeding behavior is a specific topic of study] (see Table I).

The second (Tomiyama *et al.*, 2001; Waddington *et al.*, 2005) accesses and quantifies several distinct topographies of orofacial movement that can be resolved only in a restrictor; this approach captures these specific forms of orofacial movement [i.e. vertical jaw movements, horizontal jaw movements, tongue protrusions and rapid movements of the incisors, together with movements of the head and of the vibrissae] (see Table II), but at the expense of those other behaviors constituting the *ethogram*.

Table I

General Behaviors in Mice that Involve Orofacial Movements, as Assessed Ethologically.

Behavior	Abbreviation	Description
Sniffing	Sn	Movements of the vibrissae and flairing of the nostrils, in the air, over the floor or along the cage wall
Grooming - total	Gr_t	Grooming of any form
Grooming - syntactic	Gr_s	Characteristic grooming syntax of sequential grooming of the snout and then the face with the forepaws, followed by vigoror grooming of the flank/anogenital region with the snout
Chewing	Ch	Chewing directed onto any physical material without consumption

Table II
SPECIFIC OROFACIAL MOVEMENTS IN MICE, AS ASSESSED IN A RESTRICTOR.

Movement	Abbreviation	Description
Jaw - vertical	Jv	Jaw movements in vertical plane
Jaw - horizontal	Jh	Jaw movements in horizontal plane
Tongue protrusions	Tg	Protrusion of tongue outside of mouth
Chattering of incisors	Ct	High-frequency rhythmical jaw movements with tapping of the incisors
Head	Hd	Movements of the head
Vibrissae	Vb	Movements of the vibrissae

Orofacial movements can be measured spontaneously as: (i) Part of the *ethogram* over an initial 60 min period of exploration, followed by several hours of subsequent habituation to the environment, and: (ii) Over a 180 min period of habituation to the restrictor. After habituation in either paradigm, orofacial movements can also be measured following acute challenge with dopaminergic agonists or other psychopharmacological agents. In systematic studies (Tomiyama *et al.*, 2001; Waddington *et al.*, 2005; O'Sullivan *et al.*, 2010) we have utilized: (i) The D1-like agonist SKF 83959, which acts selectively at D1-like receptors coupled to phosphoinositide hydrolysis; previous evidence has indicated that orofacial movements are induced preferentially by this putative subtype of D1-like receptors, rather than by those coupled to adenylate cyclase; (ii) The D2-like agonist RU 24213, which acts selectively at D2, D3 and D4 receptors to induce locomotion and other hyperactivities but is less active to induce orofacial movements.

II. Orofacial Movements in Mice with "Knockout" of D1-like Receptors

A. OROFACIAL MOVEMENTS IN MICE WITH "KNOCKOUT" OF D1 RECEPTORS

1. *Spontaneous Orofacial Movements*

Within the *ethogram* (McNamara *et al.*, 2003), total grooming over initial exploration is reduced in D1 KO relative to WT (Table III); subsequently sniffing habituates in WT but not in D1 KO, such that sniffing occurs to excess, with enduring reduction in total grooming (Table IV). D1 KO does not influence syntactic grooming or chewing relative to WT.

Table III
General Phenotypic Behaviors in Mutant Mice that Involve Orofacial Movements, as Assessed Ethologically over Initial Exploration.

Mutant	Sn	Gr_t	Gr_s	Ch
D1	=	↓	=	=
D5	=	=	=	=
D2	=	=	=	=
D3	=	=	=	=
D4	↓	=	=	=
DARPP-32	=	↓	=	=

Orofacial behaviors are as defined in Table I.
↓ decrease in KO.
= unaltered in KO.

Table IV
General Phenotypic Behaviors in Mutant Mice that Involve Orofacial Movements, as Assessed Ethologically over Subsequent Habituation.

Mutant	Sn	Gr_t	Gr_s	Ch
D1	↑ (h)	↓	=	=
D5	=	↓	=	=
D2	=	=	=	=
D3	=	=	=	=
D4	=	=	=	=
DARPP-32	=	↑↓ (h)	=	=

Orofacial behaviors are as defined in Table I.
↑ increase in KO.
↓ decrease in KO.
↑↓ effect of KO varies over habituation.
= unaltered in KO.
(h) KO phenotype involves disruption to habituation.

In the restrictor (Tomiyama *et al.*, 2002), vertical jaw movements are initially prominent in WT but then decline over subsequent habituation; in D1 KO, total vertical jaw movements are unaltered, though there is a small reduction in rate of habituation to the restrictor. Conversely, horizontal jaw movements in WT are initially uncommon but then increase over subsequent habituation; in D1 KO, these movements are markedly reduced. The low rate of tongue protrusions in WT is even lower in D1 KO throughout habituation. The low rate of incisor chattering in WT is also lower initially in D1 KO but increases over habituation to ultimately

Table V
OROFACIAL MOVEMENT PHENOTYPE IN MUTANT MICE, AS ASSESSED DURING HABITUATION TO A RESTRICTOR.

Mutant	Jv	Jh	Tg	Ct	Hd	Vb
D1	↑↓ (h)	↓ (h)	↓	↓ (h)	↑ (h)	↑ (h)
D5	↑ (h)	↓	=	=	=	↓
D2	↑	=	↓	↓	↓ (h)	=
D3	=	=	=	↓ (h)	=	=
D4	=	=	=	=	=	=
DARPP-32	=	=	↓	=	=	=

Orofacial movements are as defined in Table II.
↑ increase in KO.
↓ decrease in KO.
↑↓ effect of KO varies over habituation.
= unaltered in KO.
(h) KO phenotype involves disruption to habituation.

attain a level aproaching that of WT. Head and vibrissae movements are initially prominent in WT but decline over habituation; in D1 KO, head and vibrissae movements are little altered, other than a slower rate of habituation, such that they occur ultimately to slight excess (Table V).

2. *Orofacial Movements Induced by D1-like Agonist Challenge*

Within the *ethogram* (McNamara *et al.*, 2003), SKF 83959 induces sniffing, total grooming and particularly syntactic grooming in WT, but not chewing. In D1 KO, elevated baseline levels of sniffing cannot be increased further by SKF 83959; induction of total grooming and particularly of syntactic grooming by SKF 83959 is reduced in D1 KO relative to WT (Table VI).

In the restrictor (Tomiyama *et al.*, 2002), SKF 83959 readily induces vertical jaw movements and tongue protrusions in WT, together with incisor chattering; these responses are essentially abolished in D1 KO. In contrast, SKF 83959 does not induce horizontal jaw movements. In WT, SKF 83959 induces some head and vibrissae movements; in D1 KO these responses are unaltered (Table VII).

3. *Orofacial Movements Induced by D2-like Agonist Challenge*

Within the *ethogram* (McNamara *et al.*, 2003), the lower doses of RU 24213 reduce sniffing and total grooming in WT, while higher doses induce stereotyped sniffing. In D1 KO, reduction in total grooming by RU 24213 is unaltered, while elevated baseline levels of sniffing cannot be increased further; RU 24213 does not induce chewing in WT but does so in D1 KO (Table VIII).

Table VI

General Phenotypic Behaviors in Mutant Mice that Involve Orofacial Movements, as Assessed Ethologically, Following Challenge with the D1-Like Agonist SKF 83959.

Mutant	Sn	Gr_t	Gr_s	Ch
D1	=	↓	↓	=
D5	=	=	↓	=
D2 (A)	=	=	=	↑ (A)
D3	=	=	=	=
D4	=	↑↓	↓	=
DARPP-32	=	=	=	=

Orofacial behaviors are as defined in Table I.
↑ effect of RU 24213 is increased in KO.
↓ effect of RU 24213 is decreased in KO.
↑↓ effect of RU 24213 varies over habituation in KO.
= effect of RU 24213 is unaltered in KO.
(A) D1-like agonist is A 68930, not SKF 83959; prominent emergence of vacuous chewing to A 68930 in KO (see text).

Table VII

Orofacial Movement Phenotype in Mutant Mice, as Assessed in a Restrictor, Following Challenge with the D1-Like Agonist SKF 83959.

Mutant	Jv	Jh	Tg	Ct	Hd	Vb
D1	↓	=	↓	↓	=	=
D5	=	=	=	=	=	=
D2	=	=	=	=	=	=
D3	=	=	=	=	=	=
D4	=	=	=	=	=	=
DARPP-32	=	=	=	=	=	=

Orofacial movements are as defined in Table II.
↓ effect of SKF 83959 is decreased in KO.
= effect of SKF 83959 is unaltered in KO.

In the restrictor (Tomiyama *et al.*, 2002), RU 24213 reduces vertical jaw movements, with this response being greater in D1 KO than in WT. In contrast, RU 24213 reduces horizontal jaw movements, tongue protrusions and incisor chattering similarly in both WT and D1 KO. RU 24213 slightly reduces head movements in WT but induces such movements in D1 KO; vibrissae movements are unaltered by RU 24213 in either WT or D1 KO (Table IX).

Table VIII
GENERAL PHENOTYPIC BEHAVIORS IN MUTANT MICE THAT INVOLVE OROFACIAL MOVEMENTS, AS ASSESSED ETHOLOGICALLY, FOLLOWING CHALLENGE WITH THE D2-LIKE AGONIST RU 24213.

Mutant	Sn	Gr_t	Gr_s	Ch
D1	=	=	=	↑
D5	=	=	=	=
D2	↓	=	=	=
D3	↓	=	=	=
D4	=	=	=	=
DARPP-32	↓	=	=	=

Orofacial behaviors are as defined in Table I.
↑ effect of RU 24213 is increased in KO.
↓ effect of RU 24213 is decreased in KO.
= effect of RU 24213 is unaltered in KO.

Table IX
OROFACIAL MOVEMENT PHENOTYPE IN MUTANT MICE, AS ASSESSED IN A RESTRICTOR, FOLLOWING CHALLENGE WITH THE D2-LIKE AGONIST RU 24213.

Mutant	Jv	Jh	Tg	Ct	Hd	Vb
D1	↑	=	=	=	↑	=
D5	=	=	=	=	=	=
D2	=	=	=	=	=	=
D3	=	=	=	↑	=	=
D4	=	=	=	=	=	=
DARPP-32	=	=	=	=	=	=

Orofacial movements are as defined in Table II.
↑ effect of RU 24213 is increased in KO.
= effect of RU 24213 is unaltered in KO.

B. Orofacial Movements in Mice with "Knockout" of D5 Receptors

1. *Spontaneous Orofacial Movements*

Within the *ethogram* (O'Sullivan *et al.*, 2005), orofacial behaviors over initial exploration are unaltered in D5 KO relative to WT (Table III); over subsequent habituation, total grooming is reduced in D5 KO relative to WT (Table IV).

In the restrictor (Tomiyama *et al.*, 2006), vertical jaw movements are increased and habituate more slowly in D5 KO relative to WT. Conversely, horizontal jaw movements and vibrissae movements are decreased. Other topographies of orofacial movement are unaltered in D5 KO relative to WT (Table V).

2. *Orofacial Movements Induced by D1-like Agonist Challenge*

Within the *ethogram* (O'Sullivan *et al.*, 2005), induction by SKF 83959 of total grooming, particularly syntactic grooming, is reduced in D5 KO relative to WT; under challenge with SKF 83959, D5 KO does not influence sniffing or chewing relative to WT (Table VI).

In the restrictor (Tomiyama *et al.*, 2006), the effects of SKF 83959 on orofacial movements are unaltered in D5 KO relative to WT (Table VII).

3. *Orofacial Movements Induced by D2-like Agonist Challenge*

Within the *ethogram* (O'Sullivan *et al.*, 2005), the effects of RU 24213 on orofacial behaviors are unaltered in D5 KO relative to WT (Table VIII).

In the restrictor (Tomiyama *et al.*, 2006), the effects of RU 24213 on orofacial movements are unaltered in D5 KO relative to WT (Table IX).

C. Overview

At the level of the *ethogram*, Tables III and IV indicate that phenotypes of orofacial behavior in D1-like KOs involve shifts over time between the individual elements of behavior in the natural mouse repertoire that are associated with orofacial movements. Phenotypic effects are most evident for grooming, for which there appears to be an enduring role for D1 receptors, with some involvement of D5 receptors also revealed over habituation; thus, while D1 receptors may be prepotent in regulating grooming, D5 receptors may interact with the neuronal substrate(s) of habituation to play distinct modulatory roles in the expression of both grooming and sniffing. While there is dense D1 receptor expression in the striatum, these findings complement anatomical studies indicating also modest D5 receptor expression in discrete areas of the striatum (Ciliax *et al.*, 2000; Khan *et al.*, 2000); in these areas D5 receptors appear to mediate neurophysiological processes (Baufreton *et al.*, 2003; Centonze *et al.*, 2003) in a manner suggestive of a role in processing signals relating to coordinated motor function (Rivera *et al.*, 2002a; Svenningsson and Le Moine, 2002).

As indicated in Tables VI and VIII, these profiles are reinforced by the relative effects of D1 and D5 KO on the responsivity to D1-like vs D2-like agonist stimulation; induction of chewing by stimulation of D2-like receptors only in D1 KO would be consistent with regulation of chewing by oppositional D1:D2-like rather than D5:D2-like interactions (see Waddington *et al.*, 1994, 2005).

In the restrictor, more specific topographies of orofacial movement can be resolved and quantified, though only under experimentally imposed conditions incompatible with the *ethogram.* Table V indicates that D1 receptors exert a fundamental role in regulating horizontal jaw movements and a more subtle role in relation to vertical jaw movements, tongue protrusions, incisor chattering and, in an inhibitory manner, movements of the head and vibrissae; D5 receptors appear to play lesser but not negligible, and occasionally opposite roles in regulating these orofacial movements. Apparent involvement of D1 and D5 receptors in temporal processes regulating certain orofacial movements reinforces those regulating orofacial behaviors in the *ethogram*. This suggests a broader concept of D1 and D5 receptor function than simply motoric, to involve interactions with those psychomotor processes that modulate orofacial function over time (Waddington *et al.*, 2005).

As indicated in Tables VII and IX, these profiles are reinforced by essential abolition of D1-like agonist stimulation of orofacial movements in D1 KO; enhancement of D2-like agonist effects in D1 KO further indicates disruption to D1:D2-like interactions (Waddington *et al.*, 1994, 2001), such that D1 receptors oppose the actions of D2-like receptors with respect to the inhibition of jaw movements and facilitation of head movements; D5 receptors appear to play no role in these effects of D1-like and D2-like agonists. However, two paradoxes require explanation. Firstly, what D1 mechanisms might subserve both: (i) Inhibition of spontaneous *horizontal* [but not vertical] jaw movements in D1 KO, and (ii) D1-like agonist-induced stimulation of *vertical* [but not horizontal] jaw movements in WT with abolition of that response in D1 KO. Secondly, at the level of behavior, D1 receptors [rather than D5 receptors] and D1-like receptors coupled to phosphoinositide hydrolysis [rather than those coupled to adenylate cyclase] appear prepotent in the regulation of orofacial movements (Tomiyama *et al.*, 2001; Waddington *et al.*, 2005; O'Sullivan *et al.*, 2010); however, at the cellular level, recent evidence indicates D5 receptors [rather than D1 receptors] to couple primarily to phosphoinositide hydrolysis (Sahu *et al.*, 2009). Such paradoxes emphasize diversity and complexity in the regulation of orofacial movements by D1 vs D5 receptors, associated transduction systems and their interactions with D2-like receptors, and indicate the need for further studies.

III. Orofacial Movements in Mice with "Knockout" of D2-like Receptors

A. Orofacial Movements in Mice with "Knockout" of D2 Receptors

1. *Spontaneous Orofacial Movements*

Within the *ethogram* (Clifford *et al.*, 2001), orofacial behaviors are not influenced in D2 KO relative to WT, over either initial exploration or subsequent habituation (Tables III and IV).

In the restrictor (Tomiyama *et al.*, 2004) vertical jaw movements are slightly increased in D2 KO relative to WT, while horizontal jaw movements are essentially unaltered. Low levels of tongue protrusions and incisor chattering are even lower in D2 KO throughout habituation. The head movements are reduced and habituate more rapidly, while vibrissae movements are unaltered, in D2 KO relative to WT (Table V).

2. *Orofacial Movements Induced by D1-like Agonist Challenge*

Within the *ethogram*, the effects of SKF 83959 on orofacial movements in D2 KO relative to WT are yet to be examined systematically. Using an alternative selective D1-like agonist (Clifford *et al.*, 2001), the effects of A 68930 on sniffing, total grooming and syntactic grooming are unaltered in D2 KO relative to WT (Table VI); however, in D2 KO there is prominent release of vacuous chewing (see D. OVERVIEW, below).

In the restrictor (Tomiyama *et al.*, 2004), the effects of SKF 83959 on orofacial movements are unaltered in D2 KO relative to WT (Table VII).

3. *Orofacial Movements Induced by D2-like Agonist Challenge*

Within the *ethogram* (Clifford *et al.*, 2001), the effects of RU 24213 on orofacial behaviors are unaltered in D2 KO relative to WT (Table VIII).

In the restrictor (Tomiyama *et al.*, 2004), the effects of RU 24213 on orofacial movements are unaltered in D2 KO relative to WT (Table IX).

B. Orofacial Movements in Mice with "Knockout" of D3 Receptors

1. *Spontaneous Orofacial Movements*

Within the *ethogram* (McNamara *et al.*, 2002), orofacial behaviors are unaltered in D3 KO relative to WT, over either initial exploration or subsequent habituation (Tables III and IV).

In the restrictor (Tomiyama *et al.*, 2004), vertical and horizontal jaw movements, tongue protrusions and movement of the head and vibrissae are unaltered in D3 KO relative to WT, while incisor chattering is reduced (Table V).

2. *Orofacial Movements Induced by D1-like Agonist Challenge*

Within the *ethogram* (McNamara *et al.*, 2002), the effects of SKF 83959 on orofacial behaviors are unaltered in D3 KO relative to WT (Table VI).

In the restrictor (Tomiyama *et al.*, 2004), the effects of SKF 83959 on orofacial movements are unaltered in D3 KO relative to WT (Table VII).

3. *Orofacial Movements Induced by D2-like Agonist Challenge*

Within the *ethogram* (McNamara *et al.*, 2002), inhibition of sniffing by lower doses of RU 24213 is reduced in D3 KO relative to WT; the effects of lower doses on total grooming, syntactic grooming and chewing, like the effects of higher doses on orofacial behaviors, is unaltered in D3 KO relative to WT (Table VIII).

In the restrictor (Tomiyama *et al.*, 2004), the effects of RU 24213 on vertical and horizontal jaw movements, tongue protrusions and movements of the head and vibrissae are unaltered in D3 KO relative to the profile described above for WT; the action of RU 24213 to reduce incisor chattering is greater in D3 KO relative to WT (Table IX).

C. Orofacial Movements in Mice With "Knockout" of D4 Receptors

1. *Spontaneous Orofacial Movements*

Within the *ethogram* (O'Sullivan *et al.*, 2006), sniffing is slightly reduced over initial exploration in D4 KO relative to WT, while total grooming, syntactic grooming and chewing are unaltered (Table III); over subsequent habituation, orofacial movements are unaltered in D4 KO relative to WT (Table IV).

In the restrictor (Tomiyama *et al.*, 2006), the topography of orofacial movements is unaltered in D4 KO relative to WT (Table V).

2. *Orofacial Movements Induced by D1-like Agonist Challenge*

Within the *ethogram* (O'Sullivan *et al.*, 2006), induction of both total grooming and syntactic grooming by SKF 83959 is reduced at lower doses, with an increase in total grooming at higher doses, in D4 KO relative to WT; the overall effect is thus a shift in dose-response curve to the right in D4 KO for the induction of grooming by SKF 83959 (Table VI).

In the restrictor (Tomiyama *et al.*, 2006), the effects of SKF 83959 on orofacial movements are unaltered in D4 KO relative to WT (Table VII).

3. *Orofacial Movements Induced by D2-like Agonist Challenge*

Within the *ethogram* (O'Sullivan *et al.*, 2006), the effects of RU 24213 on orofacial behaviors are unaltered in D4 KO relative to WT (Table VIII).

In the restrictor (Tomiyama *et al.*, 2006), the effects of RU 24213 on orofacial movements are unaltered in D4 KO relative to WT (Table IX).

D. Overview

At the level of the *ethogram*, Tables III and IV indicate that the phenotype of orofacial behavior in D2-like KOs is less evident and more circumscribed than in D1-like KOs; this relates primarily to a minor role for D4 receptors in the regulation of sniffing, suggesting differences in both magnitude and topography of effect relative to D1-like counterparts.

As indicated in Tables VI and VIII, this profile is accompanied by reduction of D2-like agonist stimulation of sniffing in D2 and D3 KOs, confirming topographical specificity for D2, D3, and D4 receptors in the regulation of this form of orofacial behavior and further distinguishing them from their D1 and D5 counterparts. It remains paradoxical that D4 receptors regulate spontaneous sniffing but D2/D3 receptors regulate D2-like agonist-induced sniffing; the extent to which this might reflect the relative affinities for D2, D3, and D4 receptors of endogenous DA vis-à-vis the D2-like agonist utilized, RU 24213, which shows highest affinity for D3 receptors (O'Sullivan *et al.*, 2006), remains to be determined.

There was no disruption to the effects of SKF 83959 in D3 KO and only minor disruption to induction of grooming in D4 KO. While the effects of SKF 83959 on orofacial behaviors in the *ethogram* were not investigated in D2 KO, studies with an alternative D1-like agonist, A 68930, which stimulates both phosphoinositide hydrolysis and adenylate cyclase indicated marked release of "vacuous chewing" to A 68930 in D2 KO, a response that was not evident in WT (Clifford *et al.*, 2001). This behavior has been widely studied in the rat (Waddington, 1990; Waddington *et al.*, 2005) but has proved very difficult to resolve and quantify in the mouse; that it is prominent in mice only during D1-like receptor stimulation in the absence of tonic activity through D2 receptors indicates a fundamental basis in oppositional D1-like:D2 receptor interactions (see Waddington *et al.*, 1994, 2005). While "chewing" [i.e. directed onto physical material] and "vacuous chewing" [i.e. not directed onto physical material] are at one level distinct, they involve overlapping topographies of orofacial movement; thus, findings in relation to the regulation of "vacuous chewing" appear complementary to the regulation of "chewing" by oppositional D1:D2-like interactions (see II C. OVERVIEW, above).

However, the basis of these phenomena appears complex: when the D2-like system is stimulated in the absence of tonic activity through D1 receptors, "chewing" is directed onto physical material [e.g. cage bedding, fecal pellets]; when the D1-like system is stimulated in the absence of tonic activity through D2 receptors, "vacuous chewing" involves a superficially identical pattern of orofacial movements that is *not* directed onto that same physical material. The extent to which these profiles might contain mechanistic clues to "purposeful" vs "purposeless" [involuntary?] manifestation of similar orofacial movements remains to be determined.

In the restrictor, Table V indicates that D2 receptors are involved in regulating tongue protrusions, incisor chattering, head movements and, in an inhibitory manner, vertical jaw movements; D3 receptors play a lesser role in regulating only incisor chattering, while D4 receptors do not appear to play any material role in regulating these orofacial movements.

As indicated in Tables VII and IX, the lack of effect of D2 KO on orofacial movements under D2-like [or D1-like] agonist challenge appears at variance with the above effects of D2 KO on orofacial movements in the absence of drug challenge. This anomaly cannot be explained by the involvement of other D2-like receptors in mediating the effects of RU 24213; for example, there was no material effect of D4 KO on orofacial movements under D2-like [or D1-like] agonist challenge. The effect of D3 KO only to *increase* inhibition of incisor chattering under D2-like agonist challenge [without effecting responsivity to the D1-like agonist] would also not explain the anomaly, and indeed constitutes yet another paradox. While the effect of D3 KO both to reduce spontaneous incisor chattering and to *increase* inhibition of incisor chattering under D2-like agonist challenge indicates some particular role for D3 receptors in the regulation of this orofacial movement, the mechanistic basis of these effects is unclear.

Such anomalies and paradoxes may relate to: (i) The regulatory mechanisms for any given orofacial movement being different according to whether that movement is occurring spontaneously or under drug challenge; (ii) The relative affinities of SKF 83959 for D1 vs D5 receptors and of RU 24213 for D2 vs D3 vs D4 receptors being different from those of endogenous, tonically active DA; and/or (iii) The expression of any given orofacial movement being dependent not only on its own regulatory mechanism but also on any other orofacial movement(s) that may or may not be evident concurrently, i.e. certain combinations of individual behaviors may be physiologically exclusive in accordance with a response incompatibility model. Yet again, further studies are needed.

IV. Orofacial Movements in Mice with "Knockout" of Dopamine Receptor Transduction

A. Orofacial Movements in Mice with "Knockout" of DARPP-32

1. *Spontaneous Orofacial Movements*

Within the *ethogram* (Nally *et al.*, 2003), total grooming is slightly reduced over initial exploration in DARPP-32 KO relative to WT, while sniffing, syntactic grooming and chewing are unaltered (Table III); over subsequent habituation, total grooming is labile in DARPP-32 KO relative to WT, while sniffing, syntactic grooming and chewing are unaltered (Table IV).

In the restrictor (Tomiyama *et al.*, 2006), tongue protrusions are reduced while other topographies of orofacial movement are unaltered in DARPP-32 KO relative to WT (Table V).

2. *Orofacial Movements Induced by D1-like Agonist Challenge*

Within the *ethogram* (Nally *et al.*, 2004; Waddington *et al.*, 2005), the effects of SKF 83959 on orofacial behaviors are unaltered in DARPP-32 KO relative to WT (Table VI).

In the restrictor (Tomiyama *et al.*, 2006), the effects of SKF 83959 on orofacial behaviors are unaltered in DARPP-32 KO relative to WT (Table VII).

3. *Orofacial Movements Induced by D2-like Agonist Challenge*

Within the *ethogram* (Nally *et al.*, 2004), induction by RU 24213 of sniffing is slightly reduced in DARPP-32 KO relative to WT, while total grooming, syntactic grooming and chewing are unaltered (Table VIII).

In the restrictor (Tomiyama *et al.*, 2006), the effects of RU 24213 on orofacial movements are unaltered in DARPP-32 KO relative to WT (Table IX).

B. Overview

At the level of the *ethogram*, Tables III and IV indicate only a modest, though consistent and enduring role for DARPP-32 in the regulation of total grooming. As indicated in Tables VI and VIII, this profile is in juxtaposition with no effect of DARPP-32 KO on responsivity to D1-like agonist challenge and only a modest effect of DARPP-32 KO to reduce sniffing in response to D2-like agonist challenge.

In the restrictor, Table V indicates only a modest role for DARPP-32 in the regulation of tongue protrusions. As indicated in Tables VII and IX, this profile is in juxtaposition with no effect of DARPP-32 KO on responsivity to either D1-like or D2-like agonist challenge.

With the possible exception of disruption to grooming, a behavior related particularly to D1/D5 receptor-mediated function, the DARPP-32 KO phenotype is modest and fragmentary across orofacial behaviors and movements under both spontaneous and drug-induced conditions. Such subtlety and inconsistency of phenotype in DARPP-32 KO would appear paradoxical vis-à-vis the widely espoused role of DARPP-32 as a critical regulator of DAergic function mediated via both D1-like and D2-like receptors: D1-like receptors activate phosphorylation of DARPP-32 to critically inhibit protein phosphatase-1 (PP-1), while D2-like receptors activate dephosphorylation of DARPP-32 and disinhibit PP-1, an essential mediator of the biological effects of DA (see Greengard *et al.*, 1999; Greengard, 2001).

As explanations in terms of mutant genetic background, insensitivity of the ethologically-based and restrictor-based techniques employed, or over-interpretation of the functional role of DARPP-32 do not appear likely, the operation of compensation processes consequent to the developmental absence of DARPP-32 must be considered. These issues, which may apply also to developmental absence of D1-5 receptors, are of potential methodological importance, as discussed in detail elsewhere (Nally *et al.*, 2003, 2004; Waddington *et al.*, 2005).

Another relevant factor may be phenotypic differences between vehicle-treated DARPP-32 KO in drug challenge studies and untreated DARPP-32 KO. It appears that the injection procedure can constitutes a "stressor" that is able to reveal topographically specific phenotypic effects of DARPP-32 KO that are not apparent under more naturalistic conditions; thus, developmental absence of DARPP-32 may also interact importantly with the biological substrate(s) of stress-related processes in the regulation of individual topographies of orofacial behavior (Nally *et al.*, 2003, 2004; Waddington *et al.*, 2005).

Multiple additional components in the DA receptor transduction cascade are now known (Greengard, 2001; Di Chiara, 2002; Neve, 2010); these remain essentially unexplored in relation to orofacial behaviors and specific orofacial movements, and may repay further investigation.

V. Methodological Challenges

Studies of orofacial function in genetically modified mice are powerful tools for studying aspects of orofacial function that are inaccessible using alternative techniques. However, like any technique, they have important limitations that can present significant methodological challenges.

A. Genetic Background

There is now strong evidence that background genes from one or both of the parental strains may interact with the mutated gene, and/or flanking genes proximal to it, can lead to a differential phenotype depending on strain contribution, independent of the mutation. Such findings underscore the necessity for well-defined genetic backgrounds in evaluating complex behavioral phenotypes of DA-related KOs and other mutants. All of our studies reviewed here have been performed on mutant mice congenic on a C57Bl/6 background (see Waddington *et al.*, 2005).

B. Developmental Compensation

In relation to those targets where both mutant models and conventional pharmacological approaches can be compared, KO of a given receptor can result in a phenotype distinct from, usually less profound than, that resulting from acute antagonist challenge; as a specific example, D2 KO fail to respond to a D2-like agonist, indicating the absence of D2-mediated function; yet they show substantial preservation of their *ethogram* when in WT that *ethogram* is readily attenuated by a D2 antagonist (Clifford *et al.*, 2000, 2001; McNamara *et al.* 2003). It appears that developmental absence of certain receptors can result in recruitment of compensatory processes that are able to sustain varying levels of some functions under *tonic* conditions [i.e. activation of the receptor by a physiologically relevant level of endogenous transmitter], though less so under *phasic* conditions [i.e. activation of the receptor by a physiologically excessive level of endogenous transmitter or stimulation by an agonist] conditions. All of our studies reviewed here have been performed both during the stress of initial placement in a given environment/apparatus, known to increase DAergic activity (Di Chiara, 2002), subsequent habituation to that environment/apparatus and, finally, following agonist drug challenge (see Waddington *et al.*, 2005).

Conditional and inducible KOs are becoming increasingly available and can obviate some of these concerns; they offer either spatial control [i.e. the mutation is restricted to a specific subset of cells] and/or temporal control [i.e. the mutation is manipulated to occur at a particular developmental stage] by the experimenter. However, rather than being experimental inconveniences, understanding compensatory processes may reveal novel neuronal mechanisms of orofacial regulation and therapeutic targets for dysfunction therein.

C. Sex differences

In the course of such studies, we and other investigators have noted some instances of sex differences in KO phenotype: some phenotypes may be present in one sex but not the other, while other phenotypes may be present in both sexes but to differing extents. For clarity of text and tabulation, these have not been emphasized here; however, full details are available in the individual primary sources cited. Assessments that do not take sex into account may miss material phenotypic effects. Though many studies have been carried out only in males, or sometimes in mice of "either sex" or of unspecified sex, it is clear that the phenotype of one sex cannot be assumed to apply to the other sex in the absence of systematic comparison. While all of our studies reviewed here have been performed on both sexes for the investigation of spontaneous orofacial behaviors and orofacial movements, some studies following agonist challenge were performed pragmatically on a single sex (see Waddington *et al.*, 2005). However, rather than being experimental inconveniences, sex differences in KO phenotype may be of physiological and clinical relevance; for example, in Huntington's disease (HD), a neurodegenerative disease characterized *inter alia* by orofacial dyskinesia, both its emergence (Roos *et al.*, 1991) and the involvement of genetic variation additional to pathogenetic CAG repeat expansion (Arning *et al.*, 2007) may differ between the sexes.

VI. Synthesis

Subject to the above methodological constraints, studies in DA receptor subtype KOs offer novel insights into the regulation of orofacial function. They do so at two levels: ethologically relevant behaviors, in which orofacial movements are a component of programmed motor sequences; and individual orofacial movements that, while only accessible under non-physiological conditions, represent some of the motoric "building blocks" that constitute such ethologically relevant orofacial behaviors.

However, it must be emphasized that, while they play fundamental roles, DA and its associated receptor subtypes and transduction cascades are not the sole regulators of orofacial function. Among several other implicated neurotransmitters, there appear to be important roles also for γ-aminobutyric acid (GABA) and glutamate, both independently and, more typically, through interactions with DAergic mechanisms (see Koshikawa *et al.*, 2011, this volume). Complementary studies on the use of mutant models to probe the involvement of GABA and glutamate receptors and related cellular processes in the regulation of orofacial movements are the topic of the next chapter (Tomiyama *et al.*, 2011, this volume).

While knowledge at the level of individual orofacial movements is fundamental, it is only by their integration into adaptive orofacial behaviors that an organism is capable of functionality. Critically, that functionality operates in physical, physiological, and psychosocial milieus that converge to determine the manner in which individual orofacial movements are sculpted into more adaptive orofacial behaviors. This is the deepest and most complex level of neuronal processing that we must ultimately seek to understand.

Acknowledgments

The authors' studies would be impossible without the generous collaboration of our colleagues in molecular biology who have kindly made their mutants available to us; we are indebted to: Emiliana Borrelli, John Drago, Allen Fienberg, Sara Fuchs, David Grandy, Paul Greengard, Malcolm Low, Marcelo Rubinstein, and David Sibley. The authors' studies are supported by Science Foundation Ireland Principal Investigator Grant 07/IN.1/B960, a grant for promotion of multidisciplinary research projects entitled Translational Research Network on Orofacial Neurological Disorders from the Ministry of Education, Culture, Sports, Science and Technology of Japan, and a Nihon University Multidisciplinary Grant.

References

Arning, L., Saft, C., Wieczorek, S., Andrich, J., Kraus, P.H., and Epplen, J.T. (2007). NR2A and NR2B receptor gene variations modify age at onset in Huntington disease in a sex-specific manner. *Hum. Genet.* **122**, 175–182.

Baufreton, J., Garret, M., Rivera, A., de la Calle, A., Gonon, F., Dufy, B., Bioulac, B., and Taupignon, A. (2003). D5 (not D1) dopamine receptors potentiate burst-firing in neurons of the subthalamic nucleus by modulating an L-type calcium conductance. *J. Neurosci.* **23**, 816–825.

Centonze, D., Grande, C., Saulle, E., Martin, A.B., Gubellini, P., Pavon, N., Pisani, A., Bernardi, G., Moratalla, R., and Calabresi, P. (2003). Distinct roles of D1 and D5 dopamine receptors in motor activity and striatal synaptic plasticity. *J. Neurosci.* **23**, 8506–8512.

Ciliax, B.J., Nash, N., Heilman, C., Sunahara, R., Hartney, A., Tiberi, M., Rye, D.B., Caron, M.G., Niznik, H.B., and Levey, A.I. (2000). Dopamine D (5) receptor immunolocalization in rat and monkey brain. *Synapse* **37**, 125–145.

Clifford, J.J., Tighe, O., Croke, D.T., Sibley, D.R., Drago, J., and Waddington, J.L. (1998). Topographical evaluation of the phenotype of spontaneous behaviour in mice with targeted gene deletion of the D1A dopamine receptor: paradoxical elevation of grooming syntax. *Neuropharmacology* **37**, 1595–1602.

Clifford, J.J., Usiello, A., Vallone, D., Kinsella, A., Borrelli, E., and Waddington, J.L. (2000). Topographical evaluation of behavioural phenotype in a line of mice with targeted gene deletion of the D2 dopamine receptor. *Neuropharmacology* **39**, 382–390.

Clifford, J.J., Kinsella, A., Tighe, O., Rubinstein, M., Grandy, D.K., Low, M.J., Croke, D.T., and Waddington, J.L. (2001). Comparative, topographically-based evaluation of behavioural phenotype and specification of D (1)-like:D (2) interactions in a line of incipient congenic mice with D (2) dopamine receptor 'knockout'. *Neuropsychopharmacology* **25**, 527–536.

Di Chiara, G. (2002). Handbook of Experimental Physiology: Dopamine in the CNS." Springer. *Heidelberg*

Goulding, M. (2009). Circuits controlling vertebrate locomotion: moving in a new direction. *Nat. Rev. Neurosci.* **10**, 507–518.

Greengard, P., Allen, P.B., and Nairn, A.C. (1999). Beyond the dopamine receptor: the DARPP-32/ protein phosphatase-1 cascade. *Neuron* **23**, 435–447.

Greengard, P. (2001). The neurobiology of slow synaptic transmission. *Science* **294**, 1024–1030.

Graziano, M. (2006). The organization of behavioural repertoire in motor cortex. *Annu. Rev. Neurosci.* **29**, 105–134.

Jenner, P. (2008). Molecular mechanisms of L-DOPA-induced dyskinesia. *Nat. Rev. Neurosci.* **9**, 665–677.

Kebabian, J.W., and Calne, D.B. (1979). Multiple receptors for dopamine. *Nature* **277**, 93–96.

Khan, Z.U., Gutierrez, A., Martin, R., Penafiel, A., Rivera, A., and de la Calle, A. (2000). Dopamine D5 receptors of rat and human brain. *Neuroscience* **100**, 689–699.

Koshikawa, N., Fujita, S., and Adachi, K. (2011). Behavioural pharmacology of orofacial movement disorders. *Int. Rev. Neurobiol,* in press

Lund, J.P., and Kolta, A. (2006). Brainstem circuits that control mastication. *J. Commun. Disord.* **39**, 381–390.

Margolese, H.C., Chouinard, G., Kolivakis, T.T., Beauclair, L., and Miller, R. (2005). Tardive dyskinesia in the era of typical and atypical antipsychotics. Part 1: pathophysiology and mechanisms of induction. *Can. J. Psychiatry* **50**, 541–547.

McNamara, F.N., Clifford, J.J., Tighe, O., Kinsella, A., Drago, J., Fuchs, S., Croke, D.T., and Waddington, J.L. (2002). Phenotypic, ethologically based resolution of spontaneous and D (2)-like vs D (1)-like agonist-induced behavioural topography in mice with congenic D (3) dopamine receptor "knockout". *Synapse* **46**, 19–31.

McNamara, F.N., Clifford, J.J., Tighe, O., Kinsella, A., Drago, J., Croke, D.T., and Waddington, J.L. (2003). Congenic D1A dopamine receptor mutants: ethologically based resolution of behavioural topography indicates genetic background as a determinant of knockout phenotype. *Neuropsychopharmacology* **28**, 86–99.

Nally, R.E., McNamara, F.N., Clifford, J.J., Kinsella, A., Tighe, O., Croke, D.T., Fienberg, A.A., Greengard, P., and Waddington, J.L. (2003). Topographical assessment of ethological and dopamine receptor agonist-induced behavioral phenotype in mutants with congenic DARPP-32 "knockout". *Neuropsychopharmacology* **28**, 2055–2063.

Nally, R.E., Kinsella, A., Tighe, O., Croke, D.T., Fienberg, A.A., Greengard, P., and Waddington, J.L. (2004). Ethologically based resolution of D2-like dopamine receptor agonist-versus antagonist-induced behavioral topography in dopamine- and adenosine 3',5'-monophosphate-regulated phosphoprotein of 32 kDa "knockout" mutants congenic on the C57BL/6 genetic background. *J. Pharmacol. Exp. Ther.* **310**, 1281–1287.

Neve, K.A. (2010). The Dopamine Receptors." Humana Press, Totowa. *NJ*

O'Sullivan, G., Kinsella, A., Grandy, D.K., Low, M.J., Tighe, O., Croke, D.T., and Waddington, J.L. (2006). Ethological resolution of behavioural topography and D2-like vs D1-like agonist responses in congenic D4 dopamine receptor 'knockouts': identification of D4:D1-like interactions. *Synapse* **59**, 107–118.

O'Sullivan, G.J., Kinsella, A., Sibley, D.R., Tighe, O., Croke, D.T., and Waddington, J.L. (2005). Ethological resolution of behavioural topography and D (1)-like versus D (2)-like agonist responses in congenic D (5) dopamine receptor mutants: Identification of D (5):D (2)-like interactions. *Synapse* **55**, 201–211.

O'Sullivan, G.J., O'Tuathaigh, C., Tomiyama, K., Koshikawa, N., and Waddington, J.L. (2010). Dopamine receptor subtypes and behaviour: from psychopharmacology to mutant models. In: Neve, K. (Ed.), *"The Dopamine Receptors"*. Humana Press, Totowa, NJ, pp. 323–371.

Pong, M., Horn, K.M., and Gibson, A.R. (2008). Pathways for control of face and neck musculature by the basal ganglia and cerebellum. *Brain Res. Rev.* **58**, 249–264.

Rivera, A., Alberti, I., Martin, A.B., Narvaez, J.A., de la Calle, A., and Moratalla, R. (2002). Molecular phenotype of rat striatal neurons expressing the dopamine D5 receptor subtype. *Eur. J. Neurosci* **16**, 2049–2058.

Roos, R.A., Vegter-van der Vlis, M., Hermans, J., Elshove, H.M., Moll, A.C., van de Kamp, J.J., and Bruyn, G.W. (1991). Age at onset in Huntington's disease: effect of line of inheritance and patient's sex. *J. Med. Genet.* **28**, 515–519.

Sahu, A., Tyeryar, K.R., Vongtau, H.O., Sibley, D.R., and Undie, A.S. (2009). D5 dopamine receptors are required for dopaminergic activation of phospholipase C. *Mol. Pharmacol.* **75**, 447–453.

Sessle, B.J., Adachi, K., Avivi-Arber, L., Lee, J., Nishiura, H., Yao, D., and Yoshino, K. (2007). Neuroplasticity of face primary motor cortex control of orofacial movements. *Arch. Oral Biol.* **52**, 334–337.

Svenningsson, P., Nishi, A., Fisone, G., Girault, J.A., Nairn, A.C., and Greengard, P. (2004). DARPP-32: an integrator of neurotransmission. *Annu. Rev. Pharmacol. Toxicol.* **44**, 269–296.

Svenningsson, P., and Le Moine, C. (2002). Dopamine D1/5 receptor stimulation induces c-fos expression in the subthalamic nucleus: possible involvement of local D5 receptors. *Eur. J. Neurosci.* **15**, 133–142.

Tomiyama, K., McNamara, F.N., Clifford, J.J., Kinsella, A., Koshikawa, N., and Waddington, J.L. (2001). Topographical assessment and pharmacological characterization of orofacial movements in mice: dopamine D (1)-like vs. D (2)-like receptor regulation. *Eur. J. Pharmacol.* **418**, 47–54.

Tomiyama, K., McNamara, F.N., Clifford, J.J., Kinsella, A., Drago, J., Tighe, O., Croke, D.T., Koshikawa, N., and Waddington, J.L. (2002). Phenotypic resolution of spontaneous and D (1)-like agonist-induced orofacial movement topographies in congenic dopamine D (1A) receptor 'knockout' mice. *Neuropharmacology* **42**, 644–652.

Tomiyama, K., McNamara, F.N., Clifford, J.J., Kinsella, A., Drago, J., Fuchs, S., Grandy, D.K., Low, M.J., Rubinstein, M., Tighe, O., Croke, D.T., Koshikawa, N., and Waddington, J.L. (2004). Comparative phenotypic resolution of spontaneous, D2-like and D1-like agonist-induced orofacial movement topographies in congenic mutants with dopamine D2 vs. D3 receptor "knockout". *Synapse* **51**, 71–81.

Tomiyama, K., Makihara, Y., Yamamoto, H., O'Sullivan, G., Nally, R.E., Tighe, O., Kinsella, A., Fienberg, A.A., Grandy, D.K., Sibley, D.R., Croke, D.T., Koshikawa, N., and Waddington, J.L. (2006). Disruption of orofacial movement topographies in congenic mutants with dopamine D5 but not D4 receptor or DARPP-32 transduction 'knockout'. *Eur. Neuropsychopharmacol.* **16**, 437–445.

Tomiyama, K., O'Tuathaigh, C., and Waddington, J.L. (2011). Regulation of orofacial movements: aminoacid mechanisms and mutant models. *Int. Rev. Neurobiol.* in press

van der Bilt, A., Engelen, L., Pereira, L.J., van der GLas, H.W., and Abbink, J.H. (2006). Oral physiology and mastication. *Physiol. Behav.* **89**, 22–27.

Waddington, J.L. (1990). Spontaneous orofacial movements induced in rodents by very long-term neuroleptic drug administration: phenomenology, pathophysiology and putative relationship to tardive dyskinesia. *Psychopharmacology* **101**, 431–447.

Waddington, J.L., Daly, S.A., McCauley, P.G., and O'Boyle, K.M. (1994). Levels of functional interaction between D1-like and D2-like dopamine receptor systems. In: Niznik, H.B. (Ed.), "*Dopamine Receptors and Transporters: Pharmacology, Structure and Function*". Marcel Dekker, New York, pp. 511–537.

Waddington, J.L., Daly, S.A., Downes, R.P., Deveney, A.M., McCauley, P.G., and O'Boyle, K.M. (1995). Behavioural pharmacology of 'D-1-like' dopamine receptors: further sub typing, new pharmacological probes and interactions with 'D-2-like' receptors. *Prog. Neuropsychopharmacol. Biol. Psychiatry* **19**, 811–831.

Waddington, J.L., Clifford, J.J., McNamara, F.N., Tomiyama, K., Koshikawa, N., and Croke, D.T. (2001). The psychopharmacology-molecular biology interface: exploring the behavioural roles of dopamine receptor subtypes using targeted gene deletion ('knockout'). *Prog. Neuropsychopharmacol. Biol. Psychiatry* **25**, 925–964.

Waddington, J.L., O'Tuathaigh, C., O'Sullivan, G., Tomiyama, K., Koshikawa, N., and Croke, D.T. (2005). Phenotypic studies on dopamine receptor subtype and associated signal transduction mutants: insights and challenges from 10 years at the psychopharmacology-molecular biology interface. *Psychopharmacology* **181**, 611–638.

REGULATION OF OROFACIAL MOVEMENT: AMINO ACID MECHANISMS AND MUTANT MODELS

Katsunori Tomiyama[1,2], Colm M.P. O'Tuathaigh[3,4], and John L. Waddington[3]

[1]Advanced Research Institute for the Sciences and Humanities, Nihon University, Tokyo 102, Japan
[2]Department of Pharmacology, Nihon University School of Dentistry, Tokyo 101, Japan
[3]Molecular and Cellular Therapeutics, Royal College of Surgeons in Ireland, Dublin 2, Ireland
[4]School of Medicine, University College Cork, Cork, Ireland

I. Introduction

A. Regulation of Orofacial Movements

Mammalian orofacial behavior involves complex processes: individual movements are orchestrated into functionality by pattern generators and higher centers that reflect the purpose of such movements and their physiological and psychological setting (Sawczuk, 2001; Estep, 2009; Fabbrini *et al.*, 2009). Among what are recognized to be diverse and complex mechanisms, two broad families of neurotransmitters have been particularly implicated in the regulation of orofacial movements: the catecholamines, primary dopamine (see Waddington, O'Sullivan,

INTERNATIONAL REVIEW OF
NEUROBIOLOGY, VOL. 97
DOI: 10.1016/B978-0-12-385198-7.00003-5

and Tomiyama, 2011, this volume), and the amino acids, primarily γ-aminobutyric acid (GABA) and glutamic acid (glutamate). In this chapter, we consider these roles of GABA and glutamate and how they can be better understood.

B. The Role of Amino Acids

That GABA and glutamate play important roles in regulating orofacial movements derives from: (i) The presence of GABA and glutamate in the brain regions known to be involved in the regulation of orofacial function, particularly the striatum and its efferent systems; (ii) The action of drugs that disrupts GABAergic and glutamatergic function to influence various forms of orofacial movements in several experimental models; and (iii) Abnormalities of GABAergic and glutamatergic markers in the brain tissue from individuals suffering from neuropsychiatric disorders characterized by orofacial movement disorder, most typically Huntington's disease and L-dopa dyskinesia (Inchul *et al.*, 2005; Peixoto *et al.*, 2005; Nistri *et al.*, 2006; Hikosaka, 2007; Walker, 2007; Samadi *et al.*, 2008a,b; Duty, 2010; see Koshikawa *et al.*, 2011, this volume). However, the roles of individual GABA and glutamate receptor subtypes and associated processes, in the generation and regulation of orofacial behavior and the individual motor movements that constitute such behavior remain poorly understood. Mutant mice with deletion ("knockout") of these processes provide an important tool for clarifying these issues, and are a primary focus of this article.

II. GABA Synthesis, Receptors and Associated Processes

A. GABA Synthesis

As the major inhibitory neurotransmitter in the brain, GABA is synthesized from glutamic acid via glutamic acid decarboxylase, which exists as two isoforms, GAD65 and GAD67; GAD67 is constitutively active and produces >90% of GABA in the central nervous system, while GAD65 is transiently activated and augments GABA levels for the rapid modulation of inhibitory neurotransmission (Kanaani *et al.*, 2010). Mice with "knockout" of GAD67 show deficient rhythm generation of mouth opening and tongue withdrawal at embryonic day 14; these may contribute to impaired palate formation and resultant cleft palate, with neonatal lethality (Tsunekawa *et al.*, 2005). While mice with "knockout" of GAD65 show various functional deficits (Walls *et al.*, 2010), orofacial movements have received little material investigation.

B. GABA Receptor Subtypes and Subunits

GABA mediates its physiological effects via ionotropic (ion channel-linked) $GABA_A$ and metabotropic (G-protein-coupled) $GABA_B$ receptors.

$GABA_A$ receptors are composed of five protein subunits, which involve 19 genes for subunits α1-6, β1-3, γ1-3, δ, ε, π, θ, and ρ1-3 [initially, ρ1-3 subunits were considered to constitute $GABA_C$ receptors but are now considered subtypes of $GABA_A$] (Olsen and Sieghart, 2009); $GABA_A$ receptors have received general investigation in relation to orofacial movements, using pharmacological and physiological techniques. However, while mice with targeted gene manipulation [both "knockout" and "knockin"] of $GABA_A$ receptor subunits indicate them to play diverse roles in the regulation of general motor activity, epileptogenesis, learning, memory and anxiety (Vicini and Ortinski, 2004; Olsen and Sieghart, 2009), orofacial movements have received little material investigation.

$GABA_B$ receptors involve two subunit isoforms, $GABA_{B1a}$ and $GABA_{B1b}$, both of which combine with $GABA_{B2}$ subunits to form heteromeric $GABA_{B(1a,2)}$ and $GABA_{B(1b,2)}$ receptors (Emson, 2007; Pinard *et al.*, 2010); $GABA_B$ receptors have not been extensively examined in relation to orofacial movements. While mice with "knockout" of $GABA_B$ receptors evidence hyperactivity and epileptogenesis, and mice with "knockout" of $GABA_{B(1a,2)}$ and $GABA_{B(1b,2)}$ subunits evidence differential effects on cognition and anxiety (Vigot *et al.*, 2006; Pinard *et al.*, 2010), orofacial movements have received little material investigation.

C. Orofacial Movements in Mice with "Knockout" of $GABA_A$ Receptor-Associated Processes

1. *Phospholipase C-related Catalytically Inactive Protein*

Heteropentameric $GABA_A$ receptors interact also with $GABA_A$ receptor-associated proteins (Olsen and Sieghart, 2009), among which phospholipase C-related catalytically inactive protein (PRIP) is involved in the assembly and trafficking of γ2 subunit-containing $GABA_A$ receptors (Nakayama *et al.*, 2002; Kanematsu *et al.*, 2007; Mizokami *et al.*, 2007). The family of PRIP proteins consists of PRIP-1, expressed mainly in the brain, and PRIP-2, having wider expression (Uji *et al.*, 2002; Chen and Olsen, 2007). While PRIP-1 KO disrupts several physiological processes mediated via $GABA_A$ receptors (Kanematsu *et al.*, 2007), PRIP-1 KO may also recruit compensatory changes in PRIP-2; thus, mutants with "double knockout" (DKO) of both PRIP-1 and PRIP-2 have been generated so that the investigation of PRIP-related functions might be facilitated (Mizokami *et al.*, 2007).

For evaluating the role of $GABA_A$ receptor function in orofacial movements via PRIP-1/2 DKO, in comparison with wildtype (WT) controls, we utilized a

Table I
SPECIFIC TOPOGRAPHIES OF OROFACIAL MOVEMENT IN MICE, AS ASSESSED IN A RESTRICTOR.

Movement	Abbreviation	Description
Jaw - vertical	Jv	Jaw movements in vertical plane
Jaw - horizontal	Jh	Jaw movements in horizontal plane
Tongue protrusions	Tg	Protrusion of tongue outside of mouth
Chattering of incisors	Ct	High-frequency rhythmical jaw movements with tapping of the incisors
Head	Hd	Movements of the head
Vibrissae	Vb	Movements of the vibrissae

novel assessment system (Tomiyama *et al.*, 2001); this accesses and quantifies several distinct topographies of orofacial movement that can be resolved only in a restrictor [i.e. vertical jaw movements, horizontal jaw movements, tongue protrusions, and rapid movements of the incisors, together with the movements of the head and of the vibrissae] (see Table I), but at the expense of more naturalistic behaviors that constitute the murine *ethogram* (see Waddington *et al.*, 2011, this volume). Orofacial movements are measured spontaneously over a 180 min period of habituation to the restrictor. After habituation, orofacial movements are measured following acute challenge with the $GABA_A$ergic agent diazepam or the D1-like dopamine receptor agonist SKF 83959, which acts selectively at D1-like receptors coupled to phosphoinositide hydrolysis; previous evidence has indicated that orofacial movements are induced preferentially by this putative subtype of D1-like receptors, rather than by those coupled to adenylate cyclase (Waddington *et al.*, 1995, 2005).

2. *Spontaneous Orofacial Movements*

In the restrictor (Tomiyama *et al.*, 2010), vertical jaw movements are initially prominent in WT but then decline over subsequent habituation; in PRIP-1/2 DKO, this decline in vertical jaw movements is accentuated, such that PRIP-1/2 DKO attain lower levels than WT. Conversely, horizontal jaw movements increase over assessment similarly in PRIP-1/2 DKO and WT. The low rate of tongue protrusions in WT is even lower in PRIP-1/2 DKO throughout assessment. Incisor chattering initially increases and then declines over assessment similarly in PRIP-1/2 DKO and WT. The movements of the head and vibrissae decline over habituation; in PRIP-1/2 DKO this decline in movements of the head and vibrissae is accentuated, such that PRIP-1/2 DKO attain lower levels than WT (Table II).

Table II
OROFACIAL MOVEMENT PHENOTYPE IN MUTANT MICE, AS ASSESSED DURING HABITUATION TO A RESTRICTOR.

Mutant	Jv	Jh	Tg	Ct	Hd	Vb
PRIP-1/2 DKO	↓ (h)	=	↓	=	↓ (h)	↓ (h)

PRIP-1/2 DKO: double "knockout" of phospholipase C-related catalytically inactive protein, Type I and Type 2. Orofacial movements are as defined in Table I. ↓ decrease in KO. (h) KO phenotype involves disruption to habituation. = unaltered in KO.

Table III
OROFACIAL MOVEMENT PHENOTYPE IN MUTANT MICE, AS ASSESSED IN A RESTRICTOR, FOLLOWING CHALLENGE WITH THE $GABA_A$ERGIC AGENT DIAZEPAM.

Mutant	Jv	Jh	Tg	Ct	Hd	Vb
PRIP-1/2 DKO	=	=	=	=	=	=

PRIP-1/2 DKO: double "knockout" of phospholipase C-related catalytically inactive protein, Type I and Type 2. Orofacial movements are as defined in Table I. = unaltered in KO.

3. *Orofacial Movements Induced by $GABA_A$ergic Challenge*

In the restrictor (Tomiyama *et al.*, 2010), vertical jaw movements, horizontal jaw movements, tongue protrusions and incisor chattering are not influenced by diazepam in either PRIP-1/2 DKO or WT. The head and vibrissae movements are slightly reduced by diazepam in both PRIP-1/2 DKO and WT (Table III).

4. *Orofacial Movements Induced by D1-like Agonist Challenge*

In the restrictor (Tomiyama *et al.*, 2010), SKF 83959 induces vertical jaw movements similarly in PRIP-1/2 DKO and WT, but is without material effect on horizontal jaw movements. Induction of tongue protrusions by SKF 83959 is reduced in PRIP-1/2 DKO. SKF 83959 induces incisor chattering and movements of the head and vibrissae similarly in PRIP-1/2 DKO and WT (Table IV).

D. OVERVIEW

KO of PRIP-1 and PRIP-2 is associated with reduction in the surface expression of $GABA_A$ receptors containing a $\gamma 2$ subunit and reduced sensitivity to $GABA_A$ergic drugs (Mizokami *et al.*, 2007). It has been reported that the action

Table IV
Orofacial Movement Phenotype in Mutant Mice, as Assessed in a Restrictor, Following Challenge with the D1-like Agonist SKF 83959.

Mutant	Jv	Jh	Tg	Ct	Hd	Vb
PRIP-1/2 DKO	=	=	↓	=	=	=

PRIP-1/2 DKO: double "knockout" of phospholipase C-related catalytically inactive protein, Type I and Type 2. Orofacial movements are as defined in Table I. ↓ decrease in KO. = unaltered in KO.

of the $GABA_A$ergic agent diazepam to increase $GABA_A$-elicited currents in the hippocampus and to exert anxiolytic activity, are reduced in these same PRIP-1/2 DKOs, with some reduction in ambulation (Mizokami *et al.*, 2007). Therefore, the failure of PRIP-1/2 DKO to influence effects of the $GABA_A$ergic agent diazepam on orofacial movements was unexpected.

Though non-$GABA_A$ergic actions of diazepam cannot be excluded, complex aspects of heteropentameric $GABA_A$ receptor function may be relevant. While $GABA_A$ receptors involve $\alpha:\beta:\gamma$ subunits, GABA binding to cell surface sites involves α/β subunits, PRIP regulates the assembly and trafficking of $\gamma 2$ subunit-containing $GABA_A$ receptors, and diazepam binding sites involve $\alpha/\gamma 2$ subunits (Chen and Olsen, 2007; Kanematsu *et al.*, 2007; Olsen and Sieghart, 2009). Additionally, PRIP-1/2 DKO is associated with distinct effects on $\alpha/\gamma 2$ and α/β subunits (Mizokami *et al.*, 2007). As the interactions of benzodiazepines with $GABA_A$ receptors are complex, each aspect of their diverse pharmacology may not involve a single $GABA_A$-mediated effect (Reynolds, 2008). Some of these issues may be resolved by studies in mutants with KO of individual $GABA_A$ receptor subunits in comparison with PRIP-1/2 DKO.

Orofacial movements involve particularly striatal mechanisms, with an important regulatory role for D1 receptors that interact with local $GABA_A$ergic neurons; there is also a role for extrastriatal mechanisms, particularly GABAergic efferents (Grimm and See, 2000; Adachi *et al.*, 2003; Peixoto *et al.*, 2005; see Koshikawa *et al.*, 2011, this volume). By applying our assessment system (Tomiyama *et al.*, 2001), PRIP-1/2 DKO is characterized by the intact horizontal jaw movements and incisor chattering, reduction in vertical jaw movements and tongue protrusions, with reductions in movements of the head and vibrissae. Given evidence for functional interactions between $GABA_A$ergic and D1 dopaminergic systems, it is useful to compare the phenotype of PRIP-1/2 DKO with D1 KO (Tomiyama *et al.*, 2002; see Waddington *et al.*, 2011, this volume), which are characterized by intact vertical jaw movements and movements of the head and vibrissae, reduction in tongue protrusions and marked reductions in horizontal jaw movements and incisor chattering. Thus, $GABA_A$ and D1 mechanisms exert topographically distinct regulatory effects on orofacial movements.

While induction of vertical jaw movements and incisor chattering by SKF 83959 was unaltered in PRIP-1/2 DKO, these responses were reduced in D1 KO; in contrast, induction of tongue protrusions by SKF 83959 was reduced in PRIP-1/2 DKO, as in D1 KO (Tomiyama *et al.*, 2002). This suggests that $GABA_A$ and D1 receptor-mediated processes may interact in regulating movements of the tongue. These findings reinforce the proposition that $GABA_A$ and D1 mechanisms exert topographically distinct regulatory effects on orofacial movements. Independent regulation of tongue and jaw movements can involve coordinated actions that are regulated via brainstem oromotor center, with mastication being a typical example. While limited information is available on how jaw and tongue movements are regulated differentially by the individual nuclei and receptor mechanisms, evidence suggests that a medullary-forebrain network involving different but interacting neurotransmitter systems (Berthoud, 2003; Luo *et al.*, 2006) may mediate distinct patterns of orolingual movements.

In summary, studies indicate that tongue movements appear to be co-regulated by $GABA_A$ and D1 and mechanisms, in a manner distinct from other topographies of orofacial movement. PRIP-1/2 DKO informs on the role of PRIP and $GABA_A$ receptors in regulating orofacial movements and on how the topography of orofacial movement is regulated by functional interactions between $GABA_A$ and D1 receptor systems.

III. Glutamate Receptors and Associated Processes

A. Glutamate Receptor Subtypes and Subunits

Glutamate mediates its physiological effects via two main families of receptor subtypes: ionotroptic and metabotropic receptors.

For ionotropic glutamate receptors, nomenclature has been historically diverse (Lodge, 2009) and is currently undergoing formal revision; the schema adopted here is that recommended by the International Union of Pharmacology Committee on Receptor Nomenclature and Drug Classification (Collingridge *et al.*, 2009): GluA1-4 (formerly AMPA receptor subtypes); GluK1-5 (formerly kainate receptor subtypes); GluN1, GluN2A-D and GluN3A/B (formerly NMDA receptor subtypes); GluD1/2 ("orphan" receptors); previous nomenclatures and conversion tables thereto are available (Collingridge *et al.*, 2009). For metabotropic glutamate receptors, nomenclature is as recently reviewed (Niswender and Conn, 2010): mGluR1/R5 (group I); mGluR2/3 (group II); mGluR4 and mGluR6-8 (group III).

While mice with genetic manipulation [most typically KO but also including *hypomorphs* and transgenic variants] of ionotropic and metabotropic glutamate receptor subtypes indicate them to play diverse roles in the regulation of general motor activity, epileptogenesis, sociability, cognition and information processing, anxiety, and pain (Inta *et al.*, 2010; Niswender and Conn, 2010), orofacial movements have received little material investigation.

B. Orofacial Movements in Mice with "Knockout" of Glutamate Receptor-Associated Processes

1. *Neuregulin-1*

The neuregulin-1 (NRG1) family of genes (NRG 1–4) share a common epidermal growth factor (EGF)-like domain; interaction of these domains with membrane-associated tyrosine kinases (ErbB receptors) activate intracellular signaling pathways implicated in important neurodevelopmental processes (Mei and Xiong, 2008). Among several candidate genes, NRG1 has been consistently associated with increased risk for schizophrenia (Bertram, 2008; Munafo *et al.*, 2008; Gong *et al.*, 2009). At least six different proteins and 31 isoforms of NRG1 have been described, the majority being synthesized with a transmembrane (TM)-domain (Harrison and Law, 2006; Mei and Xiong, 2008; Balu and Coyle, 2011). Delineation of the functional roles of these NRG1 isoforms is being facilitated by targeted mutation of each isoform in mice (Desbonnet *et al.*, 2009; Kirby *et al.*, 2010).

NRG1 has been shown to play a role in glutamatergic neurotransmission, specifically disruption of GluN1-3 (formerly NMDA) receptor activation in accordance with a glutamatergic hypothesis for schizophrenia (Hahn *et al.*, 2006; Bjarnadottir *et al.*, 2007; Li *et al.*, 2007; Mei and Xiong, 2008; Banerjee *et al.*, 2010), and orofacial dyskinesia is considered to be an intrinsic as well as iatrogenic aspect of schizophrenia (Whitty *et al.*, 2009). For these reasons, we have studied the orofacial movements in mutants with heterozygous deletion (HET) of NRG1 [homozygous NRG1 KO being lethal], using techniques identical to those applied in the study of PRIP-1/2 DKO.

2. *Spontaneous Orofacial Movements*

In the restrictor (Tomiyama *et al.*, 2009), while vertical and horizontal jaw movements, tongue protrusions and movements of the head and vibrissae are unaltered, incisor chattering is increased in NRG1 HET (Table V).

Table V
OROFACIAL MOVEMENT PHENOTYPE IN MUTANT MICE, AS ASSESSED DURING HABITUATION TO A RESTRICTOR.

Mutant	Jv	Jh	Tg	Ct	Hd	Vb
NRG1 HET	=	=	=	↑	=	=

NRG1 HET: heterozygous deletion of neuregulin-1. Orofacial movements are as defined in Table I. ↑ increase in NRG1 HET. = unaltered in NRG1 HET.

Table VI
OROFACIAL MOVEMENT PHENOTYPE IN MUTANT MICE, AS ASSESSED IN A RESTRICTOR, FOLLOWING CHALLENGE WITH THE D1-LIKE AGONIST SKF 83959.

Mutant	Jv	Jh	Tg	Ct	Hd	Vb
NRG1 HET	=	=	↓	=	=	=

NRG1 HET: heterozygous deletion of neuregulin-1. Orofacial movements are as defined in Table I. ↓ decrease in NRG1 HET. = unaltered in NRG1 HET.

3. *Orofacial Movements Induced by D1-like Agonist Challenge*

In the restrictor (Tomiyama *et al.*, 2009), while the effects of SKF 83959 on vertical and horizontal jaw movements, incisor chattering and movements of the head and vibrissae are unaltered, induction of tongue protrusions is reduced in NRG1 HET (Table VI).

C. OVERVIEW

This excess of incisor chattering in NRG1 HET indicates that spontaneous, topographically specific orofacial movements result from heterozygous deletion of this gene. Previous studies in NRG1 HET have indicated disruption to aspects of social behavior together with a "hyperactive" phenotype (see Desbonnet *et al.*, 2009; Kirby *et al.*, 2010) and this appears to have a circumscribed orofacial component. NRG1 is expressed in several brain regions, including the basal ganglia, and putative functional roles for NRG1 include synapse formation, neuronal migration, synaptic plasticity, and the regulation of neurotransmitter expression and release (Harrison and Law, 2006; Mei and Xiong, 2008). That NRG1 is a regulator particularly of glutamatergic function mediated through GluN1-3 (formerly NMDA) receptors (Hahn *et al.*, 2006; Bjarnadottir *et al.*, 2007; Li *et al.*, 2007; Mei and Xiong, 2008; Banerjee *et al.*, 2010) implicates glutamatergic processes in the regulation of this topography of orofacial movements.

NRG1 has been associated with the risk of schizophrenia (Bertram, 2008; Munafo *et al.*, 2008; Gong *et al.*, 2009) and increasing evidence indicates that orofacial dyskinesia is not solely an iatrogenic consequence of long-term pretreatment with antipsychotic drugs (i.e. "tardive" dyskinesia) but, rather, an intrinsic motor aspect of the network pathobiology of schizophrenia (i.e. orofacial dyskinesia) that can be further exacerbated by antipsychotics (Whitty *et al.*, 2009; Pappa, and Dazzan, 2009). As humans have a much more complex repertoire of orofacial movements than do mice, to include not just consummatory but also verbal communicative and expressive functions, specific relationships between individual topographies of orofacial movement in NRG1 HET and those constituting clinical orofacial dyskinesia, are far from clear. Nevertheless, the findings in Table V suggest at least one genetic basis for excessive orofacial movements in schizophrenia and implicate glutamatergic dysfunction as one component in their pathophysiology.

NRG1 HET shows a reduction in the induction of tongue protrusions by the D1-like agonist SKF 83959. It would appear that the topography and directionality of orofacial movement dysfunction differ according to the absence [NRG1 HET under tonic DAergic activation] or presence [NRG1 HET under phasic challenge with SKF 83959] of D1-like stimulation. This emphasizes the complexity in how distinct topographies of orofacial movements, here incisor chattering and tongue protrusions, can be regulated differentially by particular neuronal systems.

IV. Synthesis

The manifestation of orofacial movements involves the complex interplay of generators for fundamental, down-stream patterns of motor sequences with upstream basal ganglia and cortical regulatory mechanisms. The involvement of GABAergic and glutamatergic sytems in these movements is made yet more complex by the multiplicity of GABA and glutamate receptor subtypes, subunits, and associated processes, with "knockout" mice constituting a primary tools for investigating their functional roles. While the studies of orofacial function in genetically modified mice are powerful tools for studying processes that are inaccessible using alternative approaches, they present important methodological challenges that must be considered in interpreting results deriving therefrom; these include genetic background, developmental compensation and sex-specific phenotypic effects, as reviewed elsewhere (see Waddington *et al.*, 2011, this volume).

These challenges are accompanied by further opportunities, using conditional mutants that give the investigator control over the timing and anatomical localization of gene disruption. For example, we have recently investigated (Tomiyama *et al.*, 2011) individual topographies of orofacial movement in mice having progressive, postnatal loss of (a) Striatal medium spiny neuron (MSN)-specific D1 receptors [which regulate striatal $GABA_A$ receptor-mediated currents] *vs* (b) Forebrain D1 receptors. As progressive loss of MSNs and $GABA_A$ergic components is one of the hallmark features of Huntington's disease, these findings may inform on the functional role of progressive disruption to $GABA_A$/D1 processes in the orofacial pathobiology of this disorder.

The findings reviewed here indicate that regulation of orofacial movements appears to involve both GABAergic and glutamatergic sytems. These regulatory mechanisms involve the individual role of each neurotransmitter system, together with the processes by which they each interact with DAergic systems as another primary regulatory mechanism (see Koshikawa *et al.*, 2011, this volume; Waddington *et al.*, 2011, this volume); both GABA (Arias-Montaño *et al.*, 2007; Hernández-Echeagaray *et al.*, 2007; Goffin *et al.*, 2008; Towers, and Hestrin, 2008) and glutamate (Castner and Williams, 2007; Missale *et al.*, 2010) enjoy extensive interactions particularly with D1 receptor systems. The challenge is to further clarify how individual GABA and glutamate receptor subtypes and subunits, in the pontomedullary reticular formation and forebrain structures such as the striatum and cortex, contribute to the regulation of individual topographies of orofacial movement.

Acknowledgments

The authors' studies would be impossible without the generous collaboration of our colleagues in molecular biology who have kindly made their mutants available to us; we are indebted to: Richard Harvey, Masato Hirata, Takashi Kanematsu, and Donna Lai. The authors' studies are supported by a grant for promotion of multidisciplinary research projects entitled Translational Research Network on Orofacial Neurological Disorders from the Ministry of Education, Culture, Sports, Science, and Technology of Japan, a Nihon University Multidisciplinary Grant, and Science Foundation Ireland Principal Investigator Grant 07/IN.1/B960.

References

Adachi, K., Hasegawa, M., Ikeda, H., Sato, M., Koshikawa, N., and Cools, A.R. (2003). The superior colliculus contains a discrete region involved in the control of jaw movements: role of $GABA_A$ receptors. *Eur. J. Pharmacol.* **464**, 147–154.

Arias-Montaño, J.A., Floran, B., Floran, L., Aceves, J., and Young, J.M. (2007). Dopamine D (1) receptor facilitation of depolarization-induced release of gamma-amino-butyric acid in rat striatum is mediated by the cAMP/PKA pathway and involves P/Q-type calcium channels. *Synapse* **61**, 310–319.

Balu, D.T., and Coyle, J.T. (2011). Neuroplasticity signaling pathways linked to the pathophysiology of schizophrenia. *Neurosci. Biobehav. Rev.* **35**, 848–870.

Banerjee, A., Macdonald, M.L., Borgmann-Winter, K.E., and Hahn, C.G. (2010). Neuregulin 1-erbB4 pathway in schizophrenia: From genes to an interactome. *Brain Res. Bull.* **83**, 132–139.

Berthoud, H.R. (2003). Neurochemical control and reconfiguration of the medullary network controlling different oromotor behaviors. *Am. J. Physiol. Regul. Integr. Comp. Physiol.* **285**, R19–20.

Bertram, L. (2008). Genetic research in schizophrenia: new tools and future perspectives. *Schizophr. Bull.* **34**, 806–812.

Bjarnadottir, M., Misner, D.L., Haverfield-Gross, S., Bruun, S., Helgason, V.G., Stefansson, H., Sigmundsson, A., Firth, D.R., Nielsen, B., Stefansdottir, R., Novak, T.J., Stefansson, K., Gurney, M.E., and Andresson, T. (2007). Neuregulin1 (NRG1) signaling through Fyn modulates NMDA receptor phosphorylation: differential synaptic function in NRG1+/− knock-outs compared with wild-type mice. *J. Neurosci.* **27**, 4519–4529.

Castner, S.A., and Williams, G.V. (2007). Tuning the engine of cognition: a focus on NMDA/D1 receptor interactions in prefrontal cortex. *Brain Cogn.* **63**, 94–122.

Chen, Z.W., and Olsen, R.W. (2007). $GABA_A$ receptor associated proteins: a key factor regulating $GABA_A$ receptor function. *J. Neurochem.* **100**, 279–294.

Collingridge, G.L., Olsen, R.W., Peters, J., and Spedding, M. (2009). A nomenclature for ligand-gated ion channels. *Neuropharmacology* **56**, 2–5.

Desbonnet, L., Waddington, J.L., and O'Tuathaigh, C.M. (2009). Mice mutant for genes associated with schizophrenia: common phenotype or distinct endophenotypes? *Behav. Brain Res.* **204**, 258–273.

Duty, S. (2010). Therapeutic potential of targeting group III metabotropic glutamate receptors in the treatment of Parkinson's disease. *Br. J. Pharmacol.* **161**, 271–287.

Emson, P.C. (2007). GABA (B) receptors: structure and function. *Prog. Brain Res.* **160**, 43–57.

Estep, M.E. (2009). Modulation, adaptation, and control of orofacial pathways in healthy adults. *J. Commun. Disord.* **42**, 280–285.

Fabbrini, G., Defazio, G., Colosimo, C., Thompson, P.D., and Berardelli, A. (2009). Cranial movement disorders: clinical features, pathophysiology, differential diagnosis and treatment. *Nat. Clin. Pract. Neurol.* **5**, 93–105.

Goffin, D., Aarum, J., Schroeder, J.E., Jovanovic, J.N., and Chuang, T.T. (2008). D1-like dopamine receptors regulate $GABA_A$ receptor function to modulate hippocampal neural progenitor cell proliferation. *J. Neurochem.* **107**, 964–975.

Gong, Y.G., Wu, C.N., Xing, Q.H., Zhao, X.Z., Zhu, J., and He, L. (2009). A two-method meta-analysis of Neuregulin 1 (NRG1) association and heterogeneity in schizophrenia. *Schizophr. Res.* **111**, 109–114.

Grimm, J.W., and See, R.E. (2000). Chronic haloperidol-induced alterations in pallidal GABA and striatal D (1)-mediated dopamine turnover as measured by dual probe microdialysis in rats. *Neuroscience* **100**, 507–514.

Hahn, C.G., Wang, H.Y., Cho, D.S., Talbot, K., Gurm, R.E., Berrettini, W.H., Bakshi, K., Kamins, J., Borgmann-Winter, K.E., Siegel, S.J., Gallop, R.J., and Arnold, S.E. (2006). Altered neuregulin 1-erbB4 signaling contributes to NMDA receptor hypofunction in schizophrenia. *Nat. Med.* **12**, 824–828.

Harrison, P.J., and Law, A.J. (2006). Neuregulin 1 and schizophrenia: genetics, gene expression, and neurobiology. *Biol. Psychiatry* **60**, 132–140.

Hernández-Echeagaray, E., Cepeda, C., Ariano, M.A., Lobo, M.K., Sibley, D.R., and Levine, M.S. (2007). Dopamine reduction of GABA currents in striatal medium-sized spiny neurons is mediated principally by the D (1) receptor subtype. *Neurochem. Res.* **32**, 229–240.

Hikosaka, O. (2007). GABAergic output of the basal ganglia. *Prog. Brain Res.* **160**, 209–226.

Inchul, P., Amano, N., Satoda, T., Murata, T., Kawagishi, S., Yoshino, K., and Tanaka, K. (2005). Control of oro-facio-lingual movements by the substantia nigra pars reticulata: high-frequency electrical microstimulation and GABA microinjection findings in rats. *Neuroscience* **134**, 677–689.

Inta, D., Monyer, H., Sprengel, R., Meyer-Lindenberg, A., and Gass, P. (2010). Mice with genetically altered glutamate receptors as models of schizophrenia: a comprehensive review. *Neurosci. Biobehav. Rev.* **34**, 285–294.

Kanaani, J., Kolibachuk, J., Martinez, H., and Baekkeskov, S. (2010). Two distinct mechanisms target GAD67 to vesicular pathways and presynaptic clusters. *J. Cell Biol.* **190**, 911–925.

Kanematsu, T., Mizokami, A., Watanabe, K., and Hirata, M. (2007). Regulation of GABA (A)-receptor surface expression with special reference to the involvement of GABARAP (GABA (A) receptor-associated protein) and PRIP (phospholipase C-related, but catalytically inactive protein). *J. Pharmacol. Sci.* **104**, 285–292.

Kirby, B.P., Waddington, J.L., and O'Tuathaigh, C.M. (2010). Advancing a functional genomics for schizophrenia: psychopathological and cognitive phenotypes in mutants with gene disruption. *Brain Res. Bull.* **83**, 162–176.

Koshikawa, N., Fujita, S., and Adachi, K. (2011). Behavioral pharmacology of orofacial movement disorders. *Int. Rev. Neurobiol* in press.

Li, B., Woo, R.S., Mei, L., and Malinow, R. (2007). The neuregulin-1 receptor erbB4 controls glutamatergic synapse maturation and plasticity. *Neuron* **54**, 583–597.

Lodge, D. (2009). The history of the pharmacology and cloning of ionotropic glutamate receptors and the development of idiosyncratic nomenclature. *Neuropharmacology* **56**, 6–21.

Luo, P., Zhang, J., Yang, R., and Pendlebury, W. (2006). Neuronal circuitry and synaptic organization of trigeminal proprioceptive afferents mediating tongue movement and jaw-tongue coordination via hypoglossal premotor neurons. *Eur. J. Neurosci.* **23**, 269–283.

Mei, L., and Xiong, W.C. (2008). Neuregulin 1 in neural development, synaptic plasticity and schizophrenia. *Nat. Rev. Neurosci.* **9**, 437–452.

Missale, C., Fiorentini, C., Collo, G., and Spano, P. (2010). The neurobiology of dopamine receptors: evolution from the dual concept to heterodimer complexes. *J. Recept. Signal Transduct. Res.* **30**, 347–354.

Mizokami, A., Kanematsu, T., Ishibashi, H., Yamaguchi, T., Tanida, I., Takenaka, K., Nakayama, K. I., Fukami, K., Takenawa, T., Kominami, E., Moss, S.J., Yamamoto, T., Nabekura, J., and Hirata, M. (2007). Phospholipase C-related inactive protein is involved in trafficking of gamma2 subunit-containing GABA (A) receptors to the cell surface. *J. Neurosci.* **27**, 1692–1701.

Munafò, M.R., Attwood, A.S., and Flint, J. (2008). Neuregulin 1 genotype and schizophrenia. *Schizophr. Bull.* **34**, 9–12.

Nakayama, K. (2002). Role of the PLC-related, catalytically inactive protein p130 in GABA (A) receptor function. *EMBO J.* **21**, 1004–1011.

Nistri, A., Ostroumov, K., Sharifullina, E., and Taccola, G. (2006). Tuning and playing a motor rhythm: how metabotropic glutamate receptors orchestrate generation of motor patterns in the mammalian central nervous system. *J. Physiol.* **572**, 323–334.

Niswender, C.M., and Conn, P.J. (2010). Metabotropic glutamate receptors: physiology, pharmacology, and disease. *Annu. Rev. Pharmacol. Toxicol.* **50**, 295–322.

Olsen, R.W., and Sieghart, W. (2009). $GABA_A$ receptors: subtypes provide diversity of function and pharmacology. *Neuropharmacology* **56**, 141–148.

Pappa, S., and Dazzan, P. (2009). Spontaneous movement disorders in antipsychotic-naive patients with first-episode psychoses: a systematic review. *Psychol. Med.* **39**, 1065–1076.

Peixoto, M.F., Araujo, N.P., Silva, R.H., Castro, J.P., Fukushiro, D.F., Faria, R.R., Zanier-Gomes, P. H., Medrano, W.A., Frussa-Filho, R., and Abílio, V.C. (2005). Effects of gabaergic drugs on reserpine-induced oral dyskinesia. *Behav. Brain Res.* **160**, 51–59.

Pinard, A., Seddik, R., and Bettler, B. (2010). $GABA_B$ receptors: physiological functions and mechanisms of diversity. *Adv. Pharmacol.* **58**, 231–255.

Reynolds, D.S. (2008). The value of genetic and pharmacological approaches to understanding the complexities of GABA (A) receptor subtype functions. *Pharmacol. Biochem. Behav.* **90**, 37–42.

Samadi, P., Grégoire, L., Morissette, M., Calon, F., Hadj Tahar, A., Bélanger, N., Dridi, M., Bédard, P. J., and Di Paolo, T. (2008 a) Basal ganglia group II metabotropic glutamate receptors specific binding in non-human primate model of L-Dopa-induced dyskinesias. *Neuropharmacology* **54**, 258–268.

Samadi, P., Morissette, M., Calon, F., Hadj Tahar, A., Dridi, M., Belanger, N., Meltzer, L.T., Bédard, P.J., and Di Paolo, T. (2008 b) Normalization of $GABA_A$ receptor specific binding in the substantia nigra reticulata and the prevention of L-dopa-induced dyskinesias in MPTP parkinsonian monkeys. *Synapse* **62**, 101–109.

Sawczuk, A., and Mosier, K.M. (2001). Neural control of tongue movement with respect to respiration and swallowing. *Crit. Rev. Oral Biol. Med.* **12**, 18–37.

Tomiyama, K., McNamara, F.N., Clifford, J.J., Kinsella, A., Koshikawa, N., and Waddington, J.L. (2001). Topographical assessment and pharmacological characterization of orofacial movements in mice: dopamine D (1)-like vs. D (2)-like receptor regulation. *Eur. J. Pharmacol.* **418**, 47–54.

Tomiyama, K., McNamara, F.N., Clifford, J.J., Kinsella, A., Drago, J., Tighe, O., Croke, D.T., Koshikawa, N., and Waddington, J.L. (2002). Phenotypic resolution of spontaneous and D (1)-like agonist-induced orofacial movement topographies in congenic dopamine D (1A) receptor 'knockout' mice. *Neuropharmacology* **42**, 644–652.

Tomiyama, K., O'Tuathaigh, C.M., O'Sullivan, G.J., Kinsella, A., Lai, D., Harvey, R.P., Tighe, O., Croke, D.T., Koshikawa, N., and Waddington, J.L. (2009). Phenotype of spontaneous orofacial dyskinesia in neuregulin-1 'knockout' mice. *Prog. Neuropsychopharmacol. Biol. Psychiatry* **33**, 330–333.

Tomiyama, K., Song, L., Kobayashi, M., Kinsella, A., Kanematsu, T., Hirata, M., Koshikawa, N., and Waddington, J.L. (2010). Orofacial movements in phospholipase C-related catalytically inactive protein-1/2 double knockout mice: Effect of the GABAergic agent diazepam and the D (1) dopamine receptor agonist SKF 83959. *Synapse* **64**, 714–720.

Tomiyama, K., Kim, H., Kinsella, A., Ehrlich, M.E., Schütz, G., Koshikawa, N., Lawrence, A.J., Waddington, J.L., and Drago, J. (2011). Phenotypic disruption to orofacial movement topography in conditional mutants with generalised CamKIIa/Cre D1Tox *vs* striatal-specific DARPP-32/Cre D1Tox ablation of D1 dopamine receptor-expressing cells. *Synapse* in press.

Towers, S.K., and Hestrin, S. (2008). D1-like dopamine receptor activation modulates GABAergic inhibition but not electrical coupling between neocortical fast-spiking interneurons. *J. Neurosci* **28**, 2633–2641.

Tsunekawa, N., Arata, A., and Obata, K. (2005). Development of spontaneous mouth/tongue movement and related neural activity, and their repression in fetal mice lacking glutamate decarboxylase 67. *Eur. J. Neurosci.* **21**, 173–178.

Uji, A., Matsuda, M., Kukita, T., Maeda, K., Kanematsu, T., and Hirata, M. (2002). Molecules interacting with PRIP-2, a novel Ins (1,4,5) P3 binding protein type 2: Comparison with PRIP-1. *Life Sci.* **72**, 443–453.

Vicini, S., and Ortinski, P. (2004). Genetic manipulations of $GABA_A$ receptor in mice make inhibition exciting. *Pharmacol. Ther.* **103**, 109–120.

Vigot, R., Barbieri, S., Bräuner-Osborne, H., Turecek, R., Shigemoto, R., Zhang, Y.P., Luján, R., Jacobson, L.H., Biermann, B., Fritschy, J.M., Vacher, C.M., Müller, M., Sansig, G., Guetg, N., Cryan, J.F., Kaupmann, K., Gassmann, M., Oertner, T.G., and Bettler, B. (2006). Differential compartmentalization and distinct functions of $GABA_B$ receptor variants. *Neuron* **50**, 589–601.

Waddington, J.L., Daly, S.A., Downes, R.P., Deveney, A.M., McCauley, P.G., and O'Boyle, K.M. (1995). Behavioral pharmacology of 'D1-like' dopamine receptors: further subtyping, new pharmacological probes and interactions with 'D-2-like' receptors. *Prog. Neuropsychopharmacol. Biol. Psychiatry* **19**, 811–831.

Waddington, J.L., O'Tuathaigh, C., O'Sullivan, G., Tomiyama, K., Koshikawa, N., and Croke, D.T. (2005). Phenotypic studies on dopamine receptor subtype and associated signal transduction mutants: insights and challenges from 10 years at the psychopharmacology-molecular biology interface. *Psychopharmacology* **181**, 611–638.

Waddington, J.L., O'Sullivan, G.J., and Tomiyama, K. (2011). Regulation of orofacial movement: dopamine receptor mechanisms and mutant models. *Int. Rev. Neurobiol* in press.

Walker, F.O. (2007). Huntington's disease. *Lancet* **369**, 218–228.

Walls, A.B., Nilsen, L.H., Eyjolfsson, E.M., Vestergaard, H.T., Hansen, S.L., Schousboe, A., Sonnewald, U., and Waagepetersen, H.S. (2010). GAD65 is essential for synthesis of GABA destined for tonic inhibition regulating epileptiform activity. *J. Neurochem.* **115**, 1398–1408.

Whitty, P., Owoeye, O., and Waddington, J.L. (2009). Neurological signs and involuntary movements in schizophrenia: intrinsic to and informative on systems pathobiology. *Schizophr. Bull.* **35**, 415–424.

THE TRIGEMINAL CIRCUITS RESPONSIBLE FOR CHEWING

Karl-Gunnar Westberg[1] and Arlette Kolta[2]

[1]Department of Integrative Medical Biology, Section for Physiology, Umeå University, SE-901 87 Umeå, Sweden

[2]Faculté de médecine dentaire, and Groupe de Recherche sur le Système Nerveux Central du FRSQ, Université de Montréal C.P. 6128, succursale Centre-villeMontréal (Qc), Canada H3C 3J7

I. Introduction

Mastication is one of the primary behaviors expressed by the organ systems of the oro-facial region. It is the process where food is split up into smaller pieces, thus making them available for further enzymatic handling in the gastrointestinal tract. However, besides its nutritional aspect, it is also well recognized that eating and masticatory functions are of importance for social interactions and for the general well-being of humans. When mastication is impaired, health problems can arise because hard-to-chew food is avoided in favor of softer and more easily consumed products (N'gom and Woda, 2002; Hutton *et al.*, 2002). Therefore a first class chewing function is considered to be essential both because of its benefits on the nutrient balance of an individual, and on self-reported life satisfaction (Brennan *et al.*, 2008).

INTERNATIONAL REVIEW OF NEUROBIOLOGY, VOL. 97
DOI: 10.1016/B978-0-12-385198-7.00004-7

A most important goal as regards functional oral rehabilitation is to create excellent masticatory conditions by replacing missing teeth with prosthetic appliances (e.g. crowns, bridges, implants, or full dentures). Equally significant, when forming a ready-to-swallow bolus is a well balanced coordination of jaw, tongue, and facial muscle activities (Lund, 1991). This feature of mastication is governed by a variety of both peripheral and central neuronal mechanisms, which delineates the trigeminal sensory-motor control circuits of the brain.

II. Masticatory Movements

Carnivores, which feed on meat, generally chew very little or swallow their food in large chunks. However, to make vegetables, seeds, and fruits available for chemical and enzymatic digestion, it is considered an advantage if these could be broken into smaller pieces (Ellis *et al.*, 2004). This needs to handle ingested food morsels by grinding between the teeth is largely an adaptation that evolved for mammalian herbivores (Gans *et al.*, 1978; Luschei and Goodwin, 1974).

Despite dietary variation among omnivore species, a masticatory sequence (i.e. the process from the ingestion of a food morsel to its final deglutition) consists of a series of jaw movement cycles (Byrd, 1981; Morimoto *et al.*, 1985; Schwartz *et al.*, 1989; Hiiemae *et al.*, 1996; Woda *et al.*, 2006). When jaw movement profiles are analyzed in more detail, the masticatory act can be divided into three distinctive stages, each containing a series of characteristic opening and closing mandibular movement cycles (Schwartz *et al.*, 1989). Depending on species studied, several terminologies have been used for classifying and naming these (Schwartz *et al.*, 1989; Hiiemae, 2004). In primates and humans as well as in non-primates, the first stage is called "manipulative", "transport", or "preparatory" because this is when food is initially handled and reduced to chewable pieces by splitting between the anterior teeth. In the rabbit, movements of the mandible during "stage I" cycles are characterized by simple vertical opening closing orbits with little deviation away from the midline (Morimoto *et al.*, 1985; Schwartz *et al.*, 1989). The jaw-opening muscles are active during each movement cycle, while closer muscles show more intermittent activity that varies greatly according to task requirements (Weijs and Dantuma, 1975). In humans, a range of muscle activation patterns are used to generate forces that vary from gentle ones, such as those applied during precision movements needed to hold and manipulate objects between the front teeth, to powerful ones applied in large vertical compressions, needed to break solid fracture-resistant foods (Hiiemae *et al.*, 1996; Koolstra, 2002). Maximum bite forces of more that 150N have been recorded in humans (Paphangkorakit and Osborn, 1997). However, much less force is usually needed during food consumption. For instance, when cracking a peanut, forces normally vary between 20N–30N (Trulsson and Johansson, 1996).

Following the "preparatory" phase, food is transported towards the back of the mouth by movements of the cheeks and tongue, to be further split-up by grinding between the premolar and molar teeth. During this "reduction" or "chewing" phase, each jaw movement cycle can be divided into three phases [opening (O), a short fast close (FC), and a slow closing phase (SC)]. The FC phase is characterized by a crescent shaped lateral swing of the jaw, which ends up in a medially directed grinding-like transverse movement during the SC phase, that shears food between the cusps of the working side teeth (Morimoto *et al.*, 1985; Schwartz *et al.*, 1989; Lavigne *et al.*, 1987; Morimoto *et al.*, 1989; Hidaka *et al.*, 1997).

The last part of the masticatory sequence is the "pre-swallowing" or "oro-pharyngeal" stage of swallowing (Schwartz *et al.*, 1989). This is where the ready-to-swallow bolus is formed and transported towards the pharynx and upper esophagus, by concurrent activities in mylohyoid, anterior digastric, medial pterygoid, and tongue muscles (Jean, 2001). Pre-swallowing jaw movement cycles can be divided into three opening (O1–O3) and two closing phases, FC and SC. These cycles show some resemblance to those seen during the "reduction" phase of the masticatory sequence, but they are of smaller amplitude, longer duration, and contain little closing muscle activity (Schwartz *et al.*, 1989).

III. Organization of the Trigeminal Nerve

The sensory information from orofacial structures are transmitted to the trigeminal nuclei in the brainstem via the trigeminal nerve, which is divided into three branches innervating the ophthalmic, maxillary, and mandibular dermatomes, respectively (Fig. 1A). The ophthalmic and maxillary nerves are purely sensory while the mandibular nerve contains both sensory and motor axons. The latter, that innervates jaw opening and closing muscles, emerges from motoneurons in the trigeminal motor nucleus. The three branches of the trigeminal nerve converge on the trigeminal ganglion that accommodates the cell bodies of most of the sensory nerve fibers. Only those of jaw closing muscle spindle afferents (MSA) and about half of periodontal afferents have their cell bodies in the trigeminal mesencephalic nucleus (NVmes). From the trigeminal ganglion a single large sensory root enters the lateral brainstem where it forms the spinal (descending) tract of the trigeminal nerve (V; Fig. 1B). In the tract, the dorso-ventral distribution of the peripheral dermatomes is inverted (Fig. 2A). The axons which supply the ophthalmic division are now found in the ventral third of the tract, followed dorsally by those supplied by the maxillary and mandibular branches (Darian-Smith and

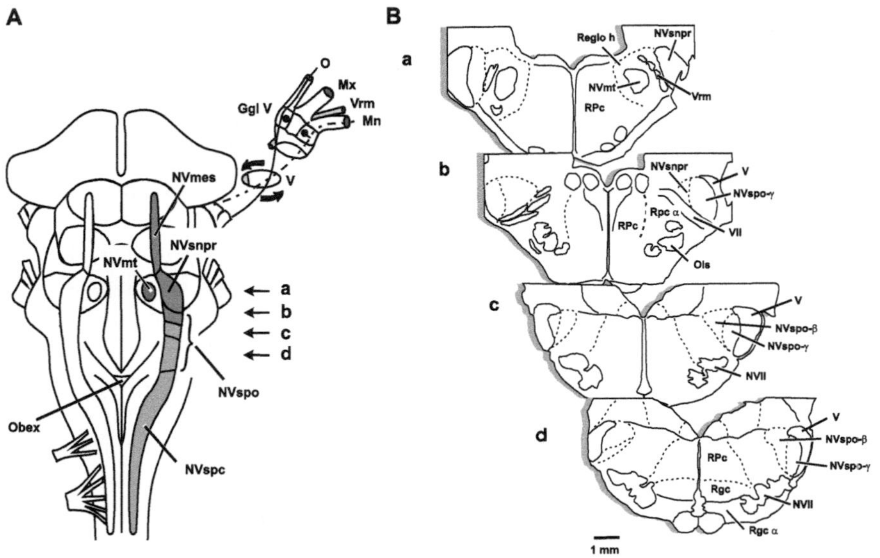

FIG. 1. Diagram showing the organization of brainstem nuclei thought to be involved in the generation of rhythmical masticatory jaw movements. A. Drawing of the brainstem seen from a dorsal view where outlines of the left and right trigeminal nuclei are indicated. The three divisions of the trigeminal nerve and the trigeminal ganglion are also indicated. Note the inversion of the divisions as they enter the trigeminal tract (Redrawn from Landgren and Olsson, 1977). B. Illustration of coronal histological sections to schematically denote the location of certain nuclei within the brainstem. The levels of the sections are marked by arrows in A. *Ggl V- trigeminal ganglion; Mn- mandibular nerve; Mx-maxillary nerve; NVsnpr - main sensory trigeminal nucleus; NVmt - trigeminal motor nucleus; NVspo-γ - subnucleus γ of the oral nucleus of the spinal trigeminal trigeminal tract; NVspo-β - subnucleus-β of the oral nucleus of the spinal trigeminal tract; O –ophthalmic nerve; Rgc-α - nucleus paragigantocellularis pars α; Rgc nucleus gigantocellularis; RPc nucleus reticularis pontis caudalis; Rpc-α nucleus reticularis parvocellularis pars α; Regio h reticular borderzone of the NVmt; NVII- facial motor nucleus; Ols Olivia superior; V- trigeminal tract; Vrm trigeminal motor root.*

Mayday, 1960; Capra and Dessem, 1992). This “inverted face” somatotopy is preserved in the subnuclei of the spinal trigeminal tact (see below).

IV. Organization of the Trigeminal Complex in the Brainstem

The trigeminal sensory nuclei extend from the midbrain through pons and medulla caudally to the level of obex (Olsson and Westberg, 1989; Capra and Dessem, 1992).

A. The Mesencephalic Trigeminal Nucleus

The NVmes begins rostrally close to the midline with a narrow column of cells formed by the somata of jaw closing MSA. This nucleus enlarges at its caudal end which holds primarily the cell bodies of mechanoreceptor afferents innervating the periodontal ligaments of the teeth (Linden, 1978; Gottlieb *et al.*, 1984; Lazarov, 2002).

B. The Main Sensory Trigeminal Nucleus

Caudal and lateral to NVmes is the main sensory trigeminal nucleus (NVsnpr; Fig. 1) which receives topographically organized inputs from primary afferents of all three branches of the trigeminal nerve with upper face regions represented ventrally and lower face regions dorsally (Eisenman *et al.*, 1963; Shigenaga *et al.*, 1986). All divisions contain sensory relay cells in the trigemino-thalamic pathway to the oro-facial primary sensory cortex (Eisenman *et al.*, 1964). However, the dorsomedial part of the NVsnpr was noted by Eisenman *et al.*, (1963) to be composed of a "round island of densely arranged cells". Later on, this particular group of neurons has been suggested to function as pre-motor interneurons (see below).

C. The Subnuclei of the Spinal Trigeminal Tract

The nucleus of the spinal trigeminal tract, caudal to the NVsnpr, is divided into two main parts; the oral (NVspo) and caudal subdivision (NVspc) (Fig. 1A). The former can be further subdivided into the three subnuclei NVspo-α, β and -γ (Meessen and Olzewski, 1949). The most rostral part, NVspo- γ, appears as a continuation of NVsnpr at the caudal end of NVmt (Fig. 1Bb). Dorsally, it contains neurons projecting to trigeminal and hypoglossal motor nuclei, while neurons in the ventral part of NVspo-γ contact cervical and upper spinal segments, the facial and abducens motor nuclei (Matsushita *et al.*, 1981; Durand *et al.*, 1983; Mizuno *et al.*, 1983; Landgren *et al.*, 1986; Kolta *et al.*, 2000).

The NVspo-β is situated approximately at the level of the facial motor nucleus (Fig. 1Bc) and it is followed by the NVspo-α, which extends to obex where it is replaced by the caudal trigeminal subnucleus (NVspc), also known as the trigeminal relay for oro-facial pain and temperature sensations (Dubner and Bennett, 1983; Sessle, 1987). Neurons within NVspo-β and -α, that roughly correspond to nucleus interpolaris in primates (Meessen and Olzewski, 1949) have been implicated, in both sensory and motor functions because of their projections to thalamus, cerebellum, spinal cord as well as to oro-facial motor nuclei (Ikeda, 1979; Hayashi *et al.*, 1984; Li *et al.*, 1995).

D. The Trigeminal Motor Nucleus

The trigeminal motor nucleus (NVmt) is situated medially to the sensory complex, roughly at the level of the NVsnpr (Fig. 1Ba). The NVmt is mainly composed of motoneurones innervating the masticatory muscles intermingled with a smaller population of commissural interneurons (see below). Motoneurons innervarting jaw closing muscles are located dorsally and laterally in the rostral and middle thirds of the NVmt, while jaw opening motoneurons are found ventromedially, in the caudal third of the nucleus. This pattern of representation has been confirmed in both anatomical and functional studies on many species (Landgren and Olsson, 1976; Mizuno *et al.*, 1981; Saad *et al.*, 1997). The motor axons innervating the jaw muscles pass between the motor and main sensory nuclei and leave the Pons as radix motoria (Fig. 1Ba; Vrm).

V. Generation of the Masticatory Jaw Movement Pattern

In the beginning of the last century Sherrington presented the first hypothesis regarding the nervous generation of masticatory movements (Sherrington, 1917). When stimulating the oral mucosa bordering the teeth or hard palate in decerebrated cats he noted that the stimulus evoked "a quick" opening of the jaw, which was "sharply followed by active return". The latter caused by a stretch reflex evoked contraction of the jaw closing muscles. Based on this observation Sherrington hypothesized that "after being started by a first bite, a rhythmic masticatory reflex tends to keep itself going so long as there is something biteable between the jaws".

However, when Sherrington made his experiments it was already known that masticatory as well as licking movements could be induced by the stimulation of a circumscribed area within the cerebral cortex in different animal species including the rabbit (Ferrier, 1886). Later Bremer (1923) identified three subregions within the rabbit's cortical "masticatory area" (CMA) from which different forms of masticatory movements could be produced by cortical surface stimulation. Further detailed experiments by Lund *et al.* (1984) confirmed this kinesiotopic-like movement representation by showing that electrical intracortical stimulation of anterior sites within the CMA elicit vertical "preparatory phase-like" jaw movements, while the stimulation of posterior sites cause "reduction phase" like movements (Lund *et al.*, 1984).

In the 1930 Rioch proposed a modified version of Sherrington's reflex-chain-theory in which she postulated that activation of cortico-fugal pathways selectively excited jaw-opening motoneurones. The rhythm of mastication would then result from a gated cyclic "subcortical inhibition" of the cortically generated drive to the jaw opening motoneurons, during the reflexly initiated jaw closing movement (Rioch, 1934).

The first solid proof that masticatory movements are generated by a central pattern generating circuit (masticatory CPG) came from experiments conducted by *Lund and Dellow* (1971). They showed that mastication could be induced by repetitive electrical stimulation of the sensory-motor cortex or descending corticobulbar pathways in paralyzed decerebrate rabbits. Thus, the basic masticatory rhythm of jaw opening and jaw closing motoneuron activities, that closely resembles the one forming the movement in the intact animal continued to be produced in a preparation deprived of all phasic sensory input. Therefore, the basic source of the motor rhythm has to reside in a "chewing center", capable of generating the chewing- like muscle activity pattern. However, as pointed out by Lund and Dellow (1971) this finding should not be taken to mean that sensory input plays no role at all. On the contrary, it is well documented that sensory feedback from peripheral sense organs is crucial to optimize masticatory bite forces (Lavigne *et al.*, 1987; Morimoto *et al.*, 1989; Inoue *et al.*, 1989; Hidaka *et al.*, 1997; Komuro *et al.*, 2001a, b; Peyron *et al.*, 2002). By using the combinations of EMG recordings and jaw movement tracking during simulated chewing in human subjects, Ottenhoff et al. (1992a, b) showed that the nervous system uses two parallel strategies to adapt the bite forces to changing properties of the food during mastication. The first, and probably most important, is a feed-forward strategy in which the muscle commands, to overcome an expected resistance is predicted already before the start of the closing movement, allowing adequate muscle force to build up ahead of tooth-food contact (van der Bilt *et al.*, 2006; Grigoriadis *et al.*, 2011) .The cortex and other supra medullary motor centers would presumably play an important role in this first anticipatory component. The second is to adjust muscle force after the onset of the jaw movement by using direct short latency feedback information from intraoral mechanoreceptors and muscle spindles about forces acting on the teeth and muscle contraction properties. The notion that both of these motor control strategies are valid has been confirmed in studies on anaesthetized rabbits during cortically induced masticatory movements (Komuro *et al.*, 2001a, b).

VI. Functional Organization of the Sensory-motor Circuitry

From studies on locomotor circuits it is known that sensory information and volleys arising from higher centers to motoneurons are integrated by populations of "last-order" pre-motor interneurons (Olsson and Landgren, 1990). In the trigeminal system such interneurons, which establish monosynaptic excitatory or inhibitory contacts with trigeminal motoneurons, were first identified by using the method of retrograde transport of wheat germ agglutinated horseradish peroxidase (WGA-HRP) deposited within the NVmt (Mizuno *et al.*, 1983; Landgren *et al.*, 1986; Li *et al.*, 1995). Neurons that have accumulated the tracer from the injection site and, thus, can be interpreted as pre-motor inter-neurons, are encountered bilaterally, mostly within dorsal (supra-trigeminal NsV), lateral (inter-trigeminal NintV) and medial (Mb) "juxta-trigeminal" parts of the border zone (Regio h) surrounding the tri-geminal motor nucleus (Fig. 2A, Ba; Lorente De No, 1922'; Meessen and Olzewski, 1949). Lateral to the motor nucleus other groups of labeled cells are confined to the dorsal part of NVsnpr mainly on the side ipsilateral to the tracer deposit (Landgren *et al.*, 1986; Yoshida *et al.*, 1998; Kolta *et al.*, 2000). Caudal to the NVsnpr, stained neurons appear dorsally in NVspo-γ with the most significant concentration on the ipsilateral side (Fig. 2Bb). Further caudal clusters of neurons are labeled bilaterally in the parvocellular part of the reticular formation (Rpc) medial to the NVspo-β (Fig. 2Bc). At the level of NVspo-α

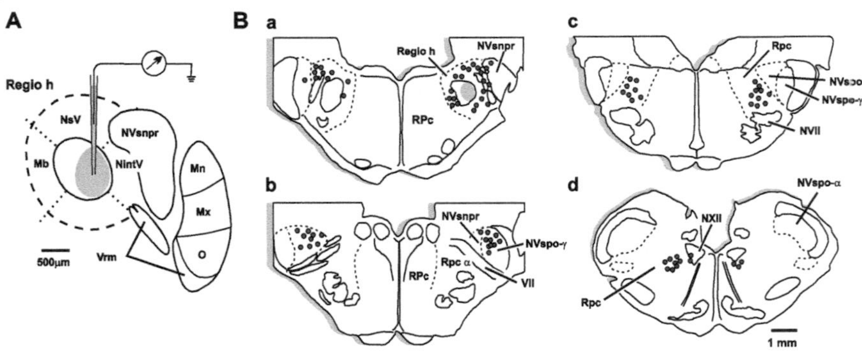

FIG. 2. Schematic illustration of a system using pressure injection of small quantities of wheat germ agglutinin-conjugated horseradish peroxidase (WGA-HRP) to identify trigeminal premotoneurons A. Tracing of a coronal histological section at the level of the NVmt. The shaded area shows the area covered by a 20nl volume of WGA-HRP tracer. The lateral (intertrigeminal, NintV) and dorsal (supratrigeminal, NsV) parts of the reticular borderzone surrounding the NVmt are indicated. B. Drawings of histological sections showing the distribution of retrogradely stained neurons with axon terminals within the NVmt. Dorsal is up. For abbreviations see Fig. 1 and text. (Redrawn from: Landgren *et al.*, 1986 and Westberg, 1990). (For interpretation of the references to color in this figure legend, the reader is referred to the Web version of the chapter.).

and rostral part of NVspc the neurons appear in the reticular formation bordering the hypoglossal motor nucleus (Fig. 2Bd). This area is also known to contain neurons projecting to the hypoglossal nucleus (Borke *et al.*, 1983).

Anatomical as well as electrophysiological evidence also suggests the existence of commissural interneurons within NVmt projecting to contralateral motoneurons (McDavid *et al.*, 2008; McDavid *et al.*, 2006). These may serve the bilateral synchronization of jaw motor activities, previously reported in electrophysiological studies (Appenteng *et al.*, 1990; Donga and Lund, 1991; Kamogawa *et al.*, 1994). The various populations of pre-motor interneurons (including those in NVmt) have been shown to be immunoreactive for glutamate, glutamic acid decarboxylase (GAD), the enzyme which synthesizes γ-aminobutyric acid (GABA), or glycine (Turman and Chandler, 1994a, b; Ginestal and Matute, 1993; Li *et al.*, 1996; Rampon *et al.*, 1996; Kolta *et al.*, 2000; McDavid *et al.*, 2006). There is also evidence that GABA and glycine are co-localized in some of the neurons (Bae *et al.*, 2002). The presence of excitatory and inhibitory transmitters in Regio h, NVspo-γ and Rpc neurons has been confirmed by the recordings of evoked monosynaptic effects on trigeminal motoneurons (Appenteng *et al.*, 1989; Appenteng *et al.*, 1990; Donga and Lund, 1991; Grimwood *et al.*, 1992; Westberg *et al.*, 1995; Kolta, 1997; Shigenaga *et al.*, 2000; Yoshida *et al.*, 2001; Inoue *et al.*, 2002), on local interneurons (Bourque and Kolta, 2001; McDavid *et al.*, 2008), and on NVsnpr neurons (Athanassiadis *et al.*, 2005b).

Regarding function, extracellular recordings from single interneurons in Regio h, NVsnpr, NVspo-γ, and Rpc show that they are activated both by primary afferent and descending central commands (Olsson *et al.*, 1986a, b; Olsson and Westberg, 1991; Westberg and Olsson, 1991; Westberg *et al.*, 1995, 1998; Inoue *et al.*, 2002; Tsuboi *et al.*, 2003). From the periphery, most respond when the inferior alveolar and/or lingual nerves are electrically stimulated at low intensity (<2T), which show that they receive inputs from mechanoreceptor afferents located in the oral mucosa, periodontal ligament, tongue, and perioral skin. Responses evoked from nerves innervating extra-oral areas (maxillary nerve) or jaw muscles (masseter, digastric) are less frequent, and often occur at stimulation strength above 2T indicating that these are evoked by inputs from nociceptive afferents. The majority of the interneurons are, in addition, activated by inputs with short latency from the cortical oral and perioral primary projection fields in cat coronal gyrus (i.e. cytoarchitectonic areas 3a and 3b), or the corresponding sensory-motor ("masticatory") area of rabbit cerebral cortex (Olsson *et al.*, 1986a, b; Westberg and Olsson, 1991; Westberg *et al.*, 1995, 1998). Many also exhibit rhythmic discharges locked to particular phases of the jaw movement cycle during feeding in conscious animals as well as during mastication evoked in anesthetized and paralyzed rabbits and rats (Olsson *et al.*, 1986b; Donga and Lund, 1991; Inoue *et al.*, 1992; Westberg *et al.*, 1998; Tsuboi *et al.*, 2003; Athanassiadis *et al.*, 2005a). Furthermore, some interneurons start or stop their firing, change firing frequency or alter their phase of activity depending on the evoked masticatory movement pattern (Westberg *et al.*, 1998). This finding provides strong evidence that, at least a subset, contribute to the generation of not only one masticatory motor pattern but to several patterns that can be expressed during the natural behavior (Lund *et al.*, 1998).

VII. Groups of Neurons Involved in Masticatory Pattern Generation

Several current CPG models postulate the involvement of two essential neuronal components; one that accounts for rhythm generation, i.e. timing of the cycle periods that determine the onsets and offsets of involved antagonistic motoneurons during each movement cycle, and another for shaping of motoneuronal spatio-temporal activity patterns. The latter governs the amplitude of the motor outflow during a given movement task i.e. intra-cycle motor pattern generation. These two conceptual components of the GPG architecture have been viewed as either subserved by the same set of neurons or by separate groups of neurons (Grillner, 2006; McCrea and Rybak, 2008).

For years, the masticatory CPG model that prevailed had this dual component division with a rhythm generator located in the medial bulbar reticular formation (MBRF) and a pattern generator located in the lateral parvocellular reticular formation. Although different research groups had proposed this dual organization and functional division, the exact rostrocaudal localization of these different components has varied with time and species. At first, studies on the guinea pig in the 1980 suggested that the masticatory rhythm was generated in the MBRF area containing the gigantocellularis and the dorsal para-gigantocellularis nuclei (Nozaki *et al.*, 1986a, b; Chandler and Tal, 1986). This proposal was based on the fact that: 1) Injections of local anaesthetic into this area and transections around it abolish rhythmical jaw movements evoked by stimulation of the CMA and that: 2) Stimulation of the CMA evokes tonic firing at a monosynaptic latency in neurons of the contralateral para-gigantocellular nucleus (Rgc-α; Fig. 1Bd), which in turn projects to a more dorsal group located in the oral portion of the gigantocellular nucleus (Rgc; Fig. 1Bd) that fire rhythmic bursts of action potentials with the same rhythm as the trigeminal motoneurons (Chandler and Tal, 1986; Nozaki et al., 1986a, b; Chandler *et al.*, 1990). However, because this area had no direct projections to tri-geminal motoneurons, a second component, acting as a putative burst/pattern generator had to be considered and Nakamura's group proposed that this component was made of a group of pre-motor interneurons located in the caudal parvocellular reticular formation, adjacent to the hypoglossal nucleus (Fig. 2Bd). However, later it was reported that output neurons of the masticatory rhythm generating circuit in the MBRF are likely to be located in more rostral areas of the lateral reticular formation known to contain trigeminal pre-motor neurons because blocking neuronal activity in these areas, abolished rhythmic mastication (Chandler *et al.*, 1990).

Further, studies in the rabbit failed to observe any effect on mastication when deactivating the region of the gigantocellular nucleus (Scott *et al.*, 2003). Instead, the authors found that a region of the medial reticular formation slightly rostral to that containing the gigantocellular nucleus and including the nucleus pontis caudalis (RPc in Figs. 1B and 2B) seems to play an important role in masticatory pattern generation (Scott *et al.*, 2003). This region also receives cortical and peripheral inputs and injections of local anaesthetic in it alter the masticatory motor pattern (Chandler *et al.*, 1990; Scott *et al.*, 2003). This area also had very few projections to trigeminal motoneurons, but had massive projections to pre-motor inter-neurons located in the zone bordering NVmt and in the adjacent NVsnpr (Kolta *et al.*, 2000; Dal *et al.*, 2005; Athanassiadis *et al.*, 2005b) which could act as the burst generating component.

Recent evidence leads us to re-evaluate this two component CPG model. First, transections studies in "en bloc" brainstem preparations of neonate rats suggest that the minimal critical area necessary to produce rhythmic activity in the nerves innervating jaw muscles (trigeminal nerve) is a bloc extending from the rostral pole of the motor nucleus (NVmt) to the rostral pole of the facial nucleus and approximately half a millimeter from the lateral border of the brainstem (Kogo *et al.*, 1996; Tanaka *et al.*, 1999). Besides the trigeminal motoneurons, this circumscribed area also contains pre-motor inter-neurons located within the border zone of the NVmt, the NVsnpr and the rostral pole of the NVspo (Figs. 1 and 2Ba, Bb). Only a small part of the medial reticular formation, formed by the RPc is included in this area. Rhythmic activity has been recorded in neurons of all these four areas during fictive mastication *in vivo* experiments; that is mastication elicited by stimulation of the CMA in paralyzed and anaesthetized animals. However, it is still unknown which of these neurons are "generators", and which are "followers", i.e. the ones that receive rhythmic inputs from the generators.

Rhythmic output of CPGs can theoretically result from intrinsic properties of individual neurons, from interactions within a network, or from a combination of the two, a property referred to as "emergent network property". A decade ago we started using brainstem slice preparations to investigate the "rhythmogenic potential" of pre-motor interneurons both in Regio h and NVmt. It was found that these form a homogeneous population with regard to their basic electrophysiological properties. They are extensively interconnected synaptically and, except for a small population adjacent to the dorsal NVsnpr (Bourque and Kolta, 2001; Hsiao *et al.*, 2007), they seem unable to generate rhythmic activity whether by their intrinsic properties or by their reciprocal connections. However, synaptic transmission within this pre-motor network is robust and rarely fails even with high frequency stimulation or when oligosynaptic pathways are involved suggesting that inputs reaching individual neurons could be rapidly distributed to the other neurons within the network. These connections may be important to ensure a rapid and reliable distribution of rhythmic inputs received from the other populations of neurons such as those that have been recently identified in the dorso-anterior part of NVsnpr. These particular NVsnpr neurons have a number of interesting characteristics with regard to rhythm generation. They possess intrinsic bursting abilities that parallel the maturation of the masticatory motor pattern, which appears around postnatal day 12 (P12). Furthermore, the number of NVsnpr bursting neurons increases during the 2nd postanatal week when the transition in ingestive behavior from suckling to mastication occurs and stabilizes between P16–18 when the adult masticatory behavior is fully established (Westneat and Hall, 1992; Brocard *et al.*, 2006). Moreover, their bursts of action potentials occur repetitively within the frequency range of natural mastication (6–8 Hz) and are maintained and even enhanced under conditions that reduce synaptic transmission (removal of Ca^{2+} from the perfusing medium), confirming that they result from an intrinsic property.

VIII. Mechanisms of Burst Generation

As in many brain regions, including neurons of the pre-Bötzinger complex (Butera, Jr. *et al.*, 1999; Del Negro *et al.*, 2002; Del Negro *et al.*, 2005), the spinal cord (Darbon *et al.*, 2004; Zhong *et al.*, 2007; Tazerart *et al.*, 2008a), the hippocampus (Azouz *et al.*, 1996; Mattia *et al.*, 1997; Su *et al.*, 2001; Jinno *et al.*, 2003), the subthalamic nucleus (Beurrier *et al.*, 2000), the neocortex (Franceschetti *et al.*, 1995; Guatteo *et al.*, 1996; Brumberg *et al.*, 2000) and the trigeminal primary afferents of the NVmes (Wu *et al.*, 2005), bursting in NVsnpr is primarily mediated by a persistent sodium conductance (I_{NaP}). It is sensitive to riluzole and tetrodotoxin (TTX), which suppress I_{NaP} (Urbani and Belluzzi, 2000; Wu *et al.*, 2005) and inhibit bursts and the underlying plateau potentials. Both bursting and the underlying plateau potentials are seen within a voltage range that correspond to the activation and steady-state inactivation voltages typical of I_{NaP} (Crill, 1996). Within that range (roughly –65 to –50 mV), bursting frequency increases with depolarization, but firing reverts to a tonic pattern when depolarization exceeds –50 mV. The prevalence of bursting and the duration of the underlying plateau potential are also inversely related to the extracellular Ca^{2+} concentration ($[Ca^{2+}]_e$) (Brocard *et al.*, 2006). A similar relationship between $[Ca^{2+}]_e$ and the magnitude of I_{NaP} had been reported in other areas of the CNS (Azouz *et al.*, 1996; Li and Hatton, 1996; Su *et al.*, 2001; Tazerart *et al.*, 2008b). Based on this, we postulate that the Ca^{2+}-sensitivity and voltage-dependency of I_{NaP} provide a mechanism by which incoming inputs can adjust and control the output of potentially rhythmogenic neurons and determine their firing pattern (bursting vs tonic). This property would enable NVsnpr neurons to act as sensory relay cells when I_{NaP} is not active, and to become an interface converting cortical or sensory feedback into a rhythmogenic motor command when I_{NaP} is active. The conditions to activate I_{NaP} would be gathered only if inputs are activated massively or in a sustained manner, sufficient to induce both depolarization and a decrease of extra-cellular Ca^{2+}. Intense, sustained neuronal activity, (Nicholson *et al.*, 1978; Somjen, 1980; Pumain *et al.*, 1983; Pumain and Heinemann, 1985; Amzica *et al.*, 2002) as well as bursting in many brain area (Benninger *et al.*, 1980; Heinemann *et al.*, 1990; Rusakov and Fine, 2003; Cohen and Fields, 2004) has been associated to decreases of $[Ca^{2+}]_e$. For instance, $[Ca^{2+}]_e$ falls to levels as low as 0.8 mM in the cerebellar cortex of the cat during repetitive local stimulation (Nicholson *et al.*, 1978), to 0.1 mM during cortical bursting (Somjen, 1980) and to 0.08 mM in rat neocortex after local glutamate application (Amzica *et al.*, 2002). This may explain why long trains of repetitive stimulation lasting hundreds of milliseconds are required to trigger mastication by stimulation of either the CMA or the sensory tract, when sensory and cortical inputs reach most trigeminal brainstem neurons at a relatively short latency (~5 ms). In the *in vitro* slice preparation, the majority (> 90%) of dorsal NVsnpr neurons have a spontaneously bursting pattern when $[Ca^{2+}]_e$ is artificially lowered in the perfusing medium, but the majority of these cells change their firing pattern to tonic when $[Ca^{2+}]_e$ is increased to physiological levels (1.6 mM). However, even in the presence of 1.6 mM of Ca^{2+}, repetitive stimulation of the sensory tract, causes bursting in NVsnpr in about 30% of recorded cells and synchronization of units when adjacent cells are recorded (Bernier *et al.*, 2010). Interestingly, the optimal stimulation frequency to elicit bursting was found to be between 40 and 60 Hz, a value close to the natural firing frequency of intra-oral mechanoreceptors and periodontal receptors, which provide sensory inputs to neurons in the dorsal NVsnpr during mastication (Appenteng *et al.*, 1982; Trulsson, 2007; Trulsson and Johansson, 2002). Moreover, this frequency also corresponds to the optimal stimulation frequency of the cortical masticatory area that is required to elicit mastication *in vivo* (40 Hz) (Huang *et al.*, 1989; Lund and Dellow, 1971). Notably, single pulse stimulation and low frequency stimulation fail to induce bursting, which suggests that even if the dorsal NVsnpr neurons are endowed with intrinsic bursting properties, expression of these properties depends on the intensity of incoming inputs; i.e. an inadequate level of inputs does not produce sufficient $[Ca^{2+}]_e$ decrease and/or postsynaptic depolarization. On the other hand, increasing activity triggers larger depolarizations, placing the membrane potential within I_{NaP} activation range and causes larger depletion of extra-cellular Ca^{2+}. Furthermore, within the appropriate membrane potential range, bursting frequency will increase with depolarization. However, if the afferent activity becomes excessive, the membrane potential will rise above the range of activation of I_{NaP}, leading to reversal to a tonic firing pattern (Fig. 3). Thus, within

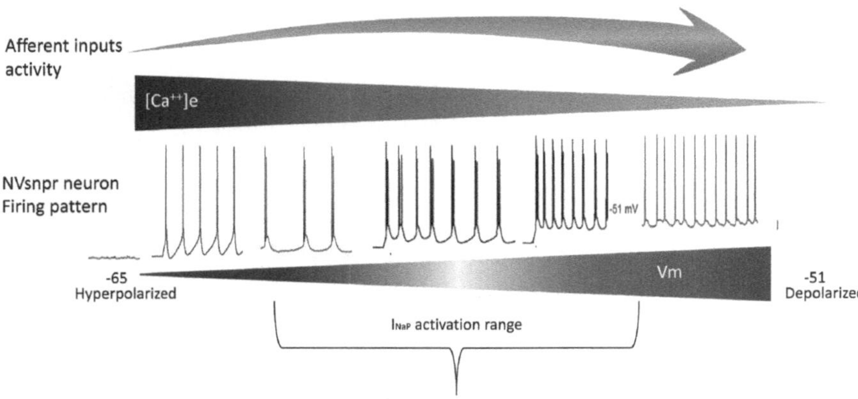

FIG. 3. Model explaining how inputs to NVsnpr neurons could interact with their intrinsic properties to induce rhythmic output. Increasing level of activity in sensory or cortical fibers would cause decreases of $[Ca^{2+}]_e$ that could lead to the activation of I_{NaP} current and rhythmic bursting. This firing pattern would be observed only within I_{NaP} activation range. (For interpretation of the references to color in this figure legend, the reader is referred to the Web version of the chapter.).

I_{NaP} activation range, the pattern of afferent inputs may directly govern the pattern of bursting.

The importance of the membrane potential becomes obvious when NMDA is used to mimic sustained activity. In this case, NMDA induces robust bursting only if the cell is hyperpolarized prior to the local NMDA application, presumably because NMDA alone without hyperpolarization depolarises the cell above I_{NaP} activation range. The fact that riluzole abolishes the NMDA-induced bursting supports the hypothesis that the latter relies on I_{NaP} activation (Kolta *et al.*, 2010). Thus, although the majority of dorsal NVsnpr neurons have intrinsic bursting abilities, only those receiving the appropriate level of inputs will fire rhythmically. This may explain why only one third of dorsal NVsnpr neurons recorded *in vivo* display a rhythmic firing pattern in phase with trigeminal motoneurons during fictive mastication. Under these experimental conditions, a fixed site on the CMA is stimulated, and sensory feedback is prevented by paralysis of the animal. Thus, the pattern of fibers activated by stimulation does not change throughout the experiment. However, in the normal functioning animal, the population of rhythmogenic neurons driving motoneurons and pre-motor interneurons are likely to be constantly changing, depending on the pattern of activity in the descending and primary afferent pathways. Although, cortical and other supra medullary commands to the masticatory CPG may be important to pre-program the pattern of masticatory movements, sensory feedback is essential to adjust these movements to changes in texture and hardness, and to counteract unexpected perturbations. During mastication, the most important primary afferent feedback is provided by periodontal receptors (Olsson *et al.*, 1988) and by jaw closing muscle spindle afferents (Goodwin and Luschei, 1975) which provide information about food hardness and elasticity and contraction properties of the jaw closing muscles, respectively (Lavigne *et al.*, 1987; Komuro *et al.*, 2001b). Interestingly, the group of NVsnpr neurons, which has an intrinsic bursting capability depending on persistent sodium channels (I_{NaP}), receive massive inputs both from periodontal receptors and muscle spindles (Tsuboi et al., 2003). Thus, we hypothesize that these neurons may function as cellular pacemaker interfaces to convert sensory feedback into appropriate rhythmogenic commands to the jaw motoneurons during mastication.

IX. Conclusions

In summary, our understanding on neuronal mechanisms involved in the control of mastication has expanded rapidly since the first ground breaking discovery of the "masticatory GPG" was made by Dellow and Lund (1971). Studies on *in vivo* models during the following decades gave important basic information on the location and connectivity of the CPG network as well as on input output properties of its constituent neurons. With the introduction of *in vitro* models it is now possible to study intrinsic membrane properties of individual circuit neurons in detail. To combine knowledge from these two levels of analysis is a great challenge for the future.

Acknowledgments

Supported by Grants from the Canadian Institutes of Health Research and an infrastructure grant from the Fonds de la Recherche en Santé du Québec.

References

Amzica, F., Massimini, M., and Manfridi, A. (2002). Spatial buffering during slow and paroxysmal sleep oscillations in cortical networks of glial cells in vivo. *J. Neurosci.* **22**, 1042–1053.

Appenteng, K., Lund, J.P., and Seguin, J.J. (1982). Intraoral mechanoreceptor activity during jaw movement in the anesthetized rabbit. *J. Neurophysiol.* **48**, 27–37.

Appenteng, K., Conyers, L., Curtis, J., and Moore, J. (1990). Monosynaptic connexions of single V interneurones to the contralateral V motor nucleus in anaesthetised rats. *Brain Res.* **514**, 128–130.

Appenteng, K., Conyers, L., and Moore, J.A. (1989). The monosynaptic excitatory connections of single trigeminal interneurones to the V motor nucleus of the rat. *J. Physiol.* **417**, 91–104.

Athanassiadis, T., Olsson, K.Å., Kolta, A. and Westberg, K-G. (2005a). Identification of c-Fos immunoreactive brainstem neurons activated during fictive mastication in the rabbit. Exp Brain Res (165): 478–489.

Athanassiadis, T., Westberg, K.G., Olsson, K.A., and Kolta, A. (2005b). Physiological characterization, localization and synaptic inputs of bursting and nonbursting neurons in the trigeminal principal sensory nucleus of the rat. *Eur. J. Neurosci.* **22**, 3099–3110.

Azouz, R., Jensen, M.S., and Yaari, Y. (1996). Ionic basis of spike after-depolarization and burst generation in adult rat hippocampal CA1 pyramidal cells. *J. Physiol.* **492**, 211–223.

Bae, Y.C., Choi, B.J., Lee, M.G., Lee, H.J., Park, K.P., Zhang, L.F., Honma, S., Fukami, H., Yoshida, A., Ottersen, O.P., and Shigenaga, Y. (2002). Quantitative ultrastructural analysis of glycine- and gamma- aminobutyric acid-immunoreactive terminals on trigeminal alpha- and gamma-motoneuron somata in the rat. *J. Comp. Neurol.* **442**, 308–319.

Benninger, C., Kadis, J., and Prince, D.A. (1980). Extracellular calcium and potassium changes in hippocampal slices. *Brain Res.* **187**, 165–182.

Bernier, A.P., Arsenault, I., Lund, J.P., and Kolta, A. (2010). Effect of the stimulation of sensory inputs on the firing of neurons of the trigeminal main sensory nucleus in the rat. *J. Neurophysiol.* **103**, 915–923.

Beurrier, C., Bioulac, B., and Hammond, C. (2000). Slowly inactivating sodium current (I(NaP)) underlies single-spike activity in rat subthalamic neurons. *J. Neurophysiol.* **83**, 1951–1957.

Borke, R.C., Nau, M.E., and Ringler Jr., R.L. (1983). Brain stem afferents of hypoglossal neurons in the rat. *Brain Res.* **269**, 47–55.

Bourque, M.J., and Kolta, A. (2001). Properties and interconnections of trigeminal interneurons of the lateral pontine reticular formation in the rat. *J. Neurophysiol.* **86**, 2583–2596.

Bremer, F. (1923). Physiologie nerveuse de la mastication chez le chat et le lapin. *Archs. Internal Physiol.* **21**, 308–352.

Brennan, D.S., Spencer, A.J., and Roberts-Thomson, K.F. (2008). Tooth loss, chewing ability and quality of life. *Qual. Life Res.* **17**, 227–235.

Brocard, F., Verdier, D., Arsenault, I., Lund, J.P., and Kolta, A. (2006). Emergence of intrinsic bursting in trigeminal sensory neurons parallels the acquisition of mastication in weanling rats. *J. Neurophysiol.* **96**, 2410–2424.

Brumberg, J.C., Nowak, L.G., and McCormick, D.A. (2000). Ionic mechanisms underlying repetitive high-frequency burst firing in supragranular cortical neurons. *J. Neurosci.* **20**, 4829–4843.

Butera, R.J., Rinzel Jr., J., and Smith, J.C. (1999). Models of respiratory rhythm generation in the pre-Botzinger complex I. Bursting pacemaker neurons. *J. Neurophysiol.* **82**, 382–397.

Byrd, K.E. (1981). Mandibular movement and muscle activity during mastication in the guinea pig (Cavia porcellus). *J. Morphol.* **170**, 147–169.

Capra, N.F., and Dessem, D. (1992). Central connections of trigeminal primary afferent neurons: topographical and functional considerations. *Crit. Rev. Oral. Biol. Med.* **4**, 1–52.

Chandler, S.H., and Tal, M. (1986). The effects of brain stem transections on the neuronal networks responsible for rhythmical jaw muscle activity in the guinea pig. *J. Neurosci.* **6**, 1831–1842.

Chandler, S.H., Turman Jr., J.E., Salem, L., and Goldberg, L.J. (1990). The effects of nanoliter ejections of lidocaine into the pontomedullary reticular formation on cortically induced rhythmical jaw movements in the guinea pig. *Brain Res.* **526**, 54–64.

Cohen, J.E., and Fields, R.D. (2004). Extracellular calcium depletion in synaptic transmission. *Neuroscientist* **10**, 12–17.

Crill, W.E. (1996). Persistent sodium current in mammalian central neurons. *Annu. Rev. Physiol.* **58**, 349–362.

Dal Bo, G., Lund, J.P., Verdier, D., and Kolta, A. (2005). Inputs to nucleus pontis caudalis from adjacent trigeminal areas. *Eur. J. Neurosci.* **22**, 1987–1996.

Darbon, P., Yvon, C., Legrand, J.C., and Streit, J. (2004). I_{NaP} underlies intrinsic spiking and rhythm generation in networks of cultured rat spinal cord neurons. *Eur. J. Neurosci.* **20**, 976–988.

Darian-Smith, I., and Mayday, G. (1960). Somatotopic organization within the brain-stem trigeminal complex of the cat. *Exp Neurol.* **2**, 290–309.

Del Negro, C.A., Koshiya, N., Butera Jr., R.J., and Smith, J.C. (2002). Persistent sodium current, membrane properties and bursting behavior of pre-botzinger complex inspiratory neurons in vitro. *J. Neurophysiol.* **88**, 2242–2250.

Del Negro, C.A., Morgado-Valle, C., Hayes, J.A., Mackay, D.D., Pace, R.W., Crowder, E.A., and Feldman, J.L. (2005). Sodium and calcium current-mediated pacemaker neurons and respiratory rhythm generation. *J. Neurosci.* **25**, 446–453.

Donga, R., and Lund, J.P. (1991). Discharge patterns of trigeminal commissural last-order interneurons during fictive mastication in the rabbit. *J. Neurophysiol.* **66**, 1564–1578.

Dubner, R., and Bennett, G.J. (1983). Spinal and trigeminal mechanisms of nociception. *Annu. Rev. Neurosci.* **6**, 381–418.

Durand, J., Gogan, P., Gueritaud, J.P., Horcholle-Bossavit, G., and Tyc-Dumont, S. (1983). Morphological and electrophysiological properties of trigeminal neurones projecting to the accessory abducens nucleus of the cat. *Exp. Brain Res.* **53**, 118–128.

Eisenman, J., Fromm, G., Landgren, S., and Novin, D. (1964). The ascending projections of trigeminal neurons in the cat, investigated by antidromic stimulation. *Acta. Physiol. Scand.* **60**, 337–350.

Eisenman, J., Landgren, S., and Novin, D. (1963). Functional organisation in the main sensory trigeminal nucleus and in the rostral subdivision of the nucleus of the spinal trigeminal tract in the cat. *Acta. Physiol. Scand.* **214**, 44.

Ellis, P.R., Kendall, C.W.C., Ren, Y., Parker, C., Pacy, J.F., Waldron, K.W., and Jenkins, D.J.A. (2004). Role of cell walls in the bioaccessibility of lipids in almond seeds. *Am. J. Clin. Nutr.* **80**, 604–613.

Ferrier, D. (1886). The Function of the Brain. London.

Franceschetti, S., Guatteo, E., Panzica, F., Sancini, G., Wanke, E., and Avanzini, G. (1995). Ionic mechanisms underlying burst firing in pyramidal neurons: intracellular study in rat sensorimotor cortex. *Brain Res.* **696**, 127–139.

Gans, C., De, V.F., and Gorniak, G.C. (1978). Analysis of mammalian masticatory mechanisms: progress and problems. *Anat. Histol. Embryol.* **7**, 226–244.

Ginestal, E., and Matute, C. (1993). Gamma-aminobutyric acid-immunoreactive neurons in the rat trigeminal nuclei. *Histochemistry* **99**, 49–55.

Goodwin, G.M., and Luschei, E.S. (1975). Discharge of spindle afferents from jaw-closing muscles during chewing in alert monkeys. *J. Neurophysiol.* **38**, 560–571.

Gottlieb, S., Taylor, A., and Bosley, M.A. (1984). The distribution of afferent neurones in the mesencephalic nucleus of the fifth nerve in the cat. *J. Comp. Neurol.* **228**, 273–283.

Grigoriadis, A., Johansson, R.S., and Trulsson, M. (2011). Adaptability of mastication in people with implant-supported bridges. *J. Clin. Periodontol.* Epub ahead of print

Grillner, S. (2006). Biological pattern generation: the cellular and computational logic of networks in motion. *Neuron* **52**, 751–766.

Grimwood, P.D., Appenteng, K., and Curtis, J.C. (1992). Monosynaptic EPSPs elicited by single interneurones and spindle afferents in trigeminal motoneurones of anaesthetized rats. *J. Physiol. (Lond).* **455**, 641–662.

Guatteo, E., Franceschetti, S., Bacci, A., Avanzini, G., and Wanke, E. (1996). A TTX-sensitive conductance underlying burst firing in isolated pyramidal neurons from rat neocortex. *Brain Res.* **741**, 1–12.

Hayashi, H., Sumino, R., and Sessle, B.J. (1984). Functional organization of trigeminal subnucleus interpolaris: nociceptive and innocuous afferent inputs, projections to thalamus, cerebellum, and spinal cord, and descending modulation from periaqueductal gray. *J. Neurophysiol.* **51**, 890–905.

Heinemann, U., Stabel, J., and Rausche, G. (1990). Activity-dependent ionic changes and neuronal plasticity in rat hippocampus. *Progress in Brain Res.* **83**, 197–214.

Hidaka, O., Morimoto, T., Masuda, Y., Kato, T., Matsuo, R., Inoue, T., Kobayashi, M., and Takada, K. (1997). Regulation of masticatory force during cortically induced rhythmic jaw movements in the anesthetized rabbit. *J. Neurophysiol.* **77**, 3168–3179.

Hiiemae, K. (2004). Mechanisms of food reduction, transport and deglutition: how the texture of food affects feeding behavior. *J. Text Stud.* **35**, 171–202.

Hiiemae, K., Heath, M.R., Heath, G., Kazazoglu, E., Murray, J., Sapper, D., and Hamblett, K. (1996). Natural bites, food consistency and feeding behaviour in man. *Arch. Oral. Biol.* **41**, 175–189.

Hsiao, C.F., Gougar, K., Asai, J., and Chandler, S.H. (2007). Intrinsic membrane properties and morphological characteristics of interneurons in the rat supratrigeminal region. *J. Neurosci. Res.* **85**, 3673–3686.

Huang, C.S., Hiraba, H., Murray, G.M., and Sessle, B.J. (1989). Topographical distribution and functional properties of cortically induced rhythmical jaw movements in the monkey (Macaca Fascicularis). *J. Neurophysiol.* **61**, 635–650.

Hutton, B., Feine, J., and Morais, J. (2002). Is there an association between edentulism and nutritional state? *J. Can. Dent. Assoc.* **68**, 182–187.

Ikeda, M. (1979). Projections from the spinal and the principal sensory nuclei of the trigeminal nerve to the cerebellar cortex in the cat, as studied by retrograde transport of horseradish peroxidase. *J. Comp. Neurol.* **184**, 567–585.

Inoue, M., Nozawa-Inoue, K., Donga, R., and Yamada, Y. (2002). Convergence of selected inputs from sensory afferents to trigeminal premotor neurons with possible projections to masseter motoneurons in the rabbit. *Brain Res.* **957**, 183–191.

Inoue, T., Kato, T., Masuda, Y., Nakamura, T., Kawamura, Y., and Morimoto, T. (1989). Modifications of masticatory behavior after trigeminal deafferentation in the rabbit. *Exp. Brain Res.* **74**, 579–591.

Inoue, T., Masuda, Y., Nagashima, T., Yoshikawa, K., and Morimoto, T. (1992). Properties of rhythmically active reticular neurons around the trigeminal motor nucleus during fictive mastication in the rat. *Neurosci. Res.* **14**, 275–294.

Jean, A. (2001). Brain stem control of swallowing: neuronal network and cellular mechanisms. *Physiol. Rev.* **81**, 929–969.

Jinno, S., Ishizuka, S., and Kosaka, T. (2003). Ionic currents underlying rhythmic bursting of ventral mossy cells in the developing mouse dentate gyrus. *Eur. J. Neurosci.* **17**, 1338–1354.

Kamogawa, H., Manabe, K., Kondo, M., and Naito, K. (1994). Supra-and juxtatrigeminal inhibitory premotor neurons with bifurcating axons projecting to masseter motoneurons on both sides. *Brain Res.* **639**, 85–92.

Kolta, A. (1997). In vitro investigation of synaptic relations between interneurons surrounding the trigeminal motor nucleus and masseteric motoneurons. *J. Neurophysiol* **78**, 1720–1725.

Kolta, A., Morquette, P., Lavoie, R., Arsenault, I., and Verdier, D. (2010). Modulation of rhythmogenic properties of trigeminal neurons contributing to the masticatory CPG. *Prog. Brain Res.* **187**, 137–148.

Kolta, A., Westberg, K.G., and Lund, J.P. (2000). Identification of brainstem interneurons projecting to the trigeminal motor nucleus and adjacent structures in the rabbit. *J. Chem. Neuroanat.* **9**, 175–195.

Kogo, M., Funk, G.D., and Chandler, S.H. (1996) Rhythmical oral motor activity recorded in an in vitro brainstem preparation. Somatosens Motor. Res (13): 39–48.

Komuro, A., Masuda, Y., Iwata, K., Kobayashi, M., Kato, T., Hidaka, O., and Morimoto, T. (2001a). Influence of food thickness and hardness on possible feed-forward control of the masseteric muscle activity in the anesthetized rabbit. *Neurosci. Res* **39**, 21–29.

Komuro, A., Morimoto, T., Iwata, K., Inoue, T., Masuda, Y., Kato, T., and Hidaka, O. (2001b). Putative feed-forward control of jaw-closing muscle activity during rhythmic jaw movements in the anesthetized rabbit. *J. Neurophysiol.* **86**, 2834–2844.

Koolstra, J.H. (2002). Dynamics of the human masticatory system. *Crit. Rev. Oral. Biol. Med.* **13**, 366–376.

Landgren, S., and Olsson, K. (1977). Tuggapparatens nervösa styrmekanismer. *Studentlitteratur. Lund* (In Swedish) 1–93.

Landgren, S., and Olsson, K.A. (1976). Localization of evoked potentials in the digastric, masseteric, supra- and intertrigeminal subnuclei of the cat. *Exp. Brain Res.* **26**, 299–318.

Landgren, S., Olsson, K.A., and Westberg, K.G. (1986). Bulbar neurones with axonal projections to the trigeminal motor nucleus in the cat. *Exp. Brain Res.* **65**, 98–111.

Lavigne, G., Kim, J.S., Valiquette, C., and Lund, J.P. (1987). Evidence that periodontal pressoreceptors provide positive feedback to jaw closing muscles during mastication. *J. Neurophysiol.* **58**, 342–358.

Lazarov, N.E. (2002). Comparative analysis of the chemical neuroanatomy of the mammalian trigeminal ganglion and mesencephalic trigeminal nucleus. *Prog. Neurobiol.* **66**, 19–59.

Li, Y.Q., Takada, M., Kaneko, T., and Mizuno, N. (1995). Premotor neurons for trigeminal motor nucleus neurons innervating the jaw-closing and jaw-opening muscles: differential distribution in the lower brainstem of the rat. *J. Comp. Neurol.* **356**, 563–579.

Li, Y.Q., Takada, M., Kaneko, T., and Mizuno, N. (1996). GABAergic and glycinergic neurons projecting to the trigeminal motor nucleus: a double labeling study in the rat. *J. Comp. Neurol.* **373**, 498–510.

Li, Z., and Hatton, G.I. (1996). Oscillatory bursting of phasically firing rat supraoptic neurones in low-Ca^{2+} medium: Na^{+} influx, cytosolic Ca^{2+} and gap junctions. *J. Physiol.* **496**, 379–394.

Linden, R.W. (1978). Properties of intraoral mechanoreceptors represented in the mesencephalic nucleus of the fifth nerve in the cat. *J. Physiol.* **279**, 395–408.

Lorente de No, R. (1922). Contribution al conocimiento del nervo trigemino. Ramon, Ramon., Cajal, S. (Eds.), *Libro en honor.* **2**, Madrid, Jaminez y Molina, pp. 13–30.

Lund, J.P. (1991). Mastication and its control by the brain stem. *Crit. Rev. Oral. Biol. Med.* **2**, 33–64.

Lund, J.P., and Dellow, P.G. (1971). The influence of interactive stimuli on rhythmical masticatory movements in rabbits. *Arch. Oral. Biol.* **16**, 215–223.

Lund, J.P., Kolta, A., Westberg, K.G., and Scott, G. (1998). Brainstem mechanisms underlying feeding behaviors. *Curr. Opin. Neurobiol.* **8**, 718–724.

Lund, J.P., Sasamoto, K., Murakami, T., and Olsson, K.A. (1984). Analysis of rhythmical jaw movements produced by electrical stimulation of motor-sensory cortex of rabbits. *J. Neurophysiol.* **52**, 1014–1029.

Luschei, E.S., and Goodwin, G.M. (1974). Patterns of mandibular movement and jaw muscle activity during mastication in the monkey. *J. Neurophysiol.* **37**, 954–966.

Mattia, D., Kawasaki, H., and Avoli, M. (1997). Repetitive firing and oscillatory activity of pyramidal-like bursting neurons in the rat subiculum. *Exp. Brain Res.* **114**, 507–517.

Matsushita, M., Okado, N., Ikeda, M., and Hosoya, Y. (1981). Descending projections from the spinal and mesencephalic nuclei of the trigeminal nerve to the spinal cord in the cat. A study with the horseradish peroxidase technique. *J. Comp. Neurol.* **196**, 173–187.

McCrea, D.A., and Rybak, I.A. (2008). Organization of mammalian locomotor rhythm and pattern generation. *Brain Res. Rev.* **57**, 134–146.

McDavid, S., Lund, J.P., Auclair, F., and Kolta, A. (2006). Morphological and immunohistochemical characterization of interneurons within the rat trigeminal motor nucleus. *Neuroscience.* **139**, 1049–1059.

McDavid, S., Verdier, D., Lund, J.P., and Kolta, A. (2008). Electrical properties of interneurons found within the trigeminal motor nucleus. *Eur. J. Neurosci.* **28**, 1136–1145.

Meessen, H., and Olzewski, J. (1949). Cytoarchitekton-ischer atlas des rautenhirns des kaninchens.

Mizuno, N., Konishi, A., Matsuda, K., Nomura, S., Itoh, K., Nakamura, Y., and Sugimoto, T. (1981). Myotopical arrangement and synaptic morphology of masticatory motoneurons, with special reference to commissural interneurons. in: *Oralfacial sensory and motor functions.* (Y. Kawamura and R. Dubner Eds.), .Quintessence Publ Co Inc., Tokyo, 113–120.

Mizuno, N., Yasui, Y., Nomura, S., Itoh, K., Konishi, A., Takada, M., and Kudo, M. (1983). A light and electron microscopic study of premotor neurons for the trigeminal motor nucleus. *J. Comp. Neurol.* **215**, 290–298.

Morimoto, T., Inoue, T., Masuda, Y., and Nagashima, T. (1989). Sensory components facilitating jaw-closing muscle activities in the rabbit. *Exp. Brain Res.* **76**, 424–440.

Morimoto, T., Inoue, T., Nakamura, T., and Kawamura, Y. (1985). Characteristics of rhythmic jaw movements of the rabbit. *Arch. Oral. Biol.* **30**, 673–677.

N'gom, P.I., and Woda, A. (2002). Influence of impaired mastication on nutrition. *J. Prosthet. Dent.* **87**, 667–673.

Nicholson, C., Ten, B.G., Stockle, H., and Steinberg, R. (1978). Calcium and potassium changes in extracellular microenvironment of cat cerebellar cortex. *J. Neurophysiol.* **41**, 1026–1039.

Nozaki, S., Iriki, A., and Nakamura, Y. (1986 a) Localization of central rhythm generator involved in cortically induced rhythmical masticatory jaw-opening movement in the guinea pig. *J. Neurophysiol* **55**, 806–825.

Nozaki, S., Iriki, A., and Nakamura, Y. (1986 b) Role of corticobulbar projection neurons in cortically induced rhythmical masticatory jaw-opening movement in the guinea pig. *J. Neurophysiol* **55**, 826–845.

Olsson, K.Å., and Landgren, S. (1990). Primary afferent and descending cortical convergence on the interneurones of the borderzone of the trigeminal motor nucleus. A comparison between trigeminal and spinal interneurones. In: *Neurophysiology of the Jaws and Teeth* (Taylor M, Ed.), London 19–50.

Olsson, K.Å., Landgren, S., and Westberg, K.G. (1986 a) Location of, and peripheral convergence on, the interneuron in the disynaptic path from the coronal gyrus of the cerebral cortex to the trigeminal motoneurons in the cat. *Exp. Brain Res.* **65**, 83–97.

Olsson, K.Å., Lund, J.P., Valiquette, C., and Veilleux, D. (1988). Activity during mastication of periodontal mechanosensitive neurons of the trigeminal subnucleus oralis of the rabbit. *J. Neurophysiol.* **59**, 341–357.

Olsson, K.Å., Sasamoto, K., and Lund, J.P. (1986 b) Modulation of transmission in rostral trigeminal sensory nuclei during chewing. *J. Neurophysiol* **55**, 56–75.

Olsson, K.Å., and Westberg, K.G. (1989). Interneurones in the trigeminal motor system. In: *EMG of jaw reflexes in man.* (D. Van steenberghe and A. de Laat Eds.), (Leuven University Press, 19–50.

Olsson, K.Å., and Westberg, K.G. (1991). Integration in trigeminal premotor interneurones in the cat 2. Functional characteristics of neurones in the subnucleus-gamma of the oral nucleus of the spinal trigeminal tract with a projection to the digastric motoneurone subnucleus. *Exp. Brain Res.* **84**, 115–124.

Ottenhoff, F.A., Van der Bilt, A., Van der Glas, H.W., and Bosman, F. (1992 a) Control of elevator muscle activity during simulated chewing with varying food resistance in humans. *J. Neurophysiol.* **68**, 933–944.

Ottenhoff, F.A., Van der Bilt, A., Van der Glas, H.W., and Bosman, F. (1992 b) Peripherally induced and anticipating elevator muscle activity during simulated chewing in humans. *J. Neurophysiol.* **67**, 75–83.

Paphangkorakit, J., and Osborn, J.W. (1997). The effect of pressure on a maximum incisal bite force in man. *Arch. Oral. Biol.* **42**, 11–17.

Peyron, M.A., Lassauzay, C., and Woda, A. (2002). Effects of increased hardness on jaw movement and muscle activity during chewing of visco-elastic model foods. *Exp. Brain. Res.* **142**, 41–51.

Pumain, R., and Heinemann, U. (1985). Stimulus- and amino acid-induced calcium and potassium changes in rat neocortex. *J. Neurophysiol.* **53**, 1–16.

Pumain, R., Kurcewicz, I., and Louvel, J. (1983). Fast extracellular calcium transients: involvement in epileptic processes. *Science* **222**, 177–179.

Rampon, C., Peyron, C., Petit, J.M., Fort, P., Gervasoni, D., and Luppi, P.H. (1996). Origin of the glycinergic innervation of the rat trigeminal motor nucleus. *Neuroreport.* **7**, 3081–3085.

Rioch, J.M. (1934). The neural mechanism of mastication. *Am. J. Physiol.* **108**, 168–176.

Rusakov, D.A., and Fine, A. (2003). Extracellular Ca^{2+} depletion contributes to fast activity-dependent modulation of synaptic transmission in the brain. *Neuron* **37**, 287–297.

Saad, M., Dubuc, R., Widmer, C.G., Westberg, K.G., and Lund, J.P. (1997). Anatomical organization of efferent neurons innervating various regions of the rabbit masseter muscle. *J. Comp. Neurol.* **383**, 428–438.

Schwartz, G., Enomoto, S., Valiquette, C., and Lund, J.P. (1989). Mastication in the rabbit: a description of movement and muscle activity. *J. Neurophysiol.* **62**, 273–287.

Scott, G., Westberg, K.G., Vrentzos, N., Kolta, A., and Lund, J.P. (2003). Effect of lidocaine and NMDA injections into the medial pontobulbar reticular formation on mastication evoked by cortical stimulation in anaesthetized rabbits. *Eur. J. Neurosci.* **17**, 2156–2162.

Sessle, B.J. (1987). The neurobiology of facial and dental pain: present knowledge, future directions. *J. Dent. Res.* **66**, 962–981.

Sherrington, C.S. (1917). Reflexes elicitable in the cat from pinna vibrissae and jaws. *J. Physiol.* **51**, 404–431.

Shigenaga, Y., Hirose, Y., Yoshida, A., Fukami, H., Honma, S., and Bae, Y.C. (2000). Quantitative ultrastructure of physiologically identified premotoneuron terminals in the trigeminal motor nucleus in the cat. *J. Comp. Neurol.* **426**, 13–30.

Shigenaga, Y., Okamoto, T., Nishimori, T., Suemune, S., Nasution, I.D., Chen, I.C., Tsuru, K., Yoshida, A., Tabuchi, K., and Hosoi, M. (1986). Oral and facial representation in the trigeminal principal and rostral spinal nuclei of the cat. *J. Comp. Neurol.* **244**, 1–18.

Somjen, G.G. (1980). Stimulus-evoked and seizure-related responses of extracellular calcium activity in spinal cord compared to those in cerebral cortex. *J. Neurophysiol.* **44**, 617–632.

Su, H., Alroy, G., Kirson, E.D., and Yaari, Y. (2001). Extracellular calcium modulates persistent sodium current-dependent burst-firing in hippocampal pyramidal neurons. *J. Neurosci.* **21**, 4173–4182.

Tanaka, S., Kogo, M., Chandler, S.C., and Matsuya, T. (1999). Localization of oral-motor rhythmogenic circuits in the isolated rat brainstem preparation. Brain Res (821): 190–199.

Tazerart, S., Vinay, L., and Brocard, F. (2008 a) The persistent sodium current generates pacemaker activities in the central pattern generator for locomotion and regulates the locomotor rhythm. *J. Neurosci.* **28**, 8577–8589.

Tazerart, S., Vinay, L., and Brocard, F. (2008 b) The persistent sodium current generates pacemaker activities in the central pattern generator for locomotion and regulates the locomotor rhythm. *J. Neurosci.* **28**, 8577–8589.

Trulsson, M. (2007). Force encoding by human periodontal mechanoreceptors during mastication. *Arch. Oral. Biol.* **52**, 357–360.

Trulsson, M., and Johansson, R.S. (1996). Forces applied by the incisors and roles of periodontal afferents during food-holding and -biting tasks. *Exp. Brain Res.* **107**, 486–496.

Trulsson, M., and Johansson, R.S. (2002). Orofacial mechanoreceptors in humans: encoding characteristics and responses during natural orofacial behaviors. *Behav. Brain Res.* **135**, 27–33.

Tsuboi, A., Kolta, A., Chen, C.C., and Lund, J.P. (2003). Neurons of the trigeminal main sensory nucleus participate in the generation of rhythmic motor patterns. *Eur. J. Neurosci.* **17**, 229–238.

Turman Jr., J.E., and Chandler, S.H. (1994 a) Immunohistochemical evidence for GABA and glycine-containing trigeminal premotoneurons in the guinea pig. *Synapse.* **18**, 7–20.

Turman Jr., J.E., and Chandler, S.H. (1994 b) Immunohistochemical localization of glutamate and glutaminase in guinea pig trigeminal premotoneurons. *Brain Res.* **634**, 49–61.

Urbani, A., and Belluzzi, O. (2000). Riluzole inhibits the persistent sodium current in mammalian CNS neurons. *Eur. J. Neurosci.* **12**, 3567–3574.

Van der Bilt, A., Engelen, L., Pereira, L.J., Van der Glas, H.W., and Abbink, J.H. (2006). Oral physiology and mastication. *Physiol. Behav.* **89**, 22–27.

Weijs, W.A., and Dantuma, R. (1975). Electromyography and mechanics of mastication in the albino rat. *J. Morphol.* **146**, 1–33.

Westberg, K.G. (1990). *Interneurones in the trigeminal motor system An experimental neurobiological study in the cat.* Umeå University Odont Dissertations, Abstract No 37.

Westberg, K., Clavelou, P., Sandstrom, G., and Lund, J.P. (1998). Evidence that trigeminal brainstem interneurons form subpopulations to produce different forms of mastication in the rabbit. *J. Neurosci.* **18**, 6466–6479.

Westberg, K.G., and Olsson, K.Å. (1991). Integration in trigeminal premotor interneurones in the cat 1. Functional characteristics of neurones located in the subnucleus-gamma of the oral nucleus of the spinal trigeminal tract. *Exp. Brain Res.* **84**, 102–114.

Westberg, K.G., Sandstrom, G., and Olsson, K.A. (1995). Integration in trigeminal premotor interneurones in the cat 3. Input characteristics and synaptic actions of neurones in subnucleus-gamma of the oral nucleus of the spinal trigeminal tract with a projection to the masseteric motoneurone subnucleus. *Exp. Brain Res.* **104**, 449–461.

Westneat, M.W., and Hall, W.G. (1992). Ontogeny of feeding motor patterns in infant rats: an electromyographic analysis of suckling and chewing. *Behav. Neurosci.* **106**, 539–554.

Woda, A., Mishellany, A., and Peyron, M.A. (2006). The regulation of masticatory function and food bolus formation. *J. Oral. Rehabil* **33**, 840–849.

Wu, N., Enomoto, A., Tanaka, S., Hsiao, C.F., Nykamp, D.Q., Izhikevich, E., and Chandler, S.H. (2005). Persistent sodium currents in mesencephalic v neurons participate in burst generation and control of membrane excitability. *J. Neurophysiol.* **93**, 2710–2722.

Yoshida, A., Fukami, H., Nagase, Y., Appenteng, K., Honma, S., Zhang, L.F., Bae, Y.C., and Shigenaga, Y. (2001). Quantitative analysis of synaptic contacts made between functionally identified oralis neurons and trigeminal motoneurons in cats. *J. Neurosci.* **21**, 6298–6307.

Yoshida, A., Hiraga, T., Moritani, M., Chen, K., Takatsuki, Y., Hirose, Y., Bae, Y.C., and Shigenaga, Y. (1998). Morphologic characteristics of physiologically defined neurons in the cat trigeminal nucleus principalis. *J. Comp. Neurol.* **401**, 308–328.

Zhong, G., Masino, M.A., and Harris-Warrick, R.M. (2007). Persistent sodium currents participate in fictive locomotion generation in neonatal mouse spinal cord. *J. Neurosci.* **27**, 4507–4518.

ULTRASTRUCTURAL BASIS FOR CRANIOFACIAL SENSORY PROCESSING IN THE BRAINSTEM

Yong Chul Bae[1] and Atsushi Yoshida[2]

[1]Department of Oral Anatomy, Neurobiology, School of Dentistry, Kyungpook National University, Daegu 700-412, Korea
[2]Department of Oral Anatomy, Neurobiology, Graduate School of Dentistry, Osaka University, Suita, Osaka 565-0871, Japan

INTERNATIONAL REVIEW OF NEUROBIOLOGY, VOL. 97
DOI: 10.1016/B978-0-12-385198-7.00005-9

ABBREVIATIONS

ChAT	choline acetyltransferase
CGRP	calcitonin gene-related peptide
CNS	central nervous system
DCV	dense-cored vesicle
DRG	dorsal root ganglion
EM	electron microscope
EPSP	excitatory postsynaptic potential
FRAP	fluoride-resistant acid phosphatase
GABA	γ-aminobutyric acid
GAD	glutamic acid decarboxylase
HRP	horseradish peroxidase
HTM	high-threshold mechanoreceptive
IRt	intermediate reticular formation
IB4	isolectin B4
JC	jaw-closing
JO	jaw-opening
LTM	low-threshold mechanoreceptive
mGluR5	metabotropic glutamate receptor 5
MS	muscle spindle
NP-Y	neuropeptide Y
P2X3	P2X purinoceptor 3
PAD	primary afferent depolarization
PATs	primary afferent terminals
PC	Pacinian corpuscle
PCRt	parvocellular reticular formation
Pd	proximal dendrite
P-ending	presynaptic ending, ending presynaptic to primary afferent terminal
PL	periodontal
RA	rapidly-adapting
SA	slowly-adapting
SP	substance P
TG	trigeminal ganglion
TRPA1	transient receptor potential ankyrin 1
TRPV1	transient receptor potential vanilloid 1
TSN	trigeminal sensory nuclei
Vc	trigeminal caudal nucleus
Vdm	dorsomedial part of Vi and Vo
Vi	trigeminal interpolar nucleus

Vidm	dorsomedial part of Vi
Vmes	trigeminal mesencephalic nucleus
Vmo	trigeminal motor nucleus
Vmo.dl	dorsolateral part of Vmo
Vmo.vm	ventromedial part of Vmo
Vo	trigeminal oral nucleus
Vo.r	rostrodorsomedial part of Vo
Vodm	dorsomedial part of Vo
Vp	trigeminal principal nucleus
VPM	ventroposteromedial nucleus of thalamus
Vsup	supratrigeminal nucleus
Vtr	spinal trigeminal tract
WGA	wheat germ agglutinin
XIImo	hypoglossal nucleus

I. Introduction

Trigeminal sensory nuclei (TSN) of the brainstem receive orofacial sensory inputs and project to higher brain centers including the thalamus, reticular formation, and trigeminal motor nucleus. They are subdivided into trigeminal principal (Vp), oral (Vo), interpolar (Vi), and caudal nuclei (Vc) based on the cytoarchitectonical and functional differences (Olszewski, 1950). Whereas a single spinal nerve projects to a relatively short rostro-caudal span of the spinal dorsal horn, a single trigeminal sensory afferent branches widely and sends axon collaterals to the four TSN, suggesting that a single orofacial sensory modality is simultaneously transmitted to and processed within all TSN. In addition, previous studies have shown that the central projection patterns of the trigeminal primary afferents differ among the types of afferent fibers and among the TSN (Jacquin *et al.*, 1993; Shigenaga *et al.*, 1986a, 1989a, 1990; Takemura *et al.*, 1991). This would suggest that the trigeminal sensory information is processed differently in the different TSN, and which may reflect the functional specificity of the neural circuits that are associated with each of the fiber types and target nuclei.

Neurons communicate with one another at the synapse where neural information is processed and transmitted. So, elucidation of the synaptic organization of primary sensory afferents and the associated neurotransmitters and receptors is crucial for understanding of how the specific sensory information is processed and transmitted to the CNS. Recently, multiple electron microscopic (EM) studies have reported on the synaptic organization of various types of trigeminal primary sensory afferents or jaw muscle spindle (MS) afferents in the TSN and trigeminal motor nucleus (Vmo), which provides an anatomical substrate for processing of specific orofacial sensory or proprioceptive information at the level of the 1st relay nuclei of the brainstem. In addition, many immunocytochemical studies have investigated the neurotransmitters and receptors at the axoaxonic synapses associated with the terminals of specific trigeminal sensory afferents. Quantitative EM studies using reconstruction of serial thin sections through a bouton have also analyzed the ultrastructural features related to synaptic release. We review these recent findings below.

It is widely accepted that Vc is the principal relay nucleus for the orofacial nociceptive input. In addition, it has been shown that Vi and Vo are also involved in the transmission of intraoral nociception (Dallel *et al.*, 1988; Luccarini *et al.*, 1998; Pajot *et al.*, 2000; Sugimoto *et al.*, 1998). In contrast, it is generally assumed that Vp is involved in the processing of tactile sensation, but has no role in nociception (Sessle, 2000). However, recent findings suggest that Vp, especially its dorsal portion, is involved in the transmission of noxious stimuli from oral structures. We will review these recent findings.

Myelinated axons frequently lose their myelin, become thinner, and branch before reaching the organ they innervate (Peng *et al.*, 1999). The dental pulp, which is a preferred model for the study of peripheral pain mechanism, is richly innervated by nociceptive afferents; most intradental axons are unmyelinated and a small fraction are small myelinated fibers of Aδ type (for review, see Byers, 1984; Hildebrand *et al.*, 1995; Sessle, 1987). However, little is known about the parent axons that give rise to these intradental axons, which may provide important clues as to the nature of the primary sensory neurons that innervate the dental pulp; we here present recent findings on the parent pulpal axons in the trigeminal ganglion (TG) and the morphological changes they undergo during their peripheral course to the pulp.

II. Trigeminal Sensory Nuclei and Ultrastructure of Primary Afferent Terminals

A. Cytoarchitectonic Organization of TSN

The group of trigeminal sensory nuclei is located dorsolaterally in the brainstem between the spinal cord and the rostral pons. It is subdivided, based on features of its cytoarchitecture (i.e., cell size, cell shape, and cell packing density) and neuropil (i.e., fiber size, orientation, and degree of myelination) into trigeminal principal (Vp), oral (Vo), interpolar (Vi), and caudal (Vc) nuclei (Olszewski, 1950). While most trigeminal sensory afferents, upon entering the brainstem, bifurcate into ascending and descending branches, which send axon collaterals to the Vp and the spinal trigeminal nuclei, respectively, some either descend or ascend without bifurcating. Most afferents terminate in the ipsilateral TSN; however, some ophthalmic and mandibular afferents cross the midline and terminate in the contralateral Vc (Ellrich *et al.*, 1999; Jacquin *et al.*, 1990; Marfurt and Rajchert, 1991; Pfaller and Arvidsson, 1988).

The **trigeminal principal nucleus (Vp)** is located dorsal and lateral to Vmo. It extends from the rostral pole of the Vmo to the caudal end of the Vmo: The ventral part of the Vp extends farther caudally than the dorsal part and ends at the level of the rostral pole of the facial nucleus. Vp consists of small- and medium-sized cells that are densely packed in the dorsal part but are rather loosely arranged ventrally. The dorsal part receives sensory input from intraoral structures and projects to the ipsilateral ventroposteromedial (VPM) nucleus of the thalamus in many species. The ventral part receives sensory input from the facial area and projects to the ipsilateral as well as the contralateral VPM. Vp has been considered homologous to the dorsal column nuclei (Kruger, 1979) in that it may receive exclusively tactile sensation; this has been questioned by the recent demonstration of dense projections of oral nociceptive fibers to the dorsal part of the Vp (Bae *et al.*, 2004a; Dessem *et al.*, 2007; Kim *et al.*, 2008, 2010).

The **trigeminal oral nucleus (Vo)** extends from the caudal end of Vmo rostrally, to the rostral pole of the hypoglossal nucleus caudally. It contains a loosely packed, heterogeneous population of cells, and in its ventrolateral regions, fairly large cells are scattered among small cells. The dorsomedial region of the Vo (Vodm), which receives primarily intraoral sensory input, is composed of a dense collection of small- or medium-sized cells. Vo contains a significant number of premotoneurons that project to Vmo and hypoglossal nucleus (XIImo; Olsson and Westberg, 1991; Westberg and Olsson, 1991).

The **trigeminal interpolar nucleus (Vi)** extends from the caudal pole of the facial motor nucleus rostrally to just below the obex caudally. It contains homogenously distributed small- and medium-sized cells, a few large cells and deep axonal bundles (intersubnuclear plexus of axon fascicles; Gobel and Purvis, 1972). It has the most uniform structure among all the TSN. Dorsomedial part of the Vi (Vidm) is a continuation of the Vodm. In the ventrolateral part, the cell size decreases gradually from large to medium, from rostrally to caudally. The boundary between Vi and Vc is indistinct, and the transition zone is apparent at the level of obex where a C-shaped residual part of the superficial lamina of Vc swings into the Vi. At the transition zone, a bulb like thickening of the dorsal and ventral ends of the superficial lamina of Vc extend slightly further rostrally into the Vi.

The **trigeminal caudal nucleus (Vc)** extends from the level of obex caudally to C2 or C3. It has laminar arrangement and is structurally very similar to the dorsal horn of the spinal cord, and is therefore referred to as medullary dorsal horn (Gobel *et al.*, 1977, 1981). It consists of a marginal layer (lamina I), gelatinous layer (lamina II), and magnocellular layer (laminae III/IV). **Lamina I** is very thin and consists of two or three rows of mediolaterally-elongated mainly trigeminothalamic neurons. **Lamina II** contains densely packed small round cells, including stalked cells, which are presumably excitatory, and islet cells, which are inhibitory intrinsic neurons (Gobel, 1975, 1978). It is subdivided into a thin outer zone (IIo) containing densely packed cells, and thick inner zone (IIi) where cells are less densely packed. Substance P (SP)-positive (+) and calcitonin gene related peptide (CGRP) + peptidergic C-fiber afferents are dense in laminae I and IIo (Martin-Schild *et al.*, 1999; Sugimoto *et al.*, 1997), whereas isolectin B4 (IB4)+ or P2X purinoceptor 3 (P2X3)+ non-peptidergic C-fiber afferents are dense in IIi (Ambalavanar and Morris, 1992; Kim *et al.*, 2008). These afferents form many synaptic glomeruli of type I and few synaptic glomeruli of type II in IIi, whereas synaptic glomeruli are absent in IIo in the rat (Ribeiro-da-Silva and Coimbra, 1982). Aδ-fibers innervating high threshold mechanoreceptors also terminate in laminae I and II. **Laminae III/IV** contains mostly medium-sized cells and few large cells, which are irregularly and loosely arranged, and a dense network of small myelinated fibers (deep bundles) connecting Vc to the rostral trigeminal nuclei. It contains intrinsic neurons and a few trigeminothalamic neurons. **Laminae V/VI** contain cells which are more heterogeneous in size and shape than those in lamina IV, and is characterized by the presence of large cell bodies. Space limitations prevent us from providing further detail in this text on the cytoarchitectonical and functional features of TSN and their species differences.

B. Ultrastructural Features of Primary Afferent Terminal (PAT)

1. *PAT*

EM studies of functionally-identified primary afferents have shown that central terminals of Aβ-low-threshold mechanoreceptive afferents (Bae *et al.*, 1993, 1994, 2005a, b; Nakagawa *et al.*, 1997; Sugimoto *et al.*, 1991), tooth pulp afferents (Bae *et al.*, 2003, 2004b), D-hair and Aδ-high-threshold mechanoreceptive afferents (Alvarez *et al.*, 1992; Réthelyi *et al.*, 1982), myelinated afferents (Bae *et al.*, 2000; Falls, 1986), mesencephalic periodontal afferents (Bae *et al.*, 1996, 1997), and MS afferents (Kishimoto *et al.*, 1998), contain many clear round vesicles (40–60 nm in diameter) and few large dense-cored vesicles (DCV: 80–110 nm in diameter). In addition, Alvarez *et al.* (1993), using a combination of postembedding immunogold staining and intra-axonal labeling in the monkey spinal cord, reported that C-fiber terminals contain a large number of DCV, which display SP or CGRP immunoreactivity. Based on these multiple EM studies, it is now widely accepted that PATs arising from Aβ-, Aδ-, and non-peptidergic C-fibers contain clear round vesicles and few DCV, whereas PATs arising from peptidergic C-fibers contain clear round vesicles and many DCV. PATs participate in synaptic contacts of asymmetrical type with postsynaptic dendrites, spines or somata, and sometimes in synaptic contacts of symmetrical type with presynaptic endings containing pleomorphic vesicles (p-endings); while most p-endings are axon terminals, some may be vesicle-containing dendrites. PATs with round, elongated, sinusoid shape usually form simple synapses, whereas those with scalloped shape usually form glomeruli and show complex synaptic connectivity. The shape and synaptic connectivity of PATs differ among various fiber types and their target regions; they also differ among boutons arising from a single axon or axon collateral.

2. *Synapse*

The synapse is morphologically composed of: 1) Presynaptic density, consisting of synaptic proteins involved in the priming, docking, and recycling of synaptic vesicles, 2) Postsynaptic density, consisting of various receptors and scaffolding proteins that mediate receptor clustering, regulate receptor function, and link the postsynaptic membrane to the cytoskeleton, and, 3) Synaptic cleft, where the neurotransmitter is released (for review, see Craig *et al.*, 2006; Sudhof, 2004). Gray (1959) distinguished type I and type II synapses based on characteristics of synapses in the cerebral cortex. Thereafter, Colonnier (1968) classified the synapse, based on the symmetry of the pre- and post-synaptic density, as symmetric and asymmetric, which roughly correspond to type I and type II, respectively. Type I or asymmetrical synapse has thicker postsynaptic density and wider synaptic cleft compared to type II or symmetric synapse, which has a less well developed post-synaptic density that is as thick as the presynaptic density. These structural differences generally correlate with the functional differences: type I synapses being usually excitatory and type II synapses being inhibitory. The shape of synaptic vesicles is considered less reliable as a determinant of the type of the synapse because it may vary with the osmolarity of the fixative. Thus, synaptic vesicles tend to appear round in tissue that has been fixed with hypo-osmolar solution and flattened or pleomorphic after fixation with hyper-osmolar solutions (Uchizono, 1965; Valdivia, 1971). With standard EM protocols, which employ fixatives containing the usual concentration of glutaraldehyde (2–2.5%), synaptic vesicles tend to appear round in terminals that establish excitatory synapses and pleomorphic, that is, a mixture of round, oval, and flattened, in terminals that establish inhibitory synapses.

III. Synaptic Connectivity of Trigeminal Primary Sensory Afferents

A. Distribution of PATs Along the Dendritic Tree of the Postsynaptic Neurons in TSN

Most PATs arising from various types of trigeminal primary sensory afferents, including low-threshold mechanoreceptive (LTM) afferents (Bae *et al.*, 1993, 2000,

2005a,b; Nakagawa *et al.*, 1997; Sugimoto *et al.*, 1991) and tooth pulp afferents (Bae *et al.*, 2003; Matthews *et al.*, 1989) establish synapses on small- or medium-sized dendrites, which correspond to the distal and middle segments of the dendritic tree of the postsynaptic neuron, and occasionally on somata or proximal dendrites in the Vp, Vi, and Vc (Fig. 1A, C). This pattern of termination is analogous of that of the somatosensory afferents in the spinal dorsal horn, including Aβ- (Egger *et al.*, 1981;

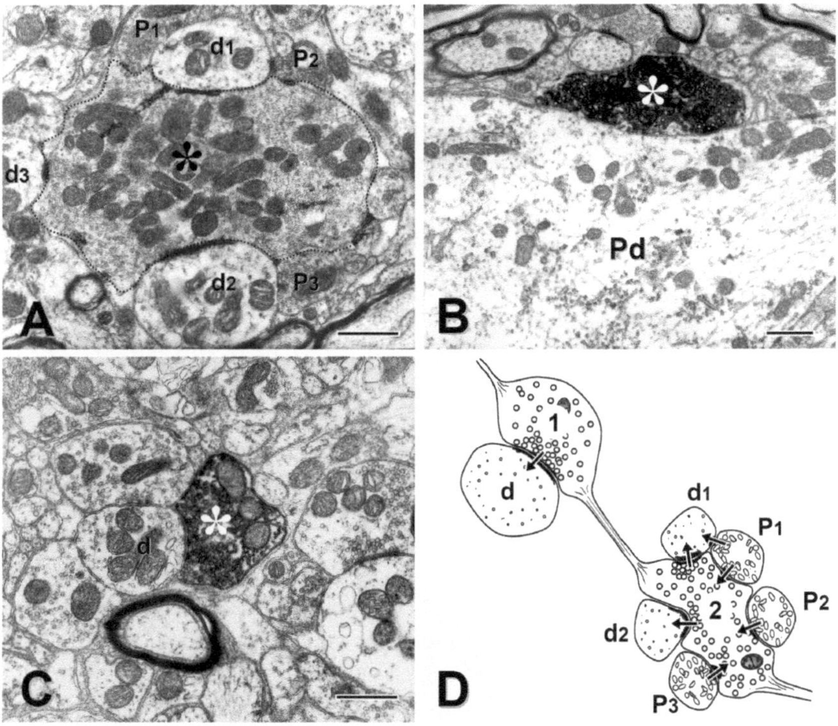

FIG. 1. **Electron micrographs (A-C) and a diagram (D) showing examples of synaptic arrangements of terminals from various types of primary afferents in the trigeminal sensory nuclei. A:** A WGA-HRP labeled terminal (asterisk) arising from a tooth pulp afferent in the trigeminal principal nucleus (Vp). The labeled terminal participates in a synaptic glomerulus by establishing asymmetric synaptic contacts with 3 dendrites (d1-d3) and receiving axoaxonic contact from 3 endings containing pleomorphic vesicles (p1-p3). **B:** An HRP-labeled terminal (asterisk), arising from a slowly adapting periodontal afferent in the trigeminal oral nucleus (Vo), forms an asymmetric synaptic contact on a proximal dendrite (Pd). **C:** An HRP-labeled terminal (asterisk), arising from a rapidly adapting vibrissa afferent in the trigeminal caudal nucleus (Vc), forms an asymmetrical axodendritic synapse on a dendrite (d). **D:** A diagram showing two different termination patterns of a primary afferent. Terminal 1 has a simple synaptic arrangement with one postsynaptic dendrite (d), whereas terminal 2 participates in a complex synaptic arrangement with two postsynaptic dendrites (d1-d2) and three presynaptic p-endings (p1-p3). Arrows indicate direction of synaptic transmission. Scale bars, 500 nm.

Maxwell *et al.*, 1982; Ralston *et al.*, 1984; Semba *et al.*, 1983, 1984, 1985), Aδ- (Alvarez *et al.*, 1992; Réthelyi *et al.*, 1982) and C-fibers (Alvarez *et al.*, 1993). In contrast, in the Vo, trigeminal PATs frequently establish synapses on the somata and proximal dendrites of the postsynaptic neurons (Bae *et al.*, 1994, 2000; Zhang *et al.*, 2001b; Fig. 1B), similar to the pattern of termination of trigeminal mesencephalic (Vmes) MS afferents in Vmo (Bae *et al.*, 1996, 1997, Kishimoto *et al.*, 1998), where a considerable fraction of the terminals (42–67%) are presynaptic to the somata or proximal dendrites of the Vmo neurons (Tables I and II). Terminals of group Ia afferents also contact far more frequently somata and proximal dendrites in the spinal ventral horn (Pierce and Mendell, 1993; Conradi *et al.*, 1983) than do the Aβ-afferents in the spinal dorsal horn (Semba *et al.*, 1983, 1984, 1985). Considering that Vmes MS afferents as well as the majority of Vo neurons project to the Vmo, and thus act as premotoneurons (Olsson and Westberg, 1991; Turman and Chandler, 1994a, b; Westberg and Olsson, 1991; Yoshida *et al.*, 2001, 2005), this synaptic connectivity may be characteristic of PATs involved in the motor function, in contrast with that involved in the somatosensory function.

Table I

FREQUENCY OF OCCURRENCE (%) OF PATS, ACCORDING TO THE NUMBER OF POSTSYNAPTIC DENDRITES (d), SHOWING AXOAXONIC SYNAPSES, OR SHOWING SYNAPSE WITH SOMA OR PROXIMAL DENDRITE (Pd) IN THE TSN AND SPINAL DORSAL HORN.

Afferent type	Termination	No. of postsynaptic dendrites (d)			Axoaxonic synapse	Soma or Pd	Reference
		1∼2d	3∼4d	≥5d			
Periodontal (SA)	Vp	70∼75	≥20 (∼6d)		91.3	5.8	Bae *et al.* (1994)
	Vo.r	97	3 (∼7d)		60	19	
Vibrissa (RA)	Vi	81	14	5 (∼7d)	79	?	Bae *et al.* (2005b)
	Vc (III/IV)	70	21	9 (∼9d)	64.6	?	
Large myelinated	Vp	86	14	0 (∼4d)	58	1.5	Bae *et al.* (2000)
	Vdm	94	5	1 (∼5d)	41	11	
	Vc	92	6	2 (∼5d)	48	3.2	
Tooth pulp	Vp	82	12	6 (∼9d)	87.9	?	Bae *et al.* (2003)
	Vdm	85	15	0 (∼7d)	53.8	?	
	Vc	61	34	5 (∼5d)	27.3	?	
HTM	Dorsal horn	35	53 (3∼6d), 12 (7∼13d)		20∼60	?	Alvarez *et al.* (1992)
C fiber	Dorsal horn	63∼64 (1d)			n.o.	?	Alvarez *et al.* (1993)

HTM: high-threshold mechanoreceptive, n.o.: not observed, RA: rapidly adapting, SA: slowly adapting.

Table II

FREQUENCY OF OCCURRENCE (%) OF TERMINALS FROM TRIGEMINAL MESENCEPHALIC (Vmes) MUSCLE SPINDLE (MS) AND PERIODONTAL (PL) AFFERENTS, ACCORDING TO THE NUMBER OF POSTSYNAPTIC DENDRITES (d), OR SHOWING SYNAPSE WITH SOMA OR PROXIMAL DENDRITE (Pd), IN THE TRIGEMINAL MOTOR (Vmo), SUPRATRIGEMINAL (Vsup) AND HYPOGLOSSAL (XIImo) NUCLEI.

Afferent type	Target nuclei	No. of postsynaptic dendrites (d)				Soma or Pd	Reference
		1d	2d	3d	4d		
MS	Vmo	82.4	15.0	2.6	0	52.1	Bae *et al.* (1996)
PL		55.4	27.7	13.8	3.1	5.8	
Ia	Vmo	88.0	8.0	4.0	0	66.7	Kishimoto *et al.* (1998)
II		83.7	11.6	4.7	0	41.7	
MS	Vsup	73.6	22.0	4.4	0	2.2	Bae *et al.* (1996)
PL		80.3	18.6	1.1	0	1.1	
Vmes	XIImo	95.0	5.0	0	0	12.0 (soma only)	Zhang *et al.* (2003)

PATs may exert different effects on the postsynaptic neuron depending on their distribution along its dendritic tree: a synapse on the soma or proximal dendrite is more likely to exert powerful or tonic effect on the activity of the postsynaptic neuron, whereas a synapse on a distal or small-sized dendrite may produce weaker and more precise effect.

B. Number of Dendrites Postsynaptic to PAT

Previous light microscopic analysis of the contacts between axon terminals of jaw-closing (JC) MS afferents or of Vo neurons and the trigeminal motoneurons in Vmo, using intraaxonal and/or intracellular labeling, showed that a single axon terminal does not contact two or more dendrites of a postsynaptic neuron, suggesting that each postsynaptic dendrite belongs to a different postsynaptic neuron (Yabuta *et al.*, 1996; Yoshida *et al.*, 1999, 2001). In the TSN, the large majority of terminals (70–97%) arising from large myelinated (Bae *et al.*, 2000) or Aβ-LTM afferents (Bae *et al.*, 1994, 2005b; Nakagawa *et al.*, 1997; Zhang *et al.*, 2001b) contact one or two postsynaptic dendrites. This suggests that, at a single bouton level, most of the orofacial tactile sensory input conveyed via trigeminal afferents is transmitted onto a specific group of postsynaptic neurons with a small degree of synaptic convergence. However, a considerable fraction of the PATs in the Vp (14–25%), Vdm (6–15%), Vi (19%), and Vc (8–30%), also contact multiple (3–9) postsynaptic dendrites, suggesting that this input can also drive multiple postsynaptic neurons projecting to various regions of the CNS and thus form a diffuse and divergent afferent system. Like the large myelinated, Aβ LTM afferents, most tooth pulp afferents, which arise mainly from small myelinated Aδ-fibers, also contact one or two dendrites in the Vp (82%) and dorsomedial part of the Vi and Vo (Vdm; 85%; Bae *et al.*, 2003). In contrast, in the Vc, a considerable fraction of tooth pulp afferent terminals (~40%) also contact three or more dendrites and participate in complex synaptic arrangements, similar to the synaptic connectivity pattern in the superficial laminae of the spinal dorsal horn, where the majority (65%) of Aδ-high threshold mechanoreceptive (HTM) afferent terminals contact more than three and up to 13 postsynaptic dendrites (Alvarez *et al.*, 1992; Table I). Considering that Vc contains a variety of neurons, including intrinsic neurons, as well as neurons projecting to thalamus, hypothalamus, parabrachial nucleus, and nucleus submedius (Allen *et al.*, 1996; Beggs *et al.*, 2003; Craig, 2003; Craig and Dostrovsky, 2001; Ding *et al.*, 1995; Gauriau and Bernard, 2004; Li *et al.*, 1997; Malick *et al.*, 2000; Newman *et al.*, 1996; Yoshida *et al.*, 1991), it is safe to assume that numbers of the pulpal afferents in Vc mediate the autonomic, affective aspect of pulpal pain, as well as its perceptual aspect.

C. Synapses of Nociceptive Afferent Terminals onto Dendritic Spines in Vc

About 61% of the tooth pulp afferents in the superficial lamina of the Vc, but only 21% in the Vp and 19% in the Vdm, make synaptic contacts with dendritic spines (Bae *et al.*, 2003). In addition, ~ 42% of terminals in the superficial lamina of the Vc that express transient receptor potential vanilloid 1 (TRPV1), a receptor involved in the mechanisms of inflammatory and neuropathic pain, are presynaptic to dendritic spines, and dendritic spines are ~ 30% of the postsynaptic targets of the TRPV1+ terminals (Yeo *et al.*, 2010). Vc is the principal relay nucleus for nociceptive information arising from the orofacial region. In addition, many studies have shown inflammation- or peripheral injury-induced neuronal plasticity in the Vc: Thus, the application of mustard oil into the rat tooth pulp (Chiang *et al.*, 1998), cutaneous application of formalin (Bernard *et al.*, 1995), and neonatal capsaicin treatment (Chiang *et al.*, 1997) all induce neuroplastic changes in the nociceptive neurons in the Vc (Chiang *et al.*, 1997, 1998). Dendritic spines show activity-dependent dynamic plasticity in their morphology and number, under various physiological and pathological conditions, which can lead to changes in synaptic connectivity and strength (for review, see Harms and Dunaevsky, 2007; Knott *et al.*, 2002). The higher frequency of synaptic contacts of nociceptive afferents with dendritic spines in Vc, than in other TSN may underlay the dynamic plasticity of the synaptic connectivity of nociceptive afferent terminals in the Vc, during inflammatory and neuropathic pain states (Chiang *et al.*, 1997, 1998).

D. Synaptic Connectivity Patterns of Trigeminal PATs in Different TSN

PATs arising from a single axon may participate in a variety of synaptic arrangements, including simple, intermediate, and complex synapses (Bae *et al.*, 1993, 1994, 2005b; Nakagawa *et al.*, 1997; Sugimoto *et al.*, 1991; Fig. 1D). However, the majority of the PATs arising from a specific axon type show a synaptic connectivity pattern that is similar within each TSN, but differs among specific nuclei. For example, highly complex synaptic glomeruli, in which PATs are associated with 5 or more pre- and post-synaptic elements, are far more frequent in Vp and Vi than in other TSN, whereas simple synaptic arrangements, in which PATs are associated with one or two pre-and post-synaptic elements, are more frequent in Vo and Vc (Bae *et al.*, 1994, 2000, 2005b; Ide and Killackey, 1985). In addition, the number of synaptic contacts per PAT is higher in the Vp or Vi, than in other TSN (slowly adapting [SA] periodontal afferents in Vp vs. Vo, 3.6 vs. 2.0; rapidly adapting [RA] vibrissa afferent in Vi vs. lamina III/IV of Vc, 4.7 vs. 3.5; tooth pulp afferents in Vp vs. lamina I/II of Vc, 5.1 vs. 2.6; Bae *et al.*, 1994, 2003, 2005b; Clements and Beitz, 1991; Ide and Killackey, 1985). In parallel with the complex synaptic arrangements being more common in Vp and Vi, the frequency of axoaxonic contacts involving PATs, i.e. PATs receiving synapses from p-endings, is higher in the Vp and Vi than in other TSN (Table I). Considering that the number of dendrites postsynaptic to PATs is fairly constant among TSN, the varying total number of contacts and frequency of complex glomeruli in different TSN appears to reflect the difference in the frequency of axoaxonic contacts.

E. Axoaxonic Synapses of Different Types of PAT

C-fiber terminals do not participate in axoaxonic contacts and thus do not receive presynaptic modulation (Knyihar-Csillik *et al.*, 1982a, 1982b; Ralston, 1979; Ruda *et al.*, 1986). In addition, Alvarez *et al.* (1993), in their EM study of physiologically-characterized primary afferents, have shown that C-fiber terminals, containing many DCV immunopositive for SP and CGRP, do not participate in axoaxonic contacts. Conversely, 40–90% of large myelinated, Aβ-LTM afferent (Bae *et al.*, 1994, 2000, 2003, 2005b), 30–90% of tooth pulp afferent terminals in the TSN (Bae *et al.*, 2003), 20–60% of Aδ-HTM afferent terminals (Alvarez *et al.*, 1992) and 50–100% of the cutaneous mechanoreceptive afferent terminals (hair follicle, Pacinian corpuscle [PC], RA and SA LTM afferents) in the spinal dorsal horn receive axoaxonic synapses (Maxwell *et al.*, 1982; Semba *et al.*, 1983, 1984, 1985; Sutherland *et al.*, 2002). Most differences in the synaptic connectivity among various types of large myelinated or Aβ-LTM afferents appear subtle in the same target nuclei, except the frequency of axoaxonic contacts: It is significantly higher in the RA than SA LTM vibrissa afferents in the Vp

(Nakagawa *et al.*, 1997) and two times higher in the RA than SA, PC LTM afferents in the spinal dorsal horn (Semba *et al.*, 1983, 1984, 1985; Sutherland *et al.*, 2002).

Axoaxonic contacts are the morphological substrate for presynaptic inhibition of PATs (Gray, 1962). It may be involved in the sharpening of sensation through lateral inhibition. The higher frequency of axoaxonic contact in the Vp and Vi than in other TSN suggests that these nuclei may be mainly involved in the processing of the discriminative aspects (location, modality, intensity, frequency, and duration of stimuli) of orofacial sensory information.

IV. Synaptic Connectivity of Trigeminal Mesencephalic Afferents

A. Jaw Muscle Spindle Afferent Terminals in the Vmo

The main features of the synaptic connectivity of jaw MS afferent terminals in the Vmo that form the monosynaptic jaw stretch-reflex circuit are that: 1) most of them (82–88%) contact a single postsynaptic target, 2) The majority of them (42–67%) contact soma or proximal dendrite, and, 3) A significant number (13–37%) receive axoaxonic contacts from 1–3 p-endings (Tables II and III; Bae *et al.*, 1996; Kishimoto *et al.*, 1998; Luo and Dessem, 1999).

Most jaw MS afferent terminals contact a single dendrite (82–88%, the remaining 12–18% contact two or three dendrites) in the Vmo, similar to the terminals of types Ia and II in the spinal cord (85–98% of terminals) contact one dendrite and 2–15% contact two or three dendrites: (Conradi *et al.*, 1983; Maxwell and Riddell, 1999; Pierce and Mendell, 1993). This suggests that a single MS afferent terminal predominantly activates a single motoneuron in the jaw stretch-reflex pathway. This is in contrast to the finding that a significant number of trigeminal somatosensory afferent terminals contact up to 9 postsynaptic dendrites in the TSN, and thus exert their excitatory effect on a multitude of postsynaptic neurons and their target regions in the CNS (Bae *et al.*, 1994, 2003, 2005b; Nakagawa *et al.*, 1997).

The majority of jaw MS afferent terminals (42–67%) contact a soma or a proximal dendrite, although their synapses may be distributed widely along the dendritic tree of the postsynaptic trigeminal motoneurons (Fig. 2). This is consistent with the pattern in the spinal cord, where a significant number of Ia afferent terminals (~20%) contact the soma of motoneurons (Pierce and Mendell, 1993), but at variance with those in the Vp, Vi, and Vc, where most somatosensory afferent terminals are presynaptic to dendritic shafts (Bae *et al.*, 1994, 2000, 2003, 2005b; Nakagawa *et al.*, 1997). These findings suggest that MS afferents, transmitting signals from stretch receptors, are likely to have a stronger influence

Table III

Frequency of Occurrence (%) of Terminals Showing Axoaxonic Contact from the Trigeminal Mesencephalic (Vmes) Muscle Spindle (ms), Periodontal (pl) Afferents and Spinal ms Afferents.

Afferent type or origin	Termination	Axoaxonic synapse	Reference
Trigeminal			
Vmes MS	Vmo	12.5	Bae *et al.* (1996)
Vmes PL	Vmo	34.8	
Vmes MS (Ia)	Vmo	36.5	Kishimoto *et al.* (1998)
Vmes MS (II)	Vmo	34.7	
Vmes MS	Vmo	28.0	Luo and Li (1991)
Vmes MS	Vmo	21.5-23.5	Luo and Dessem (1999)
Vmes	XIImo	35.0	Zhang *et al.* (2003)
Vmes MS	Vodm, Vidm, PCRt, IRt	39.0	Luo *et al.* (2006)
Vmes MS	Vsup, Vp	15.0	Luo *et al.* (1995)
Vmes MS	Vsup	53.8	Bae *et al.* (1996)
Vmes PL	Vsup	61.2	
Spinal cord			
Ia	Ventral horn	86.0	Pierce and Mendell (1993)
Ia	VI-IX	Almost all	Fyffe and Light (1984)
Ia	VI	92.0	Maxwell and Bannatyne (1983)
Ia	Clarke's column	8.0	Walmsley *et al.* (1995)
II	IV–V VI–VII	90.0	Maxwell and Riddell (1999)
Ia	IV–V	86.0	Watson and Bazzaz (2001)

IRt: intermediate reticular formation, PCRt: parvocellular reticular formation, Vidm: dorsomedial part of the trigeminal interpolar nucleus, Vmo: trigeminal motor nucleus, Vodm: dorsomedial part of the trigeminal oral nucleus, Vsup: supratrigeminal nucleus.

on the activity of postsynaptic neurons, than the sensory signals transmitted by trigeminal somatosensory afferents.

The terminals of trigeminal MS afferents receive much lower level of presynaptic input in the Vmo (13–37%) than Ia and II afferent terminals in the ventral horn of the spinal cord (86%- almost all; Table III) and also than the sensory afferent terminals in the Vp or Vi (58–91%; Table I). This suggests that the degree of presynaptic modulation at the level of PATs may be much lower for the neural circuit mediating the monosynaptic jaw stretch reflex, than that mediating spinal reflex or than that involved in the trigeminal sensory discrimination.

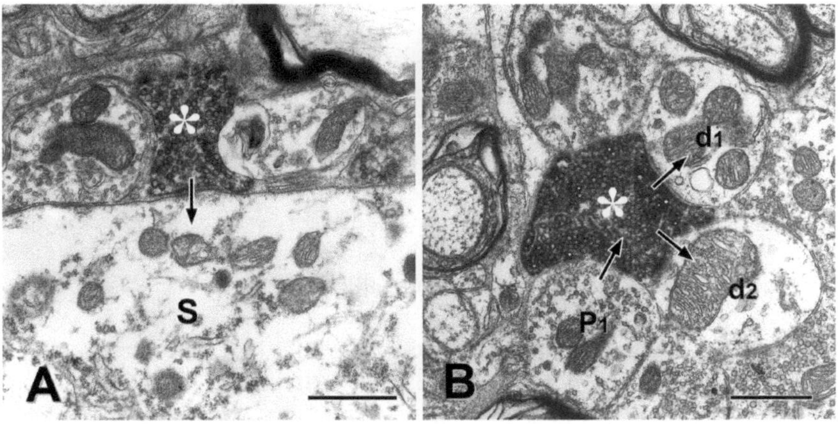

FIG. 2. **Electron micrographs of HRP-labeled terminals of jaw-closing muscle spindle afferents in the trigeminal motor nucleus. A**: An HRP-labeled terminal (asterisk) makes synaptic contact with a soma (S). **B**: An HRP-labeled terminal (asterisk) makes asymmetric synaptic contacts with two dendrites (d1, d2) and receives an axoaxonic synapse from a vesicle-containing presynaptic ending (p1). Arrows indicate direction of synaptic transmission. Scale bars, 500 nm.

B. Periodontal Vmes Afferent Terminals in the Vmo

The pattern of synaptic connectivity, including the spatial distribution of synapses along the dendritic tree of postsynaptic neurons and the number of postsynaptic dendrites per terminal, differ between Vmes periodontal (PL) and MS afferents in the Vmo (Table II; Bae *et al.*, 1996; Kishimoto *et al.*, 1998). Thus, PL afferent terminals contact soma or proximal dendrites less frequently but make 2.4 times as many contacts with dendritic shafts than the MS afferent terminals (Bae *et al.*, 1996). About 45% of PL afferent terminals are presynaptic to two upto four dendrites, whereas about 18% of MS terminals are presynaptic to two upto three dendrites (Bae *et al.*, 1996; Kishimoto *et al.*, 1998). This suggests that PL afferent terminals may exert weaker and more discrete excitatory effect on the postsynaptic neuron and may activate more motoneurons in Vmo than MS afferent terminals.

C. Jaw Muscle Spindle and Periodontal Vmes Afferent Terminals in the Vsup

The synaptic connectivity of MS afferents is similar to that of PL afferents in the Vsup, but different from that in the Vmo (Bae *et al.*, 1996; Kishimoto *et al.*, 1998; Table II), suggesting that the two types of afferents may have the same effect on the premotoneurons in Vsup but different effects on the motoneurons in the

Vmo. Synaptic connectivities of each MS and PL afferent terminals differ between in the Vmo and Vsup. Thus, the synapses of MS afferent terminals with somata or proximal dendrites are frequent in the Vmo (42–67%) and rare in the Vsup (2.2%). In addition, while about 20% of PL afferent terminals are presynaptic to two - three dendrites in the Vsup, a two times higher fraction is presynaptic to two - four dendrites in the Vmo.

Axoaxonic contacts involving Vmes MS and PL afferent terminals are also more frequent in the Vsup than in the Vmo (MS afferent terminals in the Vmo vs. Vsup: 13–37% vs. 54%, PL afferent terminals in the Vmo vs. Vsup: 35% vs. 61%; Table III), suggesting that the degree of presynaptic modulation of the Vmes afferents is different in different target nuclei. The same is true for primary afferent terminals in the spinal cord since ~ 86%, ~ 93% and ~ 98% of Ia terminals are involved in axoaxonic contact in the spinal ventral horn (Fyffe and Light, 1984; Maxwell and Riddell, 1999; Pierce and Mendell, 1993; Watson and Bazzaz, 2001), intermediate gray matter (Maxwell and Bannatyne, 1983), and the Clarke's column (Walmsley *et al.*, 1995), respectively.

D. Vmes Afferent Terminals in the XIImo

The synaptic connectivity of Vmes afferents in the XIImo, which is involved in the coordination of the jaw-tongue reflex, appears similar to that of the jaw MS afferents in the Vmo, which mediate the reflexive jaw movements. Thus, the majority (95%) of Vmes afferent terminals establish simple synapses with a single dendrite in the XIImo. They are frequently (12%) presynaptic to somata of hypoglossal motoneurons, and about one third of them receive axoaxonic contacts (Tables II and III; Zhang *et al.*, 2001a, 2003).

E. Synaptic Connectivity of Vo and Vsup Premotoneurons in the Vmo

Vo and Vsup contain inhibitory as well as excitatory premotoneurons (for Vo, Rampon *et al.*, 1996; Shigenaga *et al.*, 1988; Takata and Fujita, 1982; Turman and Chandler, 1994a; for Vsup, Kamogawa *et al.*, 1988; Kidokoro *et al.*, 1968; Kolta, 1997; Kolta *et al.*, 2000; Li *et al.*, 2002, 2005; Ohta and Moriyama, 1986; Stornetta *et al.*, 2002; Turman and Chandler, 1994a,b), which receive central as well as peripheral inputs from trigeminal somatosensory and proprioceptive MS and PL afferents, and send their axon collaterals to the Vmo (Bae *et al.*, 1996; Lingenhöhl and Friauf, 1991; Luo and Dessem, 1995; Olsson and Westberg, 1991; Shigenaga *et al.*, 1989b; Westberg *et al.*, 1995; Yoshida *et al.*, 1994). Therefore, these premotoneurons process central as well as peripheral somatosensory and proprioceptive signals, and exert direct influence onto the final output of the trigeminal

Table IV

FREQUENCY OF OCCURRENCE (%) OF PREMOTONEURON AXON TERMINALS ACCORDING TO THE SPATIAL DISTRIBUTION OF CONTACTS ON THE POSTSYNAPTIC SOMA OR PROXIMAL DENDRITE (PD), DENDRITIC SHAFT, NUMBER OF POSTSYNAPTIC DENDRITES (D), AND SHOWING AXOAXONIC SYNAPSES.

Circuit (from → to)	Soma or Pd	D. shaft	No. of postsynaptic dendrites (d)		Axoaxonic synapse	Reference
			1d	2d		
Vsup → Vmo	22	78	97	3	0	Paik *et al.* (2009a)
Vo → Vmo.dl	99	1	94	6	0	Shigenaga *et al.* (2000)
Vo → Vmo.vm	86	14	84	16	0	Shigenaga *et al.* (2000)
PCRt → XIImo	2 (soma only)	98 (including Pd)			0	Zhang and Luo (2003)
Vsup → XIImo	39 (soma only)	61 (including Pd)			0	Luo *et al.* (2001)

PCRt: parvocellular reticular formation, Pd: proximal dendrite, Vmo.dl: dorsolateral part of trigeminal motor nucleus, Vmo.vm: ventromedial part of trigeminal motor nucleus, Vsup: supratrigeminal nucleus, XIImo: hypoglossal motor nucleus.

motoneuron. The synaptic connectivity of Vo and Vsup premotoneuron axon terminals in the Vmo has some distinctive features (Paik *et al.*, 2009a; Shigenaga *et al.*, 2000): First, the premotoneuron axon terminals are not involved in axoaxonic contacts in the Vmo, consistent with the pattern of connectivity of Vsup, parvocellular reticular formation (PCRt) premotoneurons, which do not participate in axoaxonic contacts in the XIImo (Luo *et al.*, 2001; Zhang and Luo, 2003; Zhang *et al.*, 2003). This suggests that the output signals of premotoneurons are transmitted to their target motoneurons with little alteration at the level of the synapse, in contrast to the terminals of somatosensory and proprioceptive afferents, which frequently receive axoaxonic contacts and are thus a subject of significant presynaptic modulation before transmission of signals. Second, similar to the MS afferent terminals, most Vo and Vsup premotoneuron axon terminals establish a single synapse with a single dendrite; a small fraction of terminals contact two dendrites, and none contact three or more dendrites (Table IV; Paik *et al.*, 2009a; Shigenaga *et al.*, 2000).

V. Neurotransmitters in the Endings Presynaptic to PAT

A. LARGE MAJORITY OF P-ENDINGS CONTAIN BOTH GABA AND GLYCINE

Recent immunocytochemical studies of physiologically-characterized primary afferents have shown that most terminals (p-endings) presynaptic to the primary sensory and MS afferents contain γ-aminobutyric acid (GABA) and/or glycine

Table V

FREQUENCY (%) OF P-ENDINGS PRESYNAPTIC TO DIFFERENT TYPES OF PRIMARY AFFERENTS, ACCORDING TO IMMUNOREACTIVITY FOR GABA AND/OR GLYCINE (GLY).

Afferent type	Termination	Species	Immunoreactivity of p-endings				Reference
			GABA+	Both GABA+ & Gly+	Gly+	None	
Ia	IV–V	rat	58	31	11	0	Watson and Bazzaz (2001)
	VII–IX		91	9	0	0	
II	VI–VII	cat	16	84	0	0	Maxwell and Riddell (1999)
Ia	Vmo	rat	26	40	26	9	Paik *et al.* (2005)
HFA	III	rat	24	67	7	3	Watson *et al.* (2002)
Cutaneous							
HFA	III	cat	8	80	?	?	Sutherland *et al.* (2002)
RA	III		5	95	?	?	
SA	III–V		17	66	?	17	
SA (type II)	III–IV	rat	45	52	1	1	Watson (2004)
RA	III	rat	14	79	2	2	Watson (2003)
	IV–V		27	73	0	0	
Glomerulus (type II)	Dorsal horn	rat	10	86	4	0	Todd (1996)
Glomerulus	Vc	rat	17	60	18	5	Dumba *et al.* (1998)
Periodontal (SA)	Vp	cat	20	70	7	3	Bae *et al.* (2005a)
Vibrissa (RA)	Vi	cat	4	83	8	4	Moon *et al.* (2008)

HFA: hair follicle afferent, RA: rapidly-adapting, SA: slowly-adapting.

(see, Table V). The large majority of p-endings presynaptic to hair follicle afferents (67–80%), RA (73–95%) and SA (52–70%) type cutaneous afferents, to group II afferents in the intermediate gray matter (84%), and to C-boutons (central boutons) in synaptic glomeruli (60%) are immunopositive for both GABA and glycine in both the spinal dorsal horn and TSN (Table V, Fig. 3). The fraction of p-ending immunopositive for both GABA and glycine is much lower in the Ia afferents (in lamina VII–IX: 9%, in lamina IV–V: 31%, in Vmo: 40%; Table V) than in the mechanoreceptive and group II afferents (52–95%). While the fraction of p-endings containing both GABA and glycine is higher for the RA (73–95%) than for the SA type (52–70%) mechanoreceptive afferents, the fraction of those that contain GABA alone is higher for the SA (17–45%) than for the RA type (4–27%). These data suggest that the fractions of p-endings containing both GABA and glycine or GABA alone differ according to the primary afferent type, and to target region and possibly reflect functional differences.

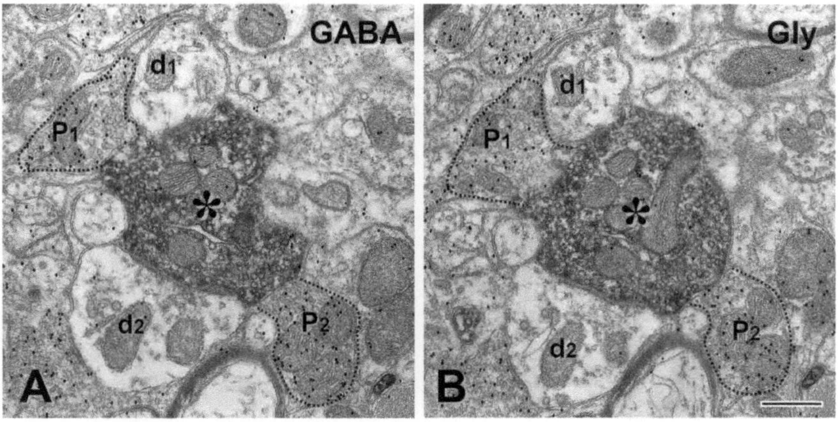

FIG. 3. **Electron micrographs of adjacent thin sections immunostained for GABA (A) and glycine (Gly; B).** An HRP-labeled terminal (asterisk) of a rapidly adapting vibrissa afferent in the trigeminal principal nucleus forms axodendritic synapses with two dendrites (d1, d2) and receives axoaxonic synapses from two p-endings (p1, p2), which are labeled for both GABA and glycine with immunogold. Scale bar, 500 nm.

B. Glycine in the Axoaxonic Contact

It is widely accepted that GABA released from the axon terminals presynaptic to the primary afferent acts on $GABA_A$ and $GABA_B$ receptors to induce primary afferent depolarization (PAD) and presynaptic inhibition (Curtis *et al.*, 1981; Edwards *et al.*, 1989; Maxwell *et al.*, 1990; Rudomin, 1990). However, the application of a very large dose of GABA antagonist reduced the height of the dorsal root potential only by one half, suggesting that neurotransmitters other than GABA contribute to the induction of PAD (Wall, 1994, 1998). At present, the functional significance of glycine in the p-endings is unknown. However, the glycine receptor antagonist strychnine did not block the dorsal root potential (Eccles *et al.*, 1963a, b), and previous studies failed to detect immunoreactivity for gephyrin, a protein associated with the β subunit of the glycine receptor, in the axoaxonic synapse between the p-ending containing glycine and its postsynaptic PAT in the spinal dorsal horn (Mitchell *et al.*, 1993; Todd *et al.*, 1995). Based on that, it has been thought that the glycine in the p-endings may not be involved in the PAD and presynaptic inhibition of the primary afferents, but that the glycine may spill over to neighboring dendrites postsynaptic to the PATs and produce postsynaptic inhibition. The existence of synaptic triads associated with various types of primary afferents in the spinal cord (Bannatyne *et al.*, 1984; Semba *et al.*, 1983; Sutherland *et al.*, 2002; Todd *et al.*, 1991; Watson, 2003, 2004) and brainstem (Bae *et al.*, 1994, 2003, 2005a, b; Zhang *et al.*, 2001), in which a p-ending presynaptic to the PAT also contacts with dendrite postsynaptic to the p-ending, supported this assumption.

However, that gephyrin is present at the axodendritic synapse associated with glycine-immunopositive endings but not at the axoaxonic synapse, may also suggest that the glycine receptor type involved in the postsynaptic inhibition may be different from that involved in the presynaptic inhibition, i.e., that some heretofore unidentified types of glycine receptor that is not associated with gephyrin, and is thus undetectable with immunohistochemistry for gephyrin, may be present in the PATs. Alternatively, the glycine receptors in the PATs may be homomeric for α subunit (Grenningloh *et al.*, 1990; Hoch *et al.*, 1989; Lynch, 2009) and/or insensitive to strychnine (Becker *et al.*, 1988; Langosch *et al.*, 1990; Mori *et al.*, 2002). In fact, the presence of $\alpha 3$ subunit of the glycine receptor in the TG and in the axoaxonic synapses associated with glycine-positive endings in the TSN, has just been reported in a preliminary study (Cho *et al.*, 2009).

C. Other Neurotransmitters in the Endings Presynaptic to PATs

A small number of endings presynaptic to glomerular and non-glomerular PATs in the spinal dorsal horn immunostain for choline acetyltransferase (ChAT) or neuropeptide Y (NPY; Doyle and Maxwell, 1994; Ribeiro-da-Silva and Cuello, 1990) and frequently coexpress GABA (Todd and Spike, 1993). Enkephalin-positive p-endings participating in the synaptic glomeruli in the spinal cord have also been reported, but apparently these are very rare (Aronin *et al.*, 1981). Recently, Yeo *et al.* (2010) reported that all enkephalin-positive terminals in the superficial lamina of Vc are involved in the axodendritic but not in axoaxonic synapses, in agreement with previous studies in the spinal cord (Glazer and Basbaum, 1981, 1984; Ruda, 1982; Sumal *et al.*, 1982). In addition, opioid receptors are expressed in nociceptive neurons that express TRPV1 or contain neuropeptides, whose central terminals are not involved in axoaxonic synapses (Endres-Becker *et al.*, 2007; Scherrer *et al.*, 2009; Wang *et al.*, 2010).

Since opioid receptors are usually localized to extrasynaptic sites of the plasma membrane (Svingos *et al.*, 1996, 1997), they may be involved in the presynaptic modulation of trigeminal nociceptive afferents through volume transmission, i.e., when released in the vicinity of nociceptive afferents, opioids may diffuse through the extracellular space and bind to receptors located in non-synaptic sites of the axonal membrane of these afferents.

VI. Quantitative Ultrastructure of PAT and their Presynaptic Endings

A. Size of PAT and the Ultrastructural Features Related to Transmitter Release

Multiple studies using EM of serial thin sections have analyzed the ultrastructural features related to synaptic release of PATs and the p-endings presynaptic to them of the trigeminal low-threshold mechanoreceptive afferents (Moon *et al.*, 2008; Nakagawa *et al.*, 1997; Zhang *et al.*, 2001b), nociceptive afferents (Bae *et al.*, 2004b), and Vmes afferents (Bae *et al.*, 1997) and showed that the bouton volume of trigeminal somatosensory and proprioceptive afferents is correlated with the size of the active zone, mitochondrial volume, apposed surface area, and vesicles number, the correlation being strong, positive, and linear. The bouton volume can be a good measure of potential synaptic efficacy considering that the size and number of active zones are closely correlated with the synaptic strength (Atwood and Marin, 1983; Propst and Ko, 1987; Yeow and Peterson, 1991). It also suggests that the "size principle", proposed by Pierce and Mendell (1993) in the Ia-motoneuron synapse in the spinal cord is applicable to the trigeminal sensory and proprioceptive afferent terminals.

B. Size of PAT and the Number of Postsynaptic Dendrites

Quantitative ultrastructural studies also showed that the size of PATs is positively correlated with the number of their postsynaptic dendrites (Bae *et al.*, 2004b; Moon *et al.*, 2008), suggesting that although larger boutons may release a larger amount of neurotransmitter overall, the amount of neurotransmitter available for the receptors of individual postsynaptic dendrites is not substantially different. In addition, the bouton size appears to be negatively correlated with the size of the postsynaptic dendrites, i.e., larger boutons tend to make synaptic contacts with smaller dendrites, reflecting a preference for the more distal parts of the dendritic tree (Nakagawa *et al.*, 1997).

C. The Size of Endings Presynaptic to PAT

The bouton volume and other ultrastructural features related to synaptic release of presynaptic p-endings are smaller than those of the PATs (Fig. 4; Bae *et al.*, 2004b; Moon *et al.*, 2008; Nakagawa *et al.*, 1997; Paik *et al.*, 2005; Zhang *et al.*, 2001b), suggesting that PAD and presynaptic inhibition exerted by p-endings may be induced by a far smaller amount of inhibitory neurotransmitter than the amount of excitatory neurotransmitter released from PATs. The smaller volume of p-endings may be important to modulate synaptic release from the PAT, but at the same time, to prevent generation of the action potential in the PAT and its retrograde propagation to the soma of the primary afferent neuron and to the periphery (Cattaert and El Manira, 1999; Dubuc *et al.*, 1985; Gossard *et al.*, 1991).

The ultrastructural features related to synaptic release are quite uniform in presynaptic p-endings whereas those of PATs of trigeminal sensory and primary afferents are widely variable. In addition, the bouton volume of PATs is positively correlated with the number of p-endings that are presynaptic to them (Bae *et al.*,

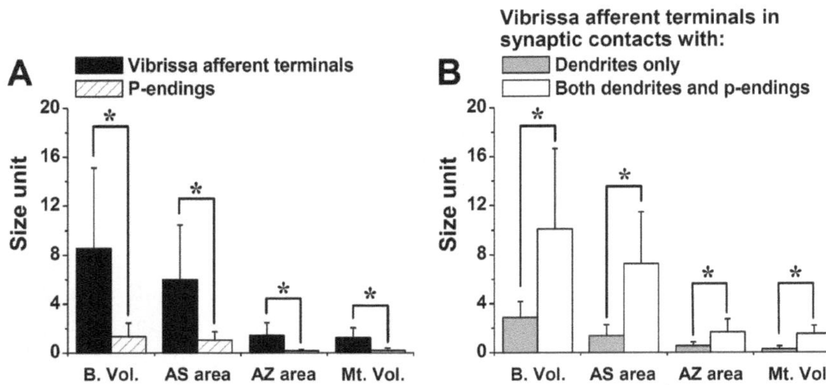

FIG. 4. **Size (mean ± SD) of ultrastructural parameters of vibrissa afferent terminals and their presynaptic endings (p-endings) in the cat trigeminal interpolar nucleus.** Bouton volume (B. Vol.; μm^3), apposed surface area (AS area; μm^2), active zone area (AZ area; μm^2) and mitochondrial volume (Mt. Vol.; μm^3) are significantly different (A) between vibrissa afferent terminals and p-endings, and (B) between vibrissa afferent terminals showing synapses with dendrites only and with both dendrites and p-endings, suggesting presynaptic modulation. Asterisks indicate statistically significant differences in each parameter at the 0.05 level (unpaired *t*-test). Modified from Moon *et al.* (2008).

2004b; Moon *et al.*, 2008; Nakagawa *et al.*, 1997; Paik *et al.*, 2005; Zhang *et al.*, 2001b); this correlation is valid for the trigeminal sensory and Ia afferents but also for the Ia-motoneuron synapse in the spinal cord (Pierce and Mendell, 1993). This suggests that the strength of presynaptic modulation of PAT may depend on the number of p-endings per PAT rather than on the diversity of synaptic strength among the p-endings. It also suggests that larger afferent boutons may receive stronger presynaptic inhibition. Supporting this notion, strong presynaptic inhibition occurs in fibers with large excitatory postsynaptic potentials (EPSPs) and in regions of large number of axoaxonic contacts in the crustacean neuromuscular junction (Tse *et al.*, 1991). Overall, PATs may receive varying degree of presynaptic inhibition depending on the number of presynaptic p-endings activated at the moment of arrival of the action potential into the PAT, thus allowing for a precise modulation of transmitter release.

D. Size of PAT has a Distinct Distribution Pattern in Different TSN

In the Vp, the bouton volume of tooth pulp afferents varies widely from small to very large and the majority of boutons are large and participate in multiple axoaxonic contacts, whereas in the Vc, the bouton volume is fairly uniform and the majority of boutons are small and are associated with few axoaxonic contacts, and in the Vdm, the bouton volume varies somewhat and the majority of boutons are of

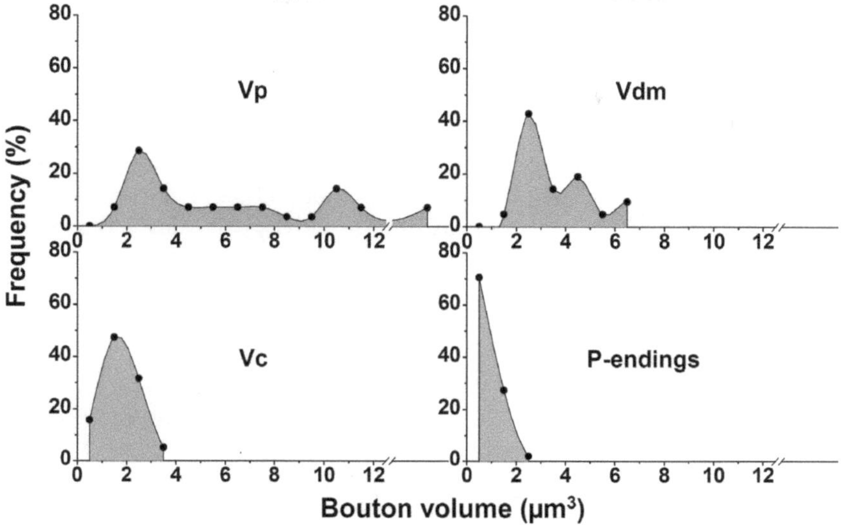

FIG. 5. **Distribution of bouton volume (μm^3) of tooth pulp afferents and p-endings in the trigeminal sensory nuclei.** The bouton volume in trigeminal principal nucleus (Vp) shows a wide range of distribution in contrast to that in dorsomedial part of trigeminal oral (Vdm) and caudal (Vc) nuclei. Closed dots and filled area indicate mean values and ranges of the distribution, respectively. P-endings analyzed are derived from Vp and Vdm. Modified from Bae *et al.* (2004b).

medium size (Fig. 5; Bae *et al.*, 2004b). The distinctive distribution of bouton size and number of axoaxonic contacts corresponds to the distinctive patterns of synaptic connectivity of PATs (Bae *et al.*, 1994, 2000, 2003, 2005b) and distinct termination pattern of primary sensory afferents in the various TSN (Marfurt, 1981; Miyoshi *et al.*, 1994; Moritani *et al.*, 1998; Shigenaga *et al.*, 1990; Takemura *et al.*, 1991, 1993), and may reflect the distinctive role of each TSN in the processing of somatosensory information.

VII. Nociceptive Afferents in the TSN

A. Projection of Nociceptive Afferents in the TSN

A variety of immunocytochemical and ultrastructural studies have focused on the synaptic connectivity of terminals in the TSN that express nociceptive-specific receptors, in an effort to elucidate where and how the specific receptor-mediated orofacial nociception is transmitted and processed within the brainstem (Bae *et al.*,

2004a; Kim *et al.*, 2008, 2010; Yeo *et al.*, 2010). Of the nociceptive receptors investigated in the TSN we will briefly summarize data regarding: 1) TRPV1, which is activated by capsaicin, noxious heat, and a variety of inflammatory mediators (Caterina *et al.*, 1999; Caterina and Julius, 2001; Tominaga *et al.*, 1998), 2) the transient receptor potential ankyrin 1 (TRPA1), which is activated by noxious cold (below 17°C) and pungent compounds, and plays a role in the development of cold and mechanical hypersensitivity following inflammation and nerve injury (Bautista *et al.*, 2005; Ji *et al.*, 2007; Petrus *et al.*, 2007; Story, 2006), and 3) the purinergic receptor P2X3, which is activated by ATP, and is involved in the mechanism of thermal and inflammatory hyperalgesia (Hamilton *et al.*, 1999; Souslova *et al.*, 2000; Tsuda *et al.*, 1999).

The TRPV1-positive (+), TRPA1+, and P2X3+ axons and terminals are all densely present in the Vc but with different distribution patterns: TRPV1 is dense in laminae I and IIo, P2X3 is dense in laminae I and IIi, and TRPA1 is dense throughout laminae I and II, implying that the specific nociceptive modalities mediated by these receptors are processed in distinct areas within Vc. At the transition between Vc and Vi, these nociceptive marker+ axons and terminals are dense in the C-shaped residual part of substantia gelatinosa that swings medially into the Vi, suggesting that this area is also largely involved in the processing of nociception (Fig. 6**B**). This area may correspond to the

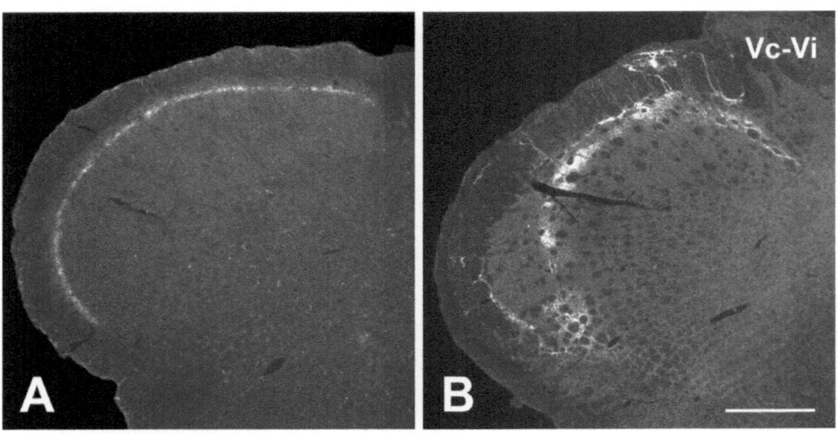

FIG. 6. **Immunofluorescent staining for P2X3 in the trigeminal caudal nucleus (Vc) at its middle level (A) and transition area between trigeminal caudal and interpolar nuclei (Vc-Vi; B). A:** P2X3-positive (+) fibers and terminals are dense in the inner part of the lamina II (IIi) throughout the dorsoventral and mediolateral aspects of Vc. **B:** A few P2X3+ fibers and terminals are visible in the ventral residual part of substantia gelatinosa, with a C-shaped curvature swinging medially into the trigeminal interpolar nucleus at the transition between the trigeminal interpolar and caudal nuclei. Scale bar, 500 μm.

"transitional zone" between Vc and Vi where many nociceptive neurons are reported to exist (Dubner and Ren, 2004; Wang *et al.*, 2006). In the Vi and Vo, nociceptive axons and terminals are few and scattered throughout the nuclei but are denser in the dorsomedial part and some middle and dorsal parts of the lateral margin of Vo and Vi, bordering the descending spinal trigeminal tract. At the Vp level, they are dense in the thin dorsal extension of the ascending tract and issue a large number of axon collaterals, which terminate in the dorsal part of Vp (Fig. 7). Traditionally, Vp is viewed as a relay for innocuous orofacial tactile information with little or no role in the transmission of nociceptive signals (for review, see Sessle, 2000). However, the dense expression of nociceptive markers in the dorsal part of Vp provides compelling evidence that this area is involved in the processing of intraoral nociception mediated by the TRPV1, TRPA1, and P2X3 receptors. That Vp may be involved in the transmission of

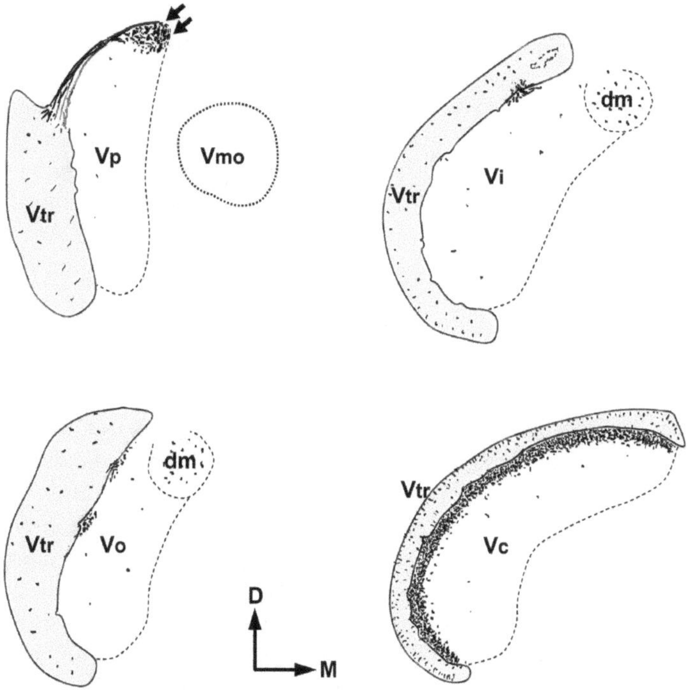

FIG. 7. **Distribution of TRPA1-positive axons and terminals in the trigeminal sensory nuclei.** TRPA1-positive axons and terminals are sparse in the trigeminal principal (Vp), oral (Vo), and interpolar (Vi) nuclei, and dense in the superficial laminae of trigeminal caudal nucleus (Vc). They are also dense in the dorsal part of Vp (arrows) and in the lateral margins of Vo and Vi, bordering the spinal trigeminal tract (Vtr). dm, dorsomedial part of Vo and Vi. D, dorsal. M, medial. Modified from Kim *et al.* (2010).

nociception is also supported by evidence that tooth pulp afferents, which are predominantly nociceptive, project to Vp (Arvidsson and Gobel, 1981; Bae *et al.*, 2003; Henry and Westrum, 1990; Marfurt and Turner, 1984; Shigenaga *et al.*, 1986b, 1989a; Takemura *et al.*, 1991; Turner and Marfurt, 1988; Westrum *et al.*, 1980, 1981), and that C-fos is expressed in the dorsal part of Vp after strong electrical stimulation of the trigeminal ganglion (Takemura *et al.*, 2000). It has also been reported that some neurons in Vp respond to noxious mechanical (pin prick) and thermal (50°C) stimuli (Eisenman *et al.*, 1963) although it is uncertain whether these neurons receive direct nociceptive input, and that high threshold, nociceptive muscle afferents project to the dorsal region of Vp (Dessem *et al.*, 2007).

B. Synaptic Connectivity of Identified Nociceptive Fiber Populations

Most TRPV1+ terminals (74%) in the Vc participate in simple synaptic arrangements with one or two dendrites, and the remaining small fraction is involved in complex synaptic arrangements with up to seven dendrites. In addition, about 13% of TRPV1+ terminals receive axoaxonic contacts from one or two glutamic acid decarboxylase (GAD) + axon terminals (Yeo *et al.*, 2010). TRPV1 is also expressed in a similar fraction of peptidergic (46%) and non-peptidergic (54%) neurons in the TG. It is expressed mostly in the unmyelinated axons (97%) and few small myelinated axons of Aδ size range (3%; Yeo *et al.*, 2010). As described early in this chapter, terminals of specific type of nociceptive afferents show distinctive synaptic connectivity pattern. For example, while most peptidergic C-fiber terminals establish synapses with one or two dendrites and rarely form synaptic glomeruli in the spinal cord (Alvarez *et al.*, 1993; Barber *et al.*, 1979; Carlton *et al.*, 1988; McNeill *et al.*, 1988), the majority of Aδ-HTM afferent terminals (65%) establish complex synaptic arrangements with four and upto thirteen postsynaptic dendrites, and frequently receive axoaxonic contact (Alvarez *et al.*, 1992). In addition, most IB4+ and fluoride-resistant acid phosphatase (FRAP)-containing non-peptidergic terminals (88%) also form glomeruli with four upto 14 dendrites and presynaptic axonal endings (Coimbra *et al.*, 1974; Gerke and Plenderleith, 2004). Considering both the pattern of synaptic connectivity of each type of nociceptive fibers and fraction of TRPV1-expressing fiber population, it is safe to deduce that the TRPV1+ terminals showing simple synaptic connectivity are derived mainly from the peptidergic C-fibers, and those showing complex synaptic connectivity are derived mainly from small myelinated Aδ and non-peptidergic C-fibers, i.e., the synaptic connectivity of specific nociceptive receptor-positive terminals is determined by their particular source of fiber population.

VIII. Morphology of Axons in the Dental Pulp

A. Parent Axons that Innervate the Dental Pulp

Many studies have investigated the types of sensory axons innervating the dental pulp to help and understand the nature of pulpal sensation. Thus, EM studies have found that 14–45% of axons in the apical part of the radicular pulp are myelinated (22–41% in rats, 20–44% in cats, 26% in dogs, 45% in marmosets, 14–28% in humans) while the remaining large majority of intradental axons are unmyelinated (Bueltmann *et al.*, 1972; Fried and Hildebrand, 1981; Hirvonen, 1987; Holje *et al.*, 1983; Holland and Robinson, 1983; Johnsen and Johns, 1978; Naftel *et al.*, 1994; Nair and Schroeder, 1995). Electrophysiological studies also reported that most of the intradental axons are nociceptive afferents with conduction velocity in the Aδ- and C-fiber range (Horiuchi and Matthews, 1974, 1976; Matthews, 1977). In addition, it has been suggested that the intradental axons may arise from larger extrapulpal parent axons because individual pulpal axons exhibit higher conduction velocity in the extrapulpal than intrapulpal regions (Cadden *et al.*, 1983; Lisney and Matthews, 1978). This was supported by the observation that the fraction of myelinated axons of all axons is higher in the inferior alveolar nerve than in the intrapulpal region (Fried and Hildebrand, 1982; Johansson *et al.*, 1992). Recently, Paik *et al.* (2010), using a combination of EM and retrograde tracing, investigated the parent axons innervating the rat permanent molar pulp and the continuously growing lower incisor pulp in the proximal sensory root of the TG, where sensory axons arise from the somata of neurons. They found that the parent axons innervating the dental pulp are mostly small myelinated fibers of Aδ size (76.8% in the parent axons innervating molar pulp and 83.0% in the parent axons innervating lower incisor pulp; Table VI). Considering that 14–45%

Table VI

Frequency (%, Mean ± SD) of HRP-labeled Parent Unmyelinated, Small Myelinated and Large Myelinated Axons, Innervating the Rat Upper Molar and Lower Incisor Pulps in the Proximal Portion of the Trigeminal Ganglion.

Target pulp	Parent axons innervating dental pulp		
	Unmyelinated axons	Small myelinated axons (<20 μm^2)	Large myelinated axons (>20 μm^2)
Upper molar pulp	$4.4 \pm 2.5^*$	76.8 ± 6.8	$19.6 \pm 7.8^*$
Lower incisor pulp	$15.3 \pm 2.1^*$	83.0 ± 1.7	$1.7 \pm 1.6^*$

* Indicates statistically significant differences ($p<0.05$, unpaired t-test) between parent axons in the molar and incisor pulp. Modified from Paik *et al.* (2009b).

of all intrapulpal axons in the apical region of the molar pulp are myelinated and that most of the axons in the lower incisor pulp are unmyelinated (Bishop, 1981; Byers, 1984; Hattyasy, 1956; Hildebrand *et al.*, 1995), these results imply that the large majority of small myelinated axons shed their myelin sheath, and become unmyelinated before entering into the dental pulp.

Previously it was shown that a small number of fibers in the dental pulp are of the Aβ type (0.9% of all intradental fibers, Naftel *et al.*, 1994). However, Paik *et al* (2010) showed that the large myelinated fibers of Aβ size (>20 μm^2 in cross-sectional area) constitute a considerable fraction of the parent axons innervating molar pulp (19.6%; Table VI). Although it has been reported that the pulpal Aβ-fibers respond to drilling and dentin probing, similar to Aδ-nociceptive fibers (Närhi, 1985, 1990) and it has been speculated that that they may mediate the innocuous sensation induced by week electrical stimulation (McGrath *et al.*, 1983; Virtanen *et al.*, 1987) or may be involved in the masticatory reflex (Cadden *et al.*, 1983; Dong *et al.*, 1985; Olgart *et al.*, 1988), the function of these fibers in the dental pulp remains poorly understood.

The continuously growing rat incisor pulp is innervated differently from the permanent molar pulp and the fraction of different axon types of all parent axons is different for these two kinds of pulp. Thus, the fraction of parent unmyelinated axons is higher for the incisor than the molar pulp, whereas the reverse is true for the fraction of parent large myelinated axons of Aβ size (Table VI; Paik *et al.*, 2009b). Also, at variance with the molar pulp, the intradental nerve fibers of the rat lower incisor are mostly unmyelinated, are usually associated with blood vessels deep in the pulp, do not usually branch, do not form plexus of Raschkow, and do not enter the dentin (Bishop, 1981; Hattyasy, 1956; for review, see Byers, 1984; Hildebrand *et al.*, 1995). These findings, at one time, have misled some researchers to believe that axons in the rat incisor pulp have exclusively autonomic function and no sensory function. The large majority of fibers in the rat incisor pulp are immunopositive for the neuropeptides CGRP and/or SP, which are believed to have roles in vasoregulation as well as nociception (for review, see Hildebrand *et al.*, 1995). In conclusion, compared to the molar teeth, sensory function associated with the dentin of the rat incisors, where dentin is continuously lost by gnawing, may be less developed but the sensory fibers may be primarily involved in the neurogenic inflammatory response and vasoregulatory function, associated with the continuous dentin formation and repair of the pulp matrix.

B. Size of Somata and Size of Axons Innervating the Dental Pulp

The large majority of sensory neurons that innervate the dental pulp have medium or large somata (Fried *et al.*, 1989; Marfurt and Turner, 1984; Sugimoto *et al.*, 1988; Sugimoto and Takemura, 1993) leading to the expectation that their

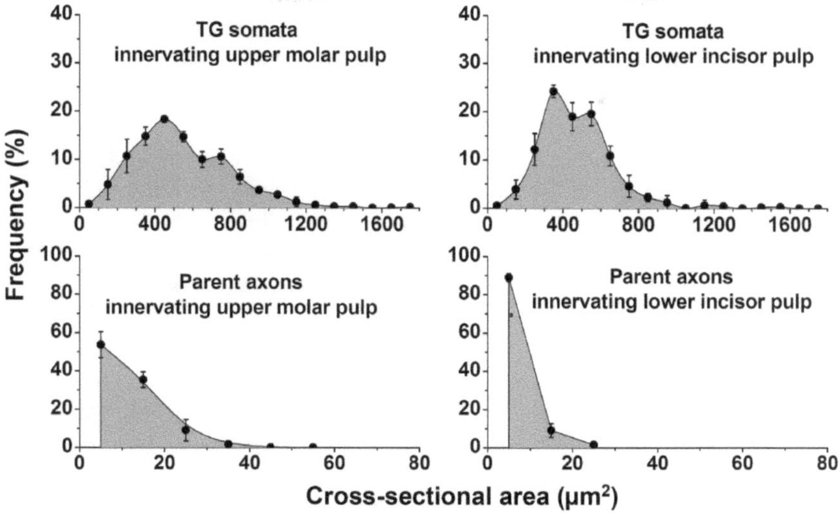

FIG. 8. **Size distribution (cross-sectional area, μm^2) of somata in the TG and of parent axons in the proximal portions of the opthalmo-maxillary and mandibular nerves that innervate upper molar and lower incisor pulp, respectively.**. Modified from Paik *et al.* (2009b).

axons would also be large. However, this is apparently not the case: most parent axons arising from these somata are small myelinated axons of Aδ type and unmyelinated axons (Paik *et al.*, 2009b). So the positive correlation between the size of somata and the size of their axons, which exists for the dorsal root ganglion (DRG) neurons (Harper and Lawson, 1985; Lawson and Waddell, 1991), may not apply for the neurons innervating the dental pulp (Table VI, Fig. 8). Since the perikaryon is responsible for the maintenance of the cytoplasm of the entire neuron, and since the primary afferent neurons do not have dendrites, the size of the soma must be proportional to the overall amount of the axoplasm, which is determined by the size of the axon, but also by its length and degree of terminal branching. Thus, extensive peripheral branching may explain the large somata but small axons of tooth pulp afferents. Indeed, tooth pulp afferents branch during their peripheral course so that a single pulpal axon innervates more than a hundred dentinal tubules (Byers, 1984; Hildebrand *et al.*, 1995; Holland and Robinson, 1983).

C. Morphological Changes of Myelinated Axons During their Intradental Course

During their peripheral course from their origin at the TG to the peripheral pulp, the myelinated axons become smaller and their myelin becomes thinner or disappears altogether, with or without tapering of the axon itself (Paik *et al.*, 2010).

The fraction of myelinated axons that lose their myelin sheath is higher in the short intradental course than in the very long extradental course from the TG to the tooth (Paik *et al.*, 2009b): up to 90% of the myelinated axons lose their myelin sheath during their intradental course from radicular to peripheral pulp, so that there are ten times more myelinated axons in the radicular pulp than in the peripheral pulp (50.3% vs. 5.2% of all fibers, respectively). In contrast, one half of the axons immunopositive for NF200, a marker for myelinated axons, are unmyelinated in the radicular pulp, suggesting that these are extensions of parent myelinated axons that have lost their myelin sheath before reaching the dental pulp (Fig. 9). Considering that myelinated axons usually lose their myelin, and become thinner with branching (Peng *et al.*, 1999), the difference in proportion of myelinated axons that become unmyelinated between extrapulpal and intrapulpal regions appears to be related to the different degrees of branching in the two regions. If the loss of myelin is related to the axonal branching, it is reasonable to expect that intrapulpal myelinated axons lose their myelin sheath in the peripheral pulp, where they branch extensively, rather than in the radicular pulp, or in the core of the coronal pulp, where they give off few axon collaterals.

The multitude of unmyelinated axons in the peripheral pulp represents the terminal segments of the myelinated axons, whose primary role may be providing larger areas of axolemma for the membrane receptors rather than fast conduction of action potentials. This assumption can be supported by a recent finding that nociceptive receptor mGluR5 is expressed much more extensively and strongly in the unmyelinated axons in the peripheral pulp than in the radicular pulp or the core of the coronal pulp, where the mGluR5+ axons are surrounded by a connective tissue sheath (Kim *et al.*, 2009).

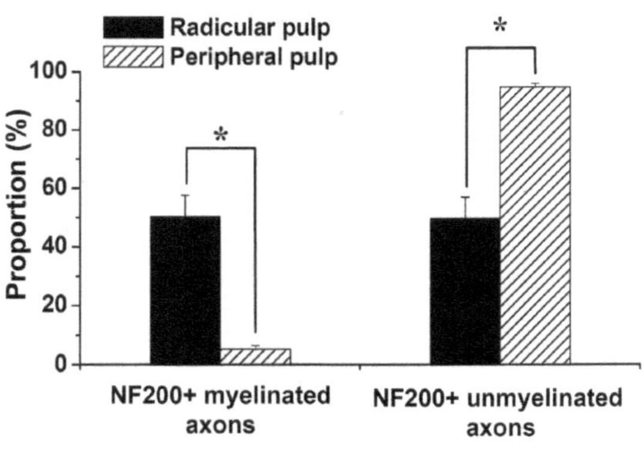

FIG. 9. **Proportion (mean ± SD, %) of NF200+ myelinated and unmyelinated axons in the radicular (50.3 ± 7.3 and 49.7 ± 7.3, respectively) and peripheral pulp (5.2 ± 1.2 and 94.8 ± 1.2, respectively) of the rat upper molar teeth.** Asterisks indicate statistically significant differences between the radicular and peripheral coronal pulp at 0.05 level (unpaired *t*-test). Modified from Paik *et al.* (2010).

IX. Summary and Conclusion

The Neurons communicate with one another at the synapse where neural information is processed and transmitted. Examination of ultrastructural synaptology of specific primary afferent terminals helps us to understand how the specific sensory information is processed and transmitted at the first relay nucleus of the CNS. Previous sections reviewed recent findings on the synaptic connectivity of various types of trigeminal somatosensory and proprioceptive afferents in the TSN and trigeminal motor nucleus: They show that neural information conveyed through trigeminal somatosensory and proprioceptive afferents is processed and transmitted in a unique manner according to the fiber types and their target nuclei. It may be closely related to the functional specificity of the neural circuit associated with each of the fiber types and target nuclei.

The next sections reviewed recent literature dealing with neurotransmitters in the endings presynaptic to PATs that may be involved in the presynaptic modulation, and quantitative ultrastructure of PATs and their presynaptic endings that are involved in the synaptic release in the TSN: Trigeminal somatosensory and proprioceptive afferents usually receive presynaptic modulation from endings containing both GABA and glycine through axonic synapse. In addition, recent findings show that glycine receptor type involved in the presynaptic inhibition may be different from that involved in the postsynaptic inhibition. Size of trigeminal PATs is positively correlated with the size of ultra structural features related to synaptic release, is widely variable and shows distinctive distribution pattern in each TSN in contrast that those of endings presynaptic to PATs are small and uniform. These findings also suggest functional heterogeneity of each TSN in processing of orofacial sensation.

The final section reviewed recent findings on the types of parent axons innervating dental pulp and their morphological changes during their peripheral course to target region: Parent axons innervating dental pulp are mostly small myelinated fibers of Aδ size, and they show extensive morphological changes such as thinning, loss of myelin, and tapering of the axon itself during their peripheral course from their origin at the TG to the peripheral pulp. Further studies on the functional significance of the extensive morphological changes of intradental axons at the peripheral pulp may be helpful to understand unique pulpal pain mechanism.

Acknowledgments

This work was supported by Basic Science Research Program through the National Research Foundation of Korea (NRF) funded by the Ministry of

Education, Science and Technology (NRF-2010-0029460; NRF-2008-314-E00213). The authors thank Dr. Juli Valtschanoff for helpful discussion and careful reading of the manuscript.

References

Allen, G.V., Barbrick, B. and Esser, M.J. (1996). Trigeminal-parabrachial connections: possible pathway for nociception-induced cardiovascular reflex responses. *Brain Res.* **715**, 125–135.

Alvarez, F.J., Kavookjian, A.M. and Light, A.R. (1992). Synaptic interactions between GABA-immunoreactive profiles and the terminals of functionally defined myelinated nociceptors in the monkey and cat spinal cord. *J. Neurosci.* **12**, 2901–2917.

Alvarez, F.J., Kavookjian, A.M. and Light, A.R. (1993). Ultrastructural morphology, synaptic relationships, and CGRP immunoreactivity of physiologically identified C-fiber terminals in the monkey spinal cord. *J. Comp. Neurol.* **329**, 472–490.

Ambalavanar, R. and Morris, R. (1992). The distribution of binding by isolectin I-B4 from Griffonia simplicifolia in the trigeminal ganglion and brainstem trigeminal nuclei in the rat. *Neuroscience* **47**, 421–429.

Aronin, N., DiFiglia, M., Liotta, A.S. and Martin, J.B. (1981). Ultrastructural localization and biochemical features of immunoreactive LEU-enkephalin in monkey dorsal horn. *J. Neurosci.* **1**, 561–577.

Arvidsson, J. and Gobel, S. (1981). An HRP study of the central projections of primary trigeminal neurons which innervate tooth pulps in the cat. *Brain Res.* **210**, 1–16.

Atwood, H.L. and Marin, L. (1983). Ultrastructure of synapses with different transmitter-releasing characteristics on motor axon terminals of a crab, Hyas arenea. *Cell. Tissue Res.* **231**, 103–115.

Bae, Y.C., Nagase, Y., Yoshida, A., Shigenaga, Y. and Sugimoto, T. (1993). Synaptic connections of a periodontal primary afferent neuron within the subnucleus oralis of the cat. *Brain Res.* **606**, 175–179.

Bae, Y.C., Nakagawa, S., Yoshida, A., Nagase, Y., Takemura, M. and Shigenaga, Y. (1994). Morphology and synaptic connections of slowly adapting periodontal afferent terminals in the trigeminal subnuclei principalis and oralis of the cat. *J. Comp. Neurol.* **348**, 121–132.

Bae, Y.C., Nakagawa, S. and Yasuda, K *et al.*, (1996). Electron microscopic observation of synaptic connections of jaw-muscle spindle and periodontal afferent terminals in the trigeminal motor and supratrigeminal nuclei in the cat. *J. Comp. Neurol.* **374**, 421–435.

Bae, Y.C., Park, K.P. and Yoshida, A *et al.*, (1997). Identification of gamma-aminobutyric acid-immunoreactive axon endings associated with mesencephalic periodontal afferent terminals and morphometry of the two types of terminals in the cat supratrigeminal nucleus. *J. Comp. Neurol.* **389**, 127–138.

Bae, Y.C., Ihn, H.J. and Park, M.J *et al.*, (2000). Identification of signal substances in synapses made between primary afferents and their associated axon terminals in the rat trigeminal sensory nuclei. *J. Comp. Neurol.* **418**, 299–309.

Bae, Y.C., Kim, J.P. and Choi, B.J *et al.*, (2003). Synaptic organization of tooth pulp afferent terminals in the rat trigeminal sensory nuclei. *J. Comp. Neurol.* **463**, 13–24.

Bae, Y.C., Oh, J.M., Hwang, S.J., Shigenaga, Y. and Valtschanoff, J.G. (2004a). Expression of vanilloid receptor TRPV1 in the rat trigeminal sensory nuclei. *J. Comp. Neurol.* **478**, 62–71.

Bae, Y.C., Paik, S.K. and Park, K.P *et al.*, (2004b). Quantitative analysis of tooth pulp afferent terminals in the rat brain stem. *Neuroreport* **15**, 2485–2489.

Bae, Y.C., Park, K.S. and Bae, J.Y *et al.*, (2005a). GABA and glycine in synaptic microcircuits associated with physiologically characterized primary afferents of cat trigeminal principal nucleus. *Exp. Brain Res.* **162**, 449–457.

Bae, Y.C., Ahn, H.J. and Park, K.P *et al.*, (2005b). The synaptic microcircuitry associated with primary afferent terminals in the interpolaris and caudalis of trigeminal sensory nuclear complex. *Brain Res.* **1060**, 118–125.

Bannatyne, B.A., Maxwell, D.J., Fyffe, R.E. and Brown, A.G. (1984). Fine structure of primary afferent axon terminals of slowly adapting cutaneous receptors in the cat. *Q. J. Exp. Physiol.* **69**, 547–557.

Barber, R.P., Vaughn, J.E., Slemmon, J.R., Salvaterra, P.M., Roberts, E. and Leeman, S.E. (1979). The origin, distribution and synaptic relationships of substance P axons in rat spinal cord. *J. Comp. Neurol.* **184**, 331–351.

Bautista, D.M., Movahed, P. and Hinman, A *et al.*, (2005). Pungent products from garlic activate the sensory ion channel TRPA1. *Proc. Natl. Acad. Sci. U. S. A.* **102**, 12248–12252.

Becker, C.M., Hoch, W. and Betz, H. (1988). Glycine receptor heterogeneity in rat spinal cord during postnatal development. *EMBO J.* **7**, 3717–3726.

Beggs, J., Jordan, S., Ericson, A.C., Blomqvist, A. and Craig, A.D. (2003). Synaptology of trigemino- and spinothalamic lamina I terminations in the posterior ventral medial nucleus of the macaque. *J. Comp. Neurol.* **459**, 334–354.

Bernard, J.F., Dallel, R., Raboisson, P., Villanueva, L. and Le Bars, D. (1995). Organization of the efferent projections from the spinal cervical enlargement to the parabrachial area and periaqueductal gray: a PHA-L study in the rat. *J. Comp. Neurol.* **353**, 480–505.

Bishop, M.A. (1981). A fine-structural survey of the pulpal innervation in the rat mandibular incisor. *Am. J. Anat.* **160**, 213–229.

Bueltmann, K.W., Karlsson, U.L. and Edie, J. (1972). Quantitative ultrastructure of intradental nerve fibres in marmosets. *Arch. Oral Biol.* **17**, 645–660.

Byers, M.R. (1984). Dental sensory receptors. *Int. Rev. Neurobiol.* **25**, 39–94.

Cadden, S.W., Lisney, S.J. and Matthews, B. (1983). Thresholds to electrical stimulation of nerves in cat canine tooth-pulp with A beta-, A delta- and C-fibre conduction velocities. *Brain Res.* **261**, 31–41.

Carlton, S.M., McNeill, D.L., Chung, K. and Coggeshall, R.E. (1988). Organization of calcitonin gene-related peptide-immunoreactive terminals in the primate dorsal horn. *J. Comp. Neurol.* **276**, 527–536.

Caterina, M.J. and Julius, D. (2001). The vanilloid receptor: a molecular gateway to the Pain pathway. *Annu. Rev. Neurosci.* **24**, 487–517.

Caterina, M.J., Rosen, T.A., Tominaga, M., Brake, A.J. and Julius, D. (1999). A capsaicin-receptor homologue with a high threshold for noxious heat. *Nature* **398**, 436–441.

Cattaert, D. and El Manira, A. (1999). Shunting versus inactivation: analysis of presynaptic inhibitory mechanisms in primary afferents of the crayfish. *J. Neurosci.* **19**, 6079–6089.

Chiang, C.Y., Hu, J.W. and Sessle, B.J. (1997). NMDA receptor involvement in neuroplastic changes induced by neonatal capsaicin treatment in trigeminal nociceptive neurons. *J. Neurophysiol.* **78**, 2799–2803.

Chiang, C.Y., Park, S.J., Kwan, C.L., Hu, J.W. and Sessle, B.J. (1998). NMDA receptor mechanisms contribute to neuroplasticity induced in caudalis nociceptive neurons by tooth pulp stimulation. *J. Neurophysiol.* **80**, 2621–2631.

Cho, Y. S., Bae J. Y., Kim, T. H., Park, M. J., Yoshida, A., Ahn, D. K., Kim, Y. S., and Bae, Y. C. (2009). Expression of the glycine receptor at the axoaxonic synapse and primary afferents in the rat trigeminal sensory nucleus and trigeminal ganglion. Abstract for 2009 Neuroscience Meeting (program#/poster#: 266.24/AA25).

Clements, J.R. and Beitz, A.J. (1991). An electron microscopic description of glutamate-like immunoreactive axon terminals in the rat principal sensory and spinal trigeminal nuclei. *J. Comp. Neurol.* **309**, 271–280.

Coimbra, A., Sodré-Borges, B.P. and Magalhães, M.M. (1974). The substantia gelatinosa Rolandi of the rat. Fine structure, cytochemistry (acid phosphatase) and changes after dorsal root section. *J. Neurocytol.* **3**, 199–217.

Colonnier, M. (1968). Synaptic patterns on different cell types in the different laminae of the cat visual cortex. An electron microscope study. *Brain Res.* **9**, 268–287.

Conradi, S., Cullheim, S., Gollvik, L. and Kellerth, J.O. (1983). Electron microscopic observations on the synaptic contacts of group I a muscle spindle afferents in the cat lumbosacral spinal cord. *Brain Res.* **265**, 31–39.

Craig, A.D. (2003). Distribution of trigeminothalamic and spinothalamic lamina I terminations in the cat. *Somatosens. Mot. Res.* **20**, 209–222.

Craig, A.D. and Dostrovsky, J.O. (2001). Differential projections of thermoreceptive and nociceptive lamina I trigeminothalamic and spinothalamic neurons in the cat. *J. Neurophysiol.* **86**, 856–870.

Craig, A.M., Graf, E.R. and Linhoff, M.W. (2006). How to build a central synapse: clues from cell culture. *Trends Neurosci.* **29**, 8–20.

Curtis, D.R., Lodge, D., Bornstein, J.C. and Peet, M.J. (1981). Selective effects of (-)-baclofen on spinal synaptic transmission in the cat. *Exp. Brain Res.* **42**, 158–170.

Dallel, R., Raboisson, P., Auroy, P. and Woda, A. (1988). The rostral part of the trigeminal sensory complex is involved in orofacial nociception. *Brain Res.* **448**, 7–19.

Dessem, D., Moritani, M. and Ambalavanar, R. (2007). Nociceptive craniofacial muscle primary afferent neurons synapse in both the rostral and caudal brain stem. *J. Neurophysiol.* **98**, 214–223.

Ding, Y.Q., Takada, M., Shigemoto, R. and Mizuno, N. (1995). Trigeminoparabrachial projection neurons showing substance P receptor-like immunoreactivity in the rat. *Neurosci. Res.* **23**, 415–418.

Dong, W.K., Chudler, E.H. and Martin, R.F. (1985). Physiological properties of intradental mechanoreceptors. *Brain Res.* **334**, 389–395.

Doyle, C.A. and Maxwell, D.J. (1994). Light- and electron-microscopic analysis of neuropeptide Y-immunoreactive profiles in the cat spinal dorsal horn. *Neuroscience* **61**, 107–121.

Dubner, R. and Ren, K. (2004). Brainstem mechanisms of persistent pain following injury. *J. Orofac. Pain* **18**, 299–305.

Dubuc, R., Cabelguen, J.M. and Rossignol, S. (1985). Rhythmic antidromic discharges of single primary afferents recorded in cut dorsal root filaments during locomotion in the cat. *Brain Res.* **359**, 375–378.

Dumba, J.S., Irish, P.S., Anderson, N.L. and Westrum, L.E. (1998). Electron microscopic analysis of gamma-aminobutyric acid and glycine colocalization in rat trigeminal subnucleus caudalis. *Brain Res.* **806**, 16–25.

Eccles, J.C., Schmidt, R.F. and Willis, W.D. (1963a). Depolarization of the central terminals of cutaneous afferent fibers. *J. Neurophysiol.* **26**, 646–661.

Eccles, J.C., Schmidt, R.F. and Willis, W.D. (1963b). Pharmacological studies on presynaptic inhibition. *J. Physiol.* **168**, 530–560.

Edwards, F.R., Harrison, P.J., Jack, J.J. and Kullmann, D.M. (1989). Reduction by baclofen of monosynaptic EPSPs in lumbosacral motoneurones of the anaesthetized cat. *J. Physiol.* **416**, 539–556.

Egger, M.D., Freeman, N.C., Malamed, S., Masarachia, P. and Proshansky, E. (1981). Electron microscopic observations of terminals of functionally identified afferent fibers in cat spinal cord. *Brain Res.* **207**, 157–162.

Eisenman, J., Landgren, S. and Novin, D. (1963). Functional organization in the main sensory trigeminal nucleus and in the rostral subdivision of the nucleus of the spinal trigeminal tract in the cat. *Acta Physiol. Scand. Suppl.* **214**, 1–44.

Ellrich, J., Andersen, O.K., Messlinger, K. and Arendt-Nielsen, L. (1999). Convergence of meningeal and facial afferents onto trigeminal brainstem neurons: an electrophysiological study in rat and man. *Pain* **82**, 229–237.

Endres-Becker, J., Heppenstall, P.A., Mousa, S.A., Labuz, D., Oksche, A., Schäfer, M., Stein, C. and Zöllner, C. (2007). Mu-opioid receptor activation modulates transient receptor potential vanilloid 1 (TRPV1) currents in sensory neurons in a model of inflammatory Pain. *Mol. Pharmacol.* **71**, 12–18.

Falls, W.M. (1986). Morphology and synaptic connections of myelinated primary axons in the ventrolateral region of rat trigeminal nucleus oralis. *J. Comp. Neurol.* **244**, 96–110.

Fried, K. and Hildebrand, C. (1981). Pulpal axons in developing, mature, and aging feline permanent incisors. A study by electron microscopy. *J. Comp. Neurol.* **203**, 23–36.

Fried, K. and Hildebrand, C. (1982). Axon number and size distribution in the developing feline inferior alveolar nerve. *J. Neurol Sci.* **53**, 169–180.

Fried, K., Arvidsson, J., Robertson, B., Brodin, E. and Theodorsson, E. (1989). Combined retrograde tracing and enzyme/immunohistochemistry of trigeminal ganglion cell bodies innervating tooth pulps in the rat. *Neuroscience* **33**, 101–109.

Fyffe, R.E. and Light, A.R. (1984). The ultrastructure of group Ia afferent fiber synapses in the lumbosacral spinal cord of the cat. *Brain Res.* **300**, 201–209.

Gauriau, C. and Bernard, J.F. (2004). A comparative reappraisal of projections from the superficial laminae of the dorsal horn in the rat: the forebrain. *J. Comp. Neurol.* **468**, 24–56.

Gerke, M.B. and Plenderleith, M.B. (2004). Ultrastructural analysis of the central terminals of primary sensory neurones labelled by transganglionic transport of Bandeiraea simplicifolia I-isolectin B4. *Neuroscience* **127**, 165–175.

Glazer, E.J. and Basbaum, A.I. (1981). Immunohistochemical localization of leucine-enkephalin in the spinal cord of the cat: enkephalin-containing marginal neurons and Pain modulation. *J. Comp. Neurol.* **196**, 377–389.

Glazer, E.J. and Basbaum, A.I. (1984). Axons which take up [3H]serotonin are presynaptic to enkephalin immunoreactive neurons in cat dorsal horn. *Brain Res.* **298**, 386–391.

Gobel, S. (1975). Golgi studies in the substantia gelatinosa neurons in the spinal trigeminal nucleus. *J. Comp. Neurol.* **162**, 397–415.

Gobel, S. (1978). Golgi studies of the neurons in layer II of the dorsal horn of the medulla (trigeminal nucleus caudalis). *J. Comp. Neurol.* **180**, 395–413.

Gobel, S. and Purvis, M.B. (1972). Anatomical studies of the organization of the spinal V nucleus: the deep bundles and the spinal V tract. *Brain Res.* **48**, 27–44.

Gobel, S., Falls, W.M. and Hockfield, S. (1977). The division of the dorsal and ventral horns of the mammalian caudal medulla into eight layers using anatomical criteria. In: Anderson, D.J., Mattews, B. (Eds.), *Pain in the Trigeminal Region.* Elsevier, Amsterdam, pp. 443–453.

Gobel, S., Falls, W.M. and Humphrey, E. (1981). Morphology and synaptic connections of ultrafine primary axons in lamina I of the spinal dorsal horn: candidates for the terminal axonal arbors of primary neurons with unmyelinated (C) axons. *J. Neurosci.* **1**, 1163–1179.

Gossard, J.P., Cabelguen, J.M. and Rossignol, S. (1991). An intracellular study of muscle primary afferents during fictive locomotion in the cat. *J. Neurophysiol.* **65**, 914–926.

Gray, E.G. (1959). Axo-somatic and axo-dendritic synapses of the cerebral cortex: an electron microscope study. *J. Anat.* **93**, 420–433.

Gray, E.G. (1962). A morphological basis for pre-synaptic inhibition? *Nature* **193**, 82–83.

Grenningloh, G., Schmieden, V., Schofield, P.R., Seeburg, P.H., Siddique, T., Mohandas, T.K., Becker, C.M. and Betz, H. (1990). Alpha subunit variants of the human glycine receptor: primary structures, functional expression and chromosomal localization of the corresponding genes. *EMBO J.* **9**, 771–776.

Hamilton, S.G., Wade, A. and McMahon, S.B. (1999). The effects of inflammation and inflammatory mediators on nociceptive behaviour induced by ATP analogues in the rat. *Br. J. Pharmacol.* **126**, 326–332.

Harms, K.J. and Dunaevsky, A. (2007). Dendritic spine plasticity: looking beyond development. *Brain Res.* **1184**, 65–71.

Harper, A.A. and Lawson, S.N. (1985). Conduction velocity is related to morphological cell type in rat dorsal root ganglion neurones. *J. Physiol.* **359**, 31–46.

Hattyasy, D. (1956). Innervation of the continuously growing incisor. *Nature* **178**, 416.

Henry, M.A. and Westrum, L.E. (1990). Central representation of dental structures in the kitten, including projections to the mesencephalic trigeminal nucleus. *Somatosens. Mot. Res.* **7**, 447–462.

Hildebrand, C., Fried, K., Tuisku, F. and Johansson, C.S. (1995). Teeth and tooth nerves. *Prog. Neurobiol.* **45**, 165–222.

Hirvonen, T.J. (1987). A quantitative electron-microscopic analysis of the axons at the apex of the canine tooth pulp in the dog. *Acta Anat. (Basel).* **128**, 134–139.

Hoch, W., Betz, H. and Becker, C.M. (1989). Primary cultures of mouse spinal cord express the neonatal isoform of the inhibitory glycine receptor. *Neuron* **3**, 339–348.

Holje, L., Hildebrand, C. and Fried, K. (1983). Proportion of unmyelinated axons in the rat inferior alveolar nerve and mandibular molar pulps after neonatal administration of capsaicin. *Brain Res.* **266**, 133–136.

Holland, G.R. and Robinson, P.P. (1983). The number and size of axons at the apex of the cat's canine tooth. *Anat. Rec.* **205**, 215–222.

Horiuchi, H. and Matthews, B. (1974). Evidence on the origin of impulses recorded from dentine in the cat. *J. Physiol.* **243**, 797–829.

Horiuchi, H. and Matthews, B. (1976). Responses of intradental nerves to chemical and osmotic stimulation of dentine in the cat. *Pain* **2**, 49–59.

Ide, L.S. and Killackey, H.P. (1985). Fine structural survey of the rat's brainstem sensory trigeminal complex. *J. Comp. Neurol.* **235**, 145–168.

Jacquin, M.F., Chiaia, N.L. and Rhoades, R.W. (1990). Trigeminal projections to contralateral dorsal horn: central extent, peripheral origins, and plasticity. *Somatosens. Mot. Res.* **7**, 153–183.

Jacquin, M.F., Renehan, W.E., Rhoades, R.W. and Panneton, W.M. (1993). Morphology and topography of identified primary afferents in trigeminal subnuclei principalis and oralis. *J. Neurophysiol.* **70**, 1911–1936.

Ji, G., Zhou, S., Kochukov, M.Y., Westlund, K.N. and Carlton, S.M. (2007). Plasticity in intact A delta- and C-fibers contributes to cold hypersensitivity in neuropathic rats. *Neuroscience* **150**, 182–193.

Johansson, C.S., Hildebrand, C. and Povlsen, B. (1992). Anatomy and developmental chronology of the rat inferior alveolar nerve. *Anat. Rec.* **234**, 144–152.

Johnsen, D. and Johns, S. (1978). Quantitation of nerve fibres in the primary and permanent canine and incisor teeth in man. *Arch. Oral Biol.* **23**, 825–829.

Kamogawa, H., Hanashima, N., Naito, K. and Kagaya, K. (1988). Candidate interneurons mediating peripherally evoked disynaptic inhibition of masseter motoneurons of both sides. *Neurosci. Lett.* **95**, 149–154.

Kidokoro, Y., Kubota, K., Shuto, S. and Sumino, R. (1968). Possible interneurons responsible for reflex inhibition of motoneurons of jaw-closing muscles from the inferior dental nerve. *J. Neurophysiol.* **31**, 709–716.

Kim, Y.S., Paik, S.K., Cho, Y.S., Shin, H.S., Bae, J.Y., Moritani, M., Yoshida, A., Ahn, D.K., Valtschanoff, J., Hwang, S.J., Moon, C. and Bae, Y.C. (2008). Expression of P2X3 receptor in the trigeminal sensory nuclei of the rat. *J. Comp. Neurol.* **506**, 627–639.

Kim, Y.S., Kim, Y.J., Paik, S.K., Cho, Y.S., Kwon, T.G., Ahn, D.K., Kim, S.K., Yoshida, A. and Bae, Y.C. (2009). Expression of metabotropic glutamate receptor mGluR5 in human dental pulp. *J. Endod.* **35**, 690–694.

Kim, Y.S., Son, J.Y., Kim, T.H., Paik, S.K., Dai, Y., Noguchi, K., Ahn, D.K. and Bae, Y.C. (2010). Expression of transient receptor potential ankyrin 1 (TRPA1) in the rat trigeminal sensory afferents and spinal dorsal horn. *J. Comp. Neurol.* **518**, 687–698.

Kishimoto, H., Bae, Y.C., Yoshida, A., Moritani, M., Takemura, M., Nakagawa, S., Nagase, Y., Wada, T., Sessle, B.J. and Shigenaga, Y. (1998). Central distribution of synaptic contacts of primary and secondary jaw muscle spindle afferents in the trigeminal motor nucleus of the cat. *J. Comp. Neurol.* **391**, 50–63.

Knott, G.W., Quairiaux, C., Genoud, C. and Welker, E. (2002). Formation of dendritic spines with GABAergic synapses induced by whisker stimulation in adult mice. *Neuron* **34**, 265–273.

Knyihar-Csillik, E., Csillik, . and Rakic, P. (1982a). Ultrastructure of normal and degenerating glomerular terminals of dorsal root axons in the substantia gelatinosa of the rhesus monkey. *J. Comp. Neurol.* **210**, 357–375.

Knyihar-Csillik, E., Csillik, B. and Rakic, P. (1982b). Periterminal synaptology of dorsal root glomerular terminals in the substantia gelatinosa of the spinal cord in the rhesus monkey. *J. Comp. Neurol.* **210**, 376–399.

Kolta, A. (1997). In vitro investigation of synaptic relations between interneurons surrounding the trigeminal motor nucleus and masseteric motoneurons. *J. Neurophysiol.* **78**, 1720–1725.

Kolta, A., Westberg, K.G. and Lund, J.P. (2000). Identification of brainstem interneurons projecting to the trigeminal motor nucleus and adjacent structures in the rabbit. *J. Chem. Neuroanat.* **19**, 175–195.

Kruger, L. (1979). Functional subdivision of the brainstem sensory trigeminal nuclear complex. In: Bonica, J.J., Liebeskind, J.C., Albe-Fessard, D.G. (Eds.), *Advances in Pain Research and Therapy.* **Vol. 3**, Raven Press, New York, pp. 127–130.

Langosch, D., Becker, C.M. and Betz, H. (1990). The inhibitory glycine receptor: a ligand-gated chloride channel of the central nervous system. *Eur. J. Biochem.* **194**, 1–8.

Lawson, S.N. and Waddell, P.J. (1991). Soma neurofilament immunoreactivity is related to cell size and fibre conduction velocity in rat primary sensory neurons. *J. Physiol.* **435**, 41–63.

Li, J.L., Kaneko, T., Shigemoto, R. and Mizuno, N. (1997). Distribution of trigeminohypothalamic and spinohypothalamic tract neurons displaying substance P receptor-like immunoreactivity in the rat. *J. Comp. Neurol.* **378**, 508–521.

Li, J.L., Wu, S.X., Tomioka, R., Okamoto, K., Nakamura, K., Kaneko, T. and Mizuno, N. (2005). Efferent and afferent connections of GABAergic neurons in the supratrigeminal and the intertrigeminal regions. An immunohistochemical tract-tracing study in the GAD67-GFP knock-in mouse. *Neurosci. Res.* **51**, 81–91.

Li, Y.Q., Tao, F.S., Okamoto, K., Nomura, S., Kaneko, T. and Mizuno, N. (2002). The supratrigeminal region of the rat sends GABA/glycine-cocontaining axon terminals to the motor trigeminal nucleus on the contralateral side. *Neurosci. Lett.* **330**, 13–16.

Lingenhöhl, K. and Friauf, E. (1991). Sensory neurons and motoneurons of the jaw-closing reflex pathway in rats: a combined morphological and physiological study using the intracellular horseradish peroxidase technique. *Exp. Brain Res.* **83**, 385–396.

Lisney, S.J. and Matthews, B. (1978). Branched afferent nerves supplying tooth-pulp in the cat. *J. Physiol.* **279**, 509–517.

Luccarini, P., Cadet, R., Duale, C. and Woda, A. (1998). Effects of lesions in the trigeminal oralis and caudalis subnuclei on different orofacial nociceptive responses in the rat. *Brain Res.* **803**, 79–85.

Luo, P.F. and Li, J.S. (1991). Monosynaptic connections between neurons of trigeminal mesencephalic nucleus and jaw-closing motoneurons in the rat: an intracellular horseradish peroxidase labeling study. *Brain Res.* **559**, 267–275.

Luo, P. and Dessem, D. (1995). Inputs from identified jaw-muscle spindle afferents to trigeminothalamic neurons in the rat: a double-labeling study using retrograde HRP and intracellular biotinamide. *J. Comp. Neurol.* **353**, 50–66.

Luo, P. and Dessem, D. (1999). Ultrastructural anatomy of physiologically identified jaw-muscle spindle afferent terminations onto retrogradely labeled jaw-elevator motoneurons in the rat. *J. Comp. Neurol.* **406**, 384–401.

Luo, P., Wong, R. and Dessem, D. (1995). Ultrastructural basis for synaptic transmission between jaw-muscle spindle afferents and trigeminothalamic neurons in the rostral trigeminal sensory nuclei of the rat. *J. Comp. Neurol.* **363**, 109–128.

Luo, P., Dessem, D. and Zhang, J. (2001). Axonal projections and synapses from the supratrigeminal region to hypoglossal motoneurons in the rat. *Brain Res.* **890**, 314–329.

Luo, P., Zhang, J., Yang, R. and Pendlebury, W. (2006). Neuronal circuitry and synaptic organization of trigeminal proprioceptive afferents mediating tongue movement and jaw-tongue coordination via hypoglossal premotor neurons. *Eur. J. Neurosci.* **23**, 3269–3283.

Lynch, J.W. (2009). Native glycine receptor subtypes and their physiological roles. *Neuropharmacology* **56**, 303–309.

Malick, A., Strassman, R.M. and Burstein, R. (2000). Trigeminohypothalamic and reticulohypothalamic tract neurons in the upper cervical spinal cord and caudal medulla of the rat. *J. Neurophysiol.* **84**, 2078–2112.

Marfurt, C.F. (1981). The central projections of trigeminal primary afferent neurons in the cat as determined by the tranganglionic transport of horseradish peroxidase. *J. Comp. Neurol.* **203**, 785–798.

Marfurt, C.F. and Rajchert, D.M. (1991). Trigeminal primary afferent projections to "non-trigeminal" areas of the rat central nervous system. *J. Comp. Neurol.* **303**, 489–511.

Marfurt, C.F. and Turner, D.F. (1984). The central projections of tooth pulp afferent neurons in the rat as determined by the transganglionic transport of horseradish peroxidase. *J. Comp. Neurol.* **223**, 535–547.

Martin-Schild, S., Gerall, A.A., Kastin, A.J. and Zadina, J.E. (1999). Differential distribution of endomorphin 1- and endomorphin 2-like immunoreactivities in the CNS of the rodent. *J. Comp. Neurol.* **405**, 450–471.

Matthews, B. (1977). Responses of intradental nerves to electrical and thermal stimulation of teeth in dogs. *J. Physiol.* **264**, 641–664.

Matthews, M.A., Hernandez, T.V., Hoffmann, K.D., Romanska, A.I. and Liles, S.L. (1989). Synaptic substrates for enkephalinergic and serotoninergic interactions with dental primary afferent terminals in trigeminal subnucleus interpolaris: an immunocytochemical study using peroxidase and colloidal gold. *Synapse* **4**, 175–195.

Maxwell, D.J. and Bannatyne, B.A. (1983). Ultrastructure of muscle spindle afferent terminations in lamina VI of the cat spinal cord. *Brain Res.* **288**, 297–301.

Maxwell, D.J. and Riddell, J.S. (1999). Axoaxonic synapses on terminals of group II muscle spindle afferent axons in the spinal cord of the cat. *Eur. J. Neurosci.* **11**, 2151–2159.

Maxwell, D.J., Bannatyne, B.A., Fyffe, R.E. and Brown, A.G. (1982). Ultrastructure of hair follicle afferent fibre terminations in the spinal cord of the cat. *J. Neurocytol.* **11**, 571–582.

Maxwell, D.J., Christie, W.M., Short, A.D. and Brown, A.G. (1990). Direct observations of synapses between GABA-immunoreactive boutons and muscle afferent terminals in lamina VI of the cat's spinal cord. *Brain Res.* **530**, 215–222.

McGrath, P.A., Gracely, R.H., Dubner, R. and Heft, M.W. (1983). Non-pain and pain sensations evoked by tooth pulp stimulation. *Pain* **15**, 377–388.

McNeill, D.L., Coggeshall, R.E. and Carlton, S.M. (1988). A light and electron microscopic study of calcitonin gene-related peptide in the spinal cord of the rat. *Exp. Neurol.* **99**, 699–708.

Mitchell, K., Spike, R.C. and Todd, A.J. (1993). An immunocytochemical study of glycine receptor and GABA in laminae I–III of rat spinal dorsal horn. *J. Neurosci.* **13**, 2371–2381.

Miyoshi, Y., Suemune, S., Yoshida, A., Takemura, M., Nagase, Y. and Shigenaga, Y. (1994). Central terminations of low-threshold mechanoreceptive afferents in the trigeminal nuclei interpolaris and caudalis of the cat. *J. Comp. Neurol.* **340**, 207–232.

Moon, Y.S., Paik, S.K., Seo, J.H., Yi, H.W., Cho, Y.S., Moritani, M., Yoshida, A., Ahn, D.K., Kim, Y. S. and Bae, Y.C. (2008). GABA- and glycine-like immunoreactivity in axonal endings presynaptic to the vibrissa afferents in the cat trigeminal interpolar nucleus. *Neuroscience* **152**, 138–145.

Mori, M., Gähwiler, B.H. and Gerber, U. (2002). Beta-alanine and taurine as endogenous agonists at glycine receptors in rat hippocampus in vitro. *J. Physiol.* **539**, 191–200.

Moritani, M., Yoshida, A., Honma, S., Nagase, Y., Takemura, M. and Shigenaga, Y. (1998). Morphological differences between fast and slowly adapting lingual afferent terminations in the principal and oral nuclei in the cat. *J. Comp. Neurol.* **396**, 64–83.

Naftel, J.P., Bernanke, J.M. and Qian, X.B. (1994). Quantitative study of the apical nerve fibers of adult and juvenile rat molars. *Anat. Rec.* **238**, 507–516.

Nair, P.N. and Schroeder, H.E. (1995). Number and size spectra of non-myelinated axons of human premolars. *Anat. Embryol. (Berl)* **192**, 35–41.

Nakagawa, S., Kurata, S., Yoshida, A., Nagase, Y., Moritani, M., Takemura, M., Bae, Y.C. and Shigenaga, Y. (1997). Ultrastructural observations of synaptic connections of vibrissa afferent terminals in cat principal sensory nucleus and morphometry of related synaptic elements. *J. Comp. Neurol.* **389**, 12–33.

Närhi, M.V. (1985). Dentin sensitivity: a review. *J. Biol. Buccale.* **13**, 75–96.

Närhi, M.V. (1990). The neurophysiology of the teeth. *Dent. Clin. North Am.* **34**, 439–448.

Newman, H.M., Stevens, R.T. and Apkarian, A.V. (1996). Direct spinal projections to limbic and striatal areas: anterograde transport studies from the upper cervical spinal cord and the cervical enlargement in squirrel monkey and rat. *J. Comp. Neurol.* **365**, 640–658.

Ohta, M. and Moriyama, Y. (1986). Supratrigeminal neurons mediate the shortest, disynaptic pathway from the central amygdaloid nucleus to the contralateral trigeminal motoneurons in the rat. *Comp. Biochem. Physiol. A Comp. Physiol.* **83**, 633–641.

Olgart, L., Gazelius, B. and Sundström, F. (1988). Intradental nerve activity and jaw-opening reflex in response to mechanical deformation of cat teeth. *Acta Physiol. Scand.* **133**, 399–406.

Olsson, K.A. and Westberg, K.G. (1991). Integration in trigeminal premotor interneurones in the cat. 2. Functional characteristics of neurones in the subnucleus-gamma of the oral nucleus of the spinal trigeminal tract with a projection to the digastric motoneurone subnucleus. *Exp. Brain Res.* **84**, 115–124.

Olszewski, J. (1950). On the anatomical and functional organization of the spinal trigeminal nucleus. *J. Comp. Neurol.* **92**, 401–413.

Paik, S.K., Oh, S.J., Son, Y.J., Ma, S.K., Ahn, C.H., Kim, S.K., Chang, Z., Moritani, M., Yoshida, A. and Bae, Y.C. (2005). Neural mechanisms controlling jaw-jerk reflex in the cat. *Neuroreport* **16**, 1565–1568.

Paik, S.K., Lee, H.J., Choi, M.K., Cho, Y.S., Park, M.J., Moritani, M., Yoshida, A., Kim, Y.S. and Bae, Y.C. (2009a). Ultrastructural analysis of glutamate-, GABA-, and glycine-immunopositive boutons from supratrigeminal premotoneurons in the rat trigeminal motor nucleus. *J. Neurosci. Res.* **87**, 1115–1122.

Paik, S.K., Park, K.P., Lee, S.K., Ma, S.K., Cho, Y.S., Kim, Y.K., Rhyu, I.J., Ahn, D.K., Yoshida, A. and Bae, Y.C. (2009b). Light and electron microscopic analysis of the somata and parent axons innervating the rat upper molar and lower incisor pulp. *Neuroscience* **162**, 1279–1286.

Paik, S.K., Lee, D.S., Kim, J.Y., Bae, J.Y., Cho, Y.S., Ahn, D.K., Yoshida, A. and Bae, Y.C. (2010). Quantitative ultrastructural analysis of the neurofilament 200-positive axons in the rat dental pulp. *J. Endod.* **36**, 1638–1642.

Pajot, J., Pelissier, T., Sierralta, F., Raboisson, P. and Dallel, R. (2000). Differential effects of trigeminal tractotomy on Adelta- and C-fiber-mediated nociceptive responses. *Brain Res.* **863**, 289–292.

Peng, Y.B., Ringkamp, M., Campbell, J.N. and Meyer, R.A. (1999). Electrophysiological assessment of the cutaneous arborization of Adelta-fiber nociceptors. *J. Neurophysiol.* **82**, 1164–1177.

Petrus, M., Peier, A.M., Bandell, M., Hwang, S.W., Huynh, T., Olney, N., Jegla, T. and Patapoutian, A. (2007). A role of TRPA1 in mechanical hyperalgesia is revealed by pharmacological inhibition. *Mol. Pain* **3**, 40.

Pfaller, K. and Arvidsson, J. (1988). Central distribution of trigeminal and upper cervical primary afferents in the rat studied by anterograde transport of horseradish peroxidase conjugated to wheat germ agglutinin. *J. Comp. Neurol.* **268**, 91–108.

Pierce, J.P. and Mendell, L.M. (1993). Quantitative ultrastructure of Ia boutons in the ventral horn: scaling and positional relationships. *J. Neurosci.* **13**, 4748–4763.

Propst, J.W. and Ko, C.P. (1987). Correlations between active zone ultrastructure and synaptic function studied with freeze-fracture of physiologically identified neuromuscular junctions. *J. Neurosci.* **7**, 3654–3664.

Ralston 3rd, H.J. (1979). The fine structure of laminae I, II, and III of the macaque spinal cord. *J. Comp. Neurol.* **184**, 619–642.

Ralston 3rd, H.J., Light, A.R., Ralston, D.D. and Perl, E.R. (1984). Morphology and synaptic relationships of physiologically identified low-threshold dorsal root axons stained with intra-axonal horseradish peroxidase in the cat and monkey. *J. Neurophysiol.* **51**, 777–792.

Rampon, C., Peyron, C., Petit, J.M., Fort, P., Gervasoni, D. and Luppi, P.H. (1996). Origin of the glycinergic innervation of the rat trigeminal motor nucleus. *Neuroreport* **7**, 3081–3085.

Réthelyi, M., Light, A.R. and Perl, E.R. (1982). Synaptic complexes formed by functionally defined primary afferent units with fine myelinated fibers. *J. Comp. Neurol.* **207**, 381–393.

Ribeiro-da-Silva, A. and Coimbra, A. (1982). Two types of synaptic glomeruli and their distribution in laminae I–III of the rat spinal cord. *J. Comp. Neurol.* **209**, 176–186.

Ribeiro-da-Silva, A. and Cuello, A.C. (1990). Choline acetyltransferase-immunoreactive profiles are presynaptic to primary sensory fibers in the rat superficial dorsal horn. *J. Comp. Neurol.* **295**, 370–384.

Ruda, M.A. (1982). Opiates and Pain pathways: demonstration of enkephalin synapses on dorsal horn projection neurons. *Science* **215**, 1523–1525.

Ruda, M.A., Bennett, G.J. and Dubner, R. (1986). Neurochemistry and neural circuitry in the dorsal horn. *Prog. Brain Res.* **66**, 219–268.

Rudomin, P. (1990). Presynaptic inhibition of muscle spindle and tendon organ afferents in the mammalian spinal cord. *Trends Neurosci.* **13**, 499–505.

Scherrer, G., Imamachi, N., Cao, Y.Q., Contet, C., Mennicken, F., O'Donnell, D., Kieffer, B.L. and Basbaum, A.I. (2009). Dissociation of the opioid receptor mechanisms that control mechanical and heat Pain. *Cell* **137**, 1148–1159.

Semba, K., Masarachia, P., Malamed, S., Jacquin, M., Harris, S., Yang, G. and Egger, M.D. (1983). An electron microscopic study of primary afferent terminals from slowly adapting type I receptors in the cat. *J. Comp. Neurol.* **221**, 466–481.

Semba, K., Masarachia, P., Malamed, S., Jacquin, M., Harris, S. and Egger, M.D. (1984). Ultrastructure of pacinian corpuscle primary afferent terminals in the cat spinal cord. *Brain Res.* **302**, 135–150.

Semba, K., Masarachia, P., Malamed, S., Jacquin, M., Harris, S., Yang, G. and Egger, M.D. (1985). An electron microscopic study of terminals of rapidly adapting mechanoreceptive afferent fibers in the cat spinal cord. *J. Comp. Neurol.* **232**, 229–240.

Sessle, B.J. (1987). The neurobiology of facial and dental Pain: present knowledge, future directions. *J. Dent. Res.* **66**, 962–981.

Sessle, B.J. (2000). Acute and chronic craniofacial Pain: brainstem mechanisms of nociceptive transmission and neuroplasticity, and their clinical correlates. *Crit. Rev. Oral Biol. Med.* **11**, 57–91.

Shigenaga, Y., Okamoto, T., Nishimori, T., Suemune, S., Nasution, I.D., Chen, I.C., Tsuru, K., Yoshida, A., Tabuchi, K., Hosoi, M. and Tsuru, H. (1986a). Oral and facial representation in the trigeminal principal and rostral spinal nuclei of the cat. *J. Comp. Neurol.* **244**, 1–18.

Shigenaga, Y., Suemune, S., Nishimura, M., Nishimori, T., Sato, H., Ishidori, H., Yoshida, A., Tsuru, K., Tsuiki, Y., Dateoka, Y., Nasution, I.D. and Hosoi, M. (1986b). Topographic representation of lower and upper teeth within the trigeminal sensory nuclei of adult cat as demonstrated by the transganglionic transport of horseradish peroxidase. *J. Comp. Neurol.* **251**, 299–316.

Shigenaga, Y., Yoshida, A., Mitsuhiro, Y., Tsuru, K. and Doe, K. (1988). Morphological and functional properties of trigeminal nucleus oralis neurons projecting to the trigeminal motor nucleus of the cat. *Brain Res.* **461**, 143–149.

Shigenaga, Y., Nishimura, M., Suemune, S., Nishimori, T., Doe, K. and Tsuru, H. (1989a). Somatotopic organization of tooth pulp primary afferent neurons in the cat. *Brain Res.* **477**, 66–89.

Shigenaga, Y., Doe, K., Suemune, S., Mitsuhiro, Y., Tsuru, K., Otani, K., Shirana, Y., Hosoi, M., Yoshida, A. and Kagawa, K. (1989b). Physiological and morphological characteristics of periodontal mesencephalic trigeminal neurons in the cat–intra-axonal staining with HRP. *Brain Res.* **505**, 91–110.

Shigenaga, Y., Otani, K. and Suemune, S. (1990). Morphology of central terminations of low-threshold trigeminal primary afferents from facial skin in the cat–intra-axonal staining with HRP. *Brain Res.* **523**, 23–50.

Shigenaga, Y., Hirose, Y., Yoshida, A., Fukami, H., Honma, S. and Bae, Y.C. (2000). Quantitative ultrastructure of physiologically identified premotoneuron terminals in the trigeminal motor nucleus in the cat. *J. Comp. Neurol.* **426**, 13–30.

Souslova, V., Cesare, P., Ding, Y., Akopian, A.N., Stanfa, L., Suzuki, R., Carpenter, K., Dickenson, A., Boyce, S., Hill, R., Nebenuis-Oosthuizen, D., Smith, A.J., Kidd, E.J. and Wood, J.N. (2000). Warm-coding deficits and aberrant inflammatory Pain in mice lacking P2X3 receptors. *Nature* **407**, 1015–1017.

Stornetta, R.L., Sevigny, C.P. and Guyenet, P.G. (2002). Vesicular glutamate transporter DNPI/VGLUT2 mRNA is present in C1 and several other groups of brainstem catecholaminergic neurons. *J. Comp. Neurol.* **444**, 191–206.

Story, G.M. (2006). The Emerging Role of TRP Channels in Mechanisms of Temperature and Pain Sensation. *Curr. Neuropharmacol.* **4**, 183–196.

Sudhof, T.C. (2004). The synaptic vesicle cycle. *Annu. Rev. Neurosci.* **27**, 509–547.

Sugimoto, T., Takemura, M. and Wakisaka, S. (1988). Cell size analysis of primary neurons innervating the cornea and tooth pulp of the rat. *Pain* **32**, 375–381.

Sugimoto, T., Nagase, Y., Nishiguchi, T., Kitamura, S. and Shigenaga, Y. (1991). Synaptic connections of a low-threshold mechanoreceptive primary neuron within the trigeminal subnucleus oralis. *Brain Res.* **548**, 338–342.

Sugimoto, T. and Takemura, M. (1993). Tooth pulp primary neurons: cell size analysis, central connection, and carbonic anhydrase activity. *Brain Res. Bull.* **30**, 221–226.

Sugimoto, T., Fujiyoshi, Y., Xiao, C., He, Y.F. and Ichikawa, H. (1997). Central projection of calcitonin gene-related peptide (CGRP)- and substance P (SP)-immunoreactive trigeminal primary neurons in the rat. *J. Comp. Neurol.* **378**, 425–442.

Sugimoto, T., He, Y.F., Xiao, C. and Ichikawa, H. (1998). c-Fos induction in the subnucleus oralis following trigeminal nerve stimulation. *Brain Res.* **783**, 158–162.

Sumal, K.K., Pickel, V.M., Miller, R.J. and Reis, D.J. (1982). Enkephalin-containing neurons in substantia gelatinosa of spinal trigeminal complex: ultrastructure and synaptic interaction with primary sensory afferents. *Brain Res.* **248**, 223–236.

Sutherland, F.I., Bannatyne, B.A., Kerr, R., Riddell, J.S. and Maxwell, D.J. (2002). Inhibitory amino acid transmitters associated with axons in presynaptic apposition to cutaneous primary afferent axons in the cat spinal cord. *J. Comp. Neurol.* **452**, 154–162.

Svingos, A.L., Moriwaki, A., Wang, J.B., Uhl, G.R. and Pickel, V.M. (1996). Ultrastructural immunocytochemical localization of mu-opioid receptors in rat nucleus accumbens: extrasynaptic plasmalemmal distribution and association with Leu5-enkephalin. *J. Neurosci.* **16**, 4162–4173.

Svingos, A.L., Moriwaki, A., Wang, J.B., Uhl, G.R. and Pickel, V.M. (1997). mu-Opioid receptors are localized to extrasynaptic plasma membranes of GABAergic neurons and their targets in the rat nucleus accumbens. *J. Neurosci.* **17**, 2585–2594.

Takata, M. and Fujita, S. (1982). The properties of excitatory postsynaptic potentials evoked in trigeminal motoneurons by trigeminal nerve stimulation. *Brain Res.* **241**, 171–175.

Takemura, M., Sugimoto, T. and Shigenaga, Y. (1991). Difference in central projection of primary afferents innervating facial and intraoral structures in the rat. *Exp. Neurol.* **111**, 324–331.

Takemura, M., Nagase, Y., Yoshida, A., Yasuda, K., Kitamura, S., Shigenaga, Y. and Matano, S. (1993). The central projections of the monkey tooth pulp afferent neurons. *Somatosens. Mot. Res.* **10**, 217–227.

Takemura, M., Shimada, T., Sugiyo, S., Nokubi, T. and Shigenaga, Y. (2000). Mapping of c-Fos in the trigeminal sensory nucleus following high- and low-intensity afferent stimulation in the rat. *Exp. Brain Res.* **130**, 113–123.

Todd, A.J. (1996). GABA and glycine in synaptic glomeruli of the rat spinal dorsal horn. *Eur. J. Neurosci.* **8**, 2492–2498.

Todd, A.J. and Spike, R.C. (1993). The localization of classical transmitters and neuropeptides within neurons in laminae I–III of the mammalian spinal dorsal horn. *Prog. Neurobiol.* **41**, 609–645.

Todd, A.J., Maxwell, D.J. and Brown, A.G. (1991). Relationships between hair-follicle afferent axons and glycine-immunoreactive profiles in cat spinal dorsal horn. *Brain Res.* **564**, 132–137.

Todd, A.J., Spike, R.C., Chong, D. and Neilson, M. (1995). The relationship between glycine and gephyrin in synapses of the rat spinal cord. *Eur. J. Neurosci.* **7**, 1–11.

Tominaga, M., Caterina, M.J., Malmberg, A.B., Rosen, T.A., Gilbert, H., Skinner, K., Raumann, B. E., Basbaum, A.I. and Julius, D. (1998). The cloned capsaicin receptor integrates multiple Pain-producing stimuli. *Neuron* **21**, 531–543.

Tse, F.W., Marin, L., Jahromi, S.S. and Atwood, H.L. (1991). Variation in terminal morphology and presynaptic inhibition at crustacean neuromuscular junctions. *J. Comp. Neurol.* **304**, 135–146.

Tsuda, M., Ueno, S. and Inoue, K. (1999). In vivo pathway of thermal hyperalgesia by intrathecal administration of alpha,beta-methylene ATP in mouse spinal cord: involvement of the glutamate-NMDA receptor system. *Br. J. Pharmacol.* **127**, 449–456.

Turman Jr, J.E. and Chandler, S.H. (1994a). Immunohistochemical evidence for GABA and glycine-containing trigeminal premotoneurons in the guinea pig. *Synapse* **18**, 7–20.

Turman Jr, J.E. and Chandler, S.H. (1994b). Immunohistochemical localization of glutamate and glutaminase in guinea pig trigeminal premotoneurons. *Brain Res.* **634**, 49–61.

Turner, D.F. and Marfurt, C.F. (1988). Uptake and transneuronal transport of horseradish peroxidase-wheat germ agglutinin by tooth pulp primary afferent neurons. *Brain Res.* **452**, 381–387.

Uchizono, K. (1965). Characteristics of excitatory and inhibitory synapses in the central nervous system of the cat. *Nature* **207**, 642–643.

Valdivia, O. (1971). Methods of fixation and the morphology of synaptic vesicles. *J. Comp. Neurol.* **142**, 257–273.

Virtanen, A.S., Huopaniemi, T., Närhi, M.V., Pertovaara, A. and Wallgren, K. (1987). The effect of temporal parameters on subjective sensations evoked by electrical tooth stimulation. *Pain* **30**, 361–371.

Wall, P.D. (1994). Impulses in the rostral branch of primary afferents in rat dorsal columns travel faster than those in the caudal branch. *Neurosci. Lett.* **165**, 75–78.

Wall, P.D. (1998). Some unanswered questions about the mechanisms and function of presynaptic inhibition. In: Rudomin, P., Romo, R., Mendell, L.M. (Eds.), *Presynaptic Inhibition and Neural Control.* Oxford University Press, New York, pp. 232.

Walmsley, B., Graham, B. and Nicol, M.J. (1995). Serial E–M and simulation study of presynaptic inhibition along a group Ia collateral in the spinal cord. *J. Neurophysiol.* **74**, 616–623.

Wang, H., Wei, F., Dubner, R. and Ren, K. (2006). Selective distribution and function of primary afferent nociceptive inputs from deep muscle tissue to the brainstem trigeminal transition zone. *J. Comp. Neurol.* **498**, 390–402.

Wang, H.B., Zhao, B., Zhong, Y.Q., Li, K.C., Li, Z.Y., Wang, Q., Lu, Y.J., Zhang, Z.N., He, S.Q., Zheng, H.C., Wu, S.X., Hökfelt, T.G., Bao, L. and Zhang, X. (2010). Coexpression of delta- and mu-opioid receptors in nociceptive sensory neurons. *Proc. Natl. Acad. Sci. U. S. A.* **107**, 13117–13122.

Watson, A.H. (2003). GABA- and glycine-like immunoreactivity in axons and dendrites contacting the central terminals of rapidly adapting glabrous skin afferents in rat spinal cord. *J. Comp. Neurol.* **464**, 497–510.

Watson, A.H. (2004). Synaptic interactions between the terminals of slow-adapting type II mechano-receptor afferents and neurones expressing gamma-aminobutyric acid- and glycine-like immuno-reactivity in the rat spinal cord. *J. Comp. Neurol.* **471**, 168–179.

Watson, A.H. and Bazzaz, A.A. (2001). GABA and glycine-like immunoreactivity at axoaxonic synapses on 1a muscle afferent terminals in the spinal cord of the rat. *J. Comp. Neurol.* **433**, 335–348.

Watson, A.H., Hughes, D.I. and Bazzaz, A.A. (2002). Synaptic relationships between hair follicle afferents and neurones expressing GABA and glycine-like immunoreactivity in the spinal cord of the rat. *J. Comp. Neurol.* **452**, 367–380.

Westberg, K.G. and Olsson, K.A. (1991). Integration in trigeminal premotor interneurones in the cat. 1. Functional characteristics of neurones in the subnucleus-gamma of the oral nucleus of the spinal trigeminal tract. *Exp. Brain Res.* **84**, 102–114.

Westberg, K.G., Sandström, G. and Olsson, K.A. (1995). Integration in trigeminal premotor interneurones in the cat. 3. Input characteristics and synaptic actions of neurones in subnucleus-gamma of the oral nucleus of the spinal trigeminal tract with a projection to the masseteric motoneurone subnucleus. *Exp. Brain Res.* **104**, 449–461.

Westrum, L.E., Canfield, R.C. and O'Connor, T.A. (1980). Projections from dental structures to the brain stem trigeminal complex as shown by transganglionic transport of horseradish peroxidase. *Neurosci. Lett.* **20**, 31–36.

Westrum, L.E., Canfield, R.C. and O'Connor, T.A. (1981). Each canine tooth projects to all brain stem trigeminal nuclei in cat. *Exp. Neurol.* **74**, 787–799.

Yabuta, N.H., Yasuda, K., Nagase, Y., Yoshida, A., Fukunishi, Y. and Shigenaga, Y. (1996). Light microscopic observations of the contacts made between two spindle afferent types and alpha-motoneurons in the cat trigeminal motor nucleus. *J. Comp. Neurol.* **374**, 436–450.

Yeo, E.J., Cho, Y.S., Paik, S.K., Yoshida, A., Park, M.J., Ahn, D.K., Moon, C., Kim, Y.S. and Bae, Y. C. (2010). Ultrastructural analysis of the synaptic connectivity of TRPV1-expressing primary afferent terminals in the rat trigeminal caudal nucleus. *J. Comp. Neurol.* **518**, 4134–4146.

Yeow, M.B. and Peterson, E.H. (1991). Active zone organization and vesicle content scale with bouton size at a vertebrate central synapse. *J. Comp. Neurol.* **307**, 475–486.

Yoshida, A., Dostrovsky, J.O., Sessle, B.J. and Chiang, C.Y. (1991). Trigeminal projections to the nucleus submedius of the thalamus in the rat. *J. Comp. Neurol.* **307**, 609–625.

Yoshida, A., Yasuda, K., Dostrovsky, J.O., Bae, Y.C., Takemura, M., Shigenaga, Y. and Sessle, B.J. (1994). Two major types of premotoneurons in the feline trigeminal nucleus oralis as demonstrated by intracellular staining with horseradish peroxidase. *J. Comp. Neurol.* **347**, 495–514.

Yoshida, A., Mukai, N., Moritani, M., Nagase, Y., Hirose, Y., Honma, S., Fukami, H., Takagi, K., Matsuya, T. and Shigenaga, Y. (1999). Physiologic and morphologic properties of motoneurons and spindle afferents innervating the temporal muscle in the cat. *J. Comp. Neurol.* **406**, 29–50.

Yoshida, A., Fukami, H., Nagase, Y., Appenteng, K., Honma, S., Zhang, L.F., Bae, Y.C. and Shigenaga, Y. (2001). Quantitative analysis of synaptic contacts made between functionally identified oralis neurons and trigeminal motoneurons in cats. *J. Neurosci.* **21**, 6298–6307.

Yoshida, A., Yamamoto, M., Moritani, M., Fukami, H., Bae, Y.C., Chang, Z., Sugiyo, S., Takemura, M., Park, K.P. and Shigenaga, Y. (2005). Bilateral projection of functionally characterized trigeminal oralis neurons to trigeminal motoneurons in cats. *Brain Res.* **1036**, 208–212.

Zhang, J. and Luo, P. (2003). Ultrastructural features of synapse from dorsal parvocellular reticular formation neurons to hypoglossal motoneurons of the rat. *Brain Res.* **963**, 262–273.

Zhang, J., Luo, P. and Pendlebury, W.W. (2001a). Light and electron microscopic observations of a direct projection from mesencephalic trigeminal nucleus neurons to hypoglossal motoneurons in the rat. *Brain Res.* **917**, 67–80.

Zhang, L.F., Moritani, M., Honma, S., Yoshida, A. and Shigenaga, Y. (2001b). Quantitative ultrastructure of slowly adapting lingual afferent terminals in the principal and oral nuclei in the cat. *Synapse* **41**, 96–111.

Zhang, J., Pendlebury, W.W. and Luo, P. (2003). Synaptic organization of monosynaptic connections from mesencephalic trigeminal nucleus neurons to hypoglossal motoneurons in the rat. *Synapse* **49**, 157–169.

MECHANISMS OF NOCICEPTIVE TRANSDUCTION AND TRANSMISSION: A MACHINERY FOR PAIN SENSATION AND TOOLS FOR SELECTIVE ANALGESIA

Alexander M. Binshtok

Department of Medical Neurobiology, Institute for Medical Research Israel Canada and Center for Research on Pain, The Hebrew University Medical School, Jerusalem, Israel

I. Introduction

Within hundred thousands of years of evolution, pain has always been absolutely important if not crucial for species survival. Recent studies on families with congenital insensitivity to pain emphasize the significance of pain phenomenon for well being if not for "being" (Indo *et al.*, 1996; Cox *et al.*, 2006). However, the agony of the dental patients in medieval times clearly demonstrates that there are states and settings, at which the cessation of the activity of the pain system is essential. How can the operational or the dental pain be targeted and selectively and reversibly blocked? In this chapter we will review the current literature describing how pain sensing peripheral nervous system detects and transmits noxious stimuli. We will also review recent findings describing the properties of the proteins that participate in pain transduction and transmission, and will introduce novel therapeutic approaches that were developed based on these findings. These novel methods of targeted delivery allow, for the first time to reach the "holy grail" of local anesthesia i.e. to produce pain-selective analgesia.

DOI: 10.1016/B978-0-12-385198-7.00006-0

0074-7742/10 $35.00

II. Nociception –the First Line of Defense

To rephrase the famous adage from Sun Tzu's Art of War, "know your enemy", biological organisms must know about danger in order to deal with it efficiently. This is what nociceptors do: These primary sensory neurons are specialized in detecting intense stimuli using a repertoire of specific high threshold heat-sensitive, mechanical-sensitive, or chemical-sensitive ion channels (Woolf and Ma, 2007). These channels, also called transducer channels, detect and quantify noxious stimuli, and report them in the form of inward currents that in turn create generator potentials. Then, after an activation threshold has been exceeded, activation of different subtypes of sodium channels lead to a flow of action potentials from the periphery toward the central nervous system (CNS), to signal the presence, location and intensity of noxious stimuli. Inflammation- or injury-mediated modulation of activation or inactivation kinetics of these channels, as well as changes in their conductance and open probability, affect the quality of transmitted information and change the output of nociceptive peripheral neurons to the CNS, thereby increasing pain (Hucho and Levine, 2007). Thus, understanding the function of transducer and voltage-sensitive channels expressed by nociceptive terminals is imperative for understanding pain perception. The identification and characterization of nociceptive specific transducers over the past decade, starting with the noxious heat sensitive TRPV1 (Caterina *et al.*, 1997), now includes detectors of noxious chemical irritants (e.g., TRPA1), noxious cold detectors (e.g., TRPM8, TRPA1), and acid sensing ion channels (e.g. ASICs) (Patapoutian *et al.*, 2009). By using this wide repertoire of transducer channels, nociceptors encode and process noxious stimuli (Loeser and Treede, 2008).

At the target organs, nociceptive neurons "compete" for the place under the sun with low-threshold sensory neurons that convey innocuous information (Meyer *et al.*, 2008). Interestingly, this co-localization does not exist in tooth pulp where the application of any (even innocuous) stimuli to the human tooth pulp produce pain and only pain (Cook *et al.*, 1997), implying that nociceptors are the only set of nerve endings that innervate this organ. These nociceptors belong to the particular class of pain-sensing neurons C-fibers the tiniest and myelin-less type of nerve fibers. Tooth dentine are innervated by another type of nociceptive neurons, thinly-myelinated (Aδ-fibers). This clear differentiation of receptive field provides a unique model to study the distinctive properties of C and Aδ-fibers (Jyvasjarvi and Kniffki, 1987).

It is clear now that the thinly-myelinated fibers are responsible for the acute well localized sharp and stinging pain, whereas C-fibers transport the dull and dragging shade of pain.

Aδ-fibers could be further classified based on the activation threshold. Type I, also called high-threshold mechanical nociceptors (HTM), respond to both mechanical and chemical stimuli. In naïve conditions, HTM neurons are likely to mediate the first pain provoked by pinprick and other intense mechanical stimuli. Relatively high heat threshold of these fibers decreases after tissue injury, thus they become sensitive to heat stimuli too. Fibers that belong to Type II of Aδ-nociceptors have a much lower heat threshold, but a very high mechanical threshold. Activity of this afferent fibers almost certainly mediates the "first" acute pain response to noxious heat (for review see (Basbaum *et al.*, 2009)).

Nociceptive C-fibers, composed of polymodal fibers are sensitive both to heat and mechanical stimuli (CMH-fibers) and selective heat-sensitive nociceptors (Perl, 2007). The latter are more sensitive to chemical stimuli (capsaicin or histamine). This group of fibers responds to mechanical stimuli only after tissue injury and comes into play when the chemical milieu of inflammation alters its properties, therefore these neurons are often called "silent" nociceptors (Schmidt *et al.*, 1995).

Despite substantial progress in identification and characterization of subtypes of nociceptive neurons, the physiology of nociception has not yet been fully revealed. A detailed understanding of the detection and processing of nociceptive stimuli is needed to comprehend peripheral aspects of pain perception and for the development of effective and selective analgesia.

III. Sodium Channels -the Old-new Target for Pain Selective Analgesia

The transmission machinery of nociceptive signals is composed of voltage gated sodium, potassium, and calcium channels ($Na_{(V)}$, $K_{(V)}$, and $Ca_{(V)}$, respectively). A barrage of recent studies demonstrate a substantial contribution of $K_{(V)}$ and $Ca_{(V)}$ both to acute nociception and to perpetuation of pain (Everill and Kocsis, 1999; Kim *et al.*, 2002; Park *et al.*, 2003; Jagodic *et al.*, 2007; Jagodic *et al.*, 2008; Takeda *et al.*, 2008). The detailed characterization of changes in $K_{(V)}$ and $Ca_{(V)}$ and their intriguing role at presynaptic terminals, at the spinal cord is beyond the scope of this review. There are several excellent reviews that summarize our understanding of the function of $K_{(V)}$ and $Ca_{(V)}$ in neuropathic and inflammatory pain (Zamponi *et al.*, 2009; Takeda *et al.*, 2011; Todorovic and Jevtovic-Todorovic, 2011). In short, the dorsal root ganglion (DRG) and trigeminal ganglion (TG) neurons express three distinct classes of potassium currents: slow inactivating sustained current (I_K), fast inactivating transient (I_A) and slow inactivating transient currents (I_D) (Everill *et al.*, 1998). The names of these currents reflect the differences in their kinetics. In addition to the differences in their inactivation rates, pharmacological tools can also distinguish between these currents. I_K current is sensitive to tetraethyl ammonium (TEA), I_A current is blocked by 4-aminopyridine and I_D current is blocked by α-dendrotoxin (α-DTX) (Everill *et al.*, 1998; Yoshida and Matsumoto, 2005). Recent studies in systematically examined changes in potassium currents following nerve injury or inflammation, demonstrated that nerve injury and inflammation produce increase of the density of I_A and I_K (Tsuboi *et al.*, 2004; Kitagawa *et al.*, 2006; Takeda *et al.*, 2006; Takeda *et al.*, 2008; Nakagawa *et al.*, 2010). Thus, chronic construction nerve injury and axotomy lead to hyperexcitability (increase in spike frequency and spike duration and decrease in threshold) in medium, and large diameter injured and uninjured TG neurons (Tsuboi *et al.*, 2004; Kitagawa *et al.*, 2006). Interestingly, proinflammatory cytokines TNFα and IL-1β, in addition to increasing sodium currents as will be described later in this chapter (see also (Binshtok *et al.*, 2008a)), also supress potassium currents in small diameter TG and DRG neurons (Takeda *et al.*, 2008). This effect of TNFα and IL-1β on potassium channels contributes to their acute effect on the excitability of nociceptive neurons.

Transient T-type voltage gated calcium channels, also called low voltage activated (LVA) are expressed in cell bodies and nerve endings of TRPV1-containing nociceptive neurons (Cardenas *et al.*, 1995; Todorovic *et al.*, 2001; Coste *et al.*, 2007; Nelson *et al.*, 2007). In these neurons, Ca(v) 3.2 is the main isoform that underlies T-type current (Talley *et al.*, 1999), since T-type current is absent in DRGs of Cav3.2 knockout mice (Nelson *et al.*, 2007; Chen *et al.*, 2010). Recently, in addition to the small nociceptive neurons that express T-type calcium channels, novel distinct sub-population of medium sized DRG neurons was described. Interestingly, these "T-rich"-neurons express selectively LVA current and not high voltage activated calcium current (Nelson *et al.*, 2005). The roles of these neurons in sensory processing is yet to be determined.

T-type calcium channels have a hyperpolarized the threshold for activation such that only a small depolarization is sufficient to activate the channels. Thus, these channels operate in a subthreshold range and consequently contribute to subthreshold neuronal excitability (Todorovic and Jevtovic-Todorovic, 2011). Activation of T-type calcium channels in nociceptive neurons affects the threshold for action potential generation and even initiates firing of action potentials (Todorovic and Jevtovic-Todorovic, 2006). The expression level of T-type channels is markedly increased in the models of neuropathic pain (Jagodic *et al.*, 2007; Jagodic *et al.*, 2008). Conversely, genetically-induced decrease in the level of the Ca (v)3.2 isoform, as well as pharmacological blockade of the T-type channel reduces excitability of nociceptive neurons and attenuates pain responses (Dogrul *et al.*, 2003; Bourinet *et al.*, 2005; Choi *et al.*, 2007).

These results point out nociceptive selective $K_{(V)}$ and $Ca_{(V)}$ channels as prime targets for the development of novel analgesics.

In this chapter, we gave more space to voltage gated $Na_{(V)}$ channels for several reasons. First, $Na_{(V)}$ activation is crucial for the generation and propagation of neuronal action potentials. The recent discovery of a direct genetic link between sodium channels and pain disorders in humans emphasizes their key role in generation of pain (Cox *et al.*, 2006). Second, there is a growing body of evidence indicating that modulation of these currents is an inflammation-activated endogenous mechanism used to control neuronal excitability (for review see (Dib-Hajj *et al.*, 2010a)). Third, historically, the blockade of sodium channels was and is the most effective way to achieve reversible blockade of pain.

$Na_{(V)}$ underlies the generation and propagation of action potential, the "1" digit of the binary code of the nervous system. The reversible blockade of these channels by sodium channel blockers is widely used for local anesthesia (Hogan *et al.*, 2009; Fredrickson *et al.*, 2010; Hawkins, 2010; Murray *et al.*, 2010; Scott, 2010).

Starting in the midst of the 19th century, using local anesthetics right at the area of injury or around the nerve innervating it was one, or mostly the only way, to block pain pathways at a peripheral, i.e. early stage of pain-development. The first local anesthetic ever to be recognized was cocaine. Albert Niemann, a German chemist, was the first person able to synthesize cocaine out of the coca-plant in 1860. Using available tools to analyze the properties of white powder he created, Niemann tasted it. The numbing of the tongue described by him was the first step into the era of local blockade of pain (Ruetsch *et al.*, 2001; Catterall and Mackie, 2007). The first thorough and systematic research on cocaine was conducted in 1880 by Vassiliy von Anrep (Yentis and Vlassakov, 1999). Following the recommendation of Sigmund Freud, its first introduction into medical procedures happened in 1884 by Carl Koller showing its topical effects when applied to the eye (Koller, 1884). Presenting his findings at a congress in Heidelberg leads to a chain reaction. Not even three months later, William Steward Halsted was able to show a cocaine-mediated nerve block of the mandibular nerve (Ruetsch *et al.*, 2001). In the following 30 years of busy research, almost all the regional anesthetic procedures and techniques still in use today, got developed in their basic layout, and a lot more local anesthetic compounds were introduced, showing better profiles of safety and efficacy. To just mention the most important ones, the first of all the synthetic drugs succeeding cocaine was procaine in 1905, followed by lidocaine in 1947, bupivicaine in 1965, and ropivacaine in 1996 (Ruetsch *et al.*, 2001). Depending on their structure, local anesthetics are divided into two subgroups, namely amino-esters, such as procaine, chloroprocaine, tetracaine and cocaine, and amino-amides, which are mostly all the others, including lidocaine and ropivacaine (Heavner, 2007). Pharmacokinetics of these two subgroups vary greatly from each other, mostly because of the fact that esters get degraded by free plasma pseudocholinesterases, while amides have to go through the whole metabolic machinery of the liver (Heavner, 2007).

The main effect of local anesthetics is the blockade of sodium channels as has been demonstrated by Taylor in his seminal paper in 1959 (Taylor, 1959). Several years after Taylor's description of the targets of local anaesthetics Fraizer *et al.* used quaternary membrane impermeant derivative of lidocaine N-ethyl-lidocaine also called QX-314. QX-314 that carries a permanent positive charge conferred by quaternary nitrogen, and therefore cannot permeate membrane lipid bilayers, was used to demonstrate that when it is applied into the cytoplasm it blocks generation of the action potential. However, if QX-314 is administered from outside of the membrane, no fast changes in membrane potential are observed (Frazier *et al.*, 1970; Strichartz, 1973). Thus, for neuronal sodium channels, local aesthetic molecules can apparently access the binding site only from the cytoplasmic end of the pore.

Lidocaine itself has a tertiary nitrogen with a pKa of 8.2, so that at pH of 7.4 $\sim$15% of the molecules will be in the unprotonated, uncharged state, which is highly permeable and provides rapid entry into the cell (Hille, 1977b). Once inside, protonation occurs to establish charged as well as uncharged forms of the molecule. It is likely that both charged and uncharged forms of the drug can bind and block the channels from the cytoplasmic surface, because benzocaine, an uncharged molecule similar to the uncharged form of lidocaine, blocks sodium channels nearly as potently as does lidocaine (Hille, 1977a, b; Schwarz *et al.*, 1977; Clapham *et al.*, 2001a). The unprotonated form of lidocaine unselectively penetrates axonal membranes and consequently, blocks the action potentials in all sensory, motor, and autonomic fibres. This lack of selectivity limits use of local anaesthetics and produces undesired side effects.

How can a selective block of nociceptors be achieved to produce a local analgesia instead of a non-specific local anaesthesia? One way would be to selectively target those $Na_{(V)}$ that are expressed only or predominantly in nociceptive neurons (Momin and Wood, 2008).

Nociceptive neurons differ from other sensory neurons not just by their small size but also by the expression of selective high threshold transducer and specific isoforms of sodium channels. In general, sodium channels are heteromultimers of large pore-forming α subunits and smaller auxiliary β subunits (Dib-Hajj *et al.*, 2009b). Nine functional α-subunits (Na(v)1.1-Na(v)1.9) of sodium channels have been identified. The sodium cannels that are composed from distinct subunits display differences in kinetics, rates of transition between different states and the dissimilarity in the voltage dependence of these transitions. Nociceptive neurons express five out of nine different isoforms of α subunits of sodium channels (Dib-Hajj *et al.*, 2010a). Remarkably, four out of five sodium channels subtypes are expressed selectively by the pain sensing neurons and play major role in the development and perpetuation of pain. (Dib-Hajj *et al.*, 2009a). The sensitivity to the micromolar concentration of the tetrodotoxin (TTX) – the deadly natural toxin from fugu fish is a property of most of the cardiac and neuronal sodium channels. Thus, seven out of nine subtypes (Na(v)1.1 Na(v)1.7) are also called TTX-sensitive (TTX-S) sodium channels. Interestingly, TTX-resistant (TTX-R) sodium channels, namely Na(v)1.8 and Na(v)1.9, are expressed almost selectively by the pain-sensing neurons. Modulation of these TTX-resistant channels by proinflammatory mediators are likely responsible for inflammation-dependent neuronal hyperexcitability and therefore inflammatory-pain hypersensitivity (Dib-Hajj *et al.*, 2010a).

Activation of Na(v)1.9 channels gives rise to a slow activating and non-inactivating persistent sodium current (Cummins *et al.*, 1999). Considering its slow kinetics, this channel has no significant contribution to the current that underlies action potentials ((Herzog *et al.*, 2001) see also (Dib-Hajj *et al.*, 2002). This assumption is well supported by the results obtained from behavioral experiments on Na(v)1.9 knockout mice. Lack of this channel has no effect on mechanical and thermal responsiveness in the absence of injury (Priest *et al.*, 2005; Amaya *et al.*, 2006). However, there are substantial differences in the responses to noxious thermal stimuli between wild type and knockout mice in the Complete Freud Adjuvant (CFA) (Amaya *et al.*, 2006), formalin, carrageenan, and prostonaids models of inflammatory pain (Priest *et al.*, 2005). Protein kinase C (PKC)-mediated potentiation of Na(v) 1.9 currents might underlie the effect of inflammation on the neuronal excitability (Baker, 2005). These data, together with results demonstrating that Na(v) 1.9 is activated by relatively small voltage deviations from resting potential (Cummins *et al.*, 1999), suggest that Na(v) 1.9 current controls subthreshold excitability of nociceptive neurons and thereby the threshold in these neurons (Cummins *et al.*, 1999; Herzog *et al.*, 2001; Baker *et al.*, 2003; Ostman *et al.*, 2008; Copel *et al.*, 2009).

Pain hypersensitivity at the site of inflammation (primary hyperalgesia) is largely the consequence of the sensitization of the peripheral terminals of nociceptors due to a reduction in their threshold and an increase in their excitability (Hucho and Levine, 2007). Multiple proinflammatory mediators are released soon after injury by the damaged tissue and infiltrating immune cells (Hucho and Levine, 2007). Interestingly, at least in the case of Na(v) 1.9, it looks like indeed it takes two to tango. Proinflammatory mediators such as bradykinin, histamine, prostaglandin E2 (PGE2), and norepinephrine applied alone failed to modulate Na(v) 1.9 current. Application of these proinflammatory factors together, substantially potentiates Na(v) 1.9 currents, and thereby increases excitability of nociceptive neurons (Maingret *et al.*, 2008). This inflammatory soup-mediated increase in nociceptive excitability acts primarily on Na(v) 1.9 channels since this effect is abolished in Na(v) 1.9 −/− animals (Maingret *et al.*, 2008). All of the above suggest that slow activation kinetics and persistence of the Na(v) 1.9 – mediated current confers upon this channel the ability of coincidence detection of multiple proinflammatory mediators. Synergistic action of these mediators, via activation of intracellular kinases, converges onto Na(v) 1.9 channels to alter nociceptive threshold, and thereby produce changes in neuronal excitability that will lead to inflammatory hyperalgesia.

Spontaneous pain during inflammation may arise either from the presence in the inflamed issue of chemicals like ATP that directly activate nociceptors via P2X ligand-gated ion channels or by indirect increase in membrane excitability, triggered by G-protein coupled, or membrane tyrosine kinase receptor mediated activation of intracellular signaling pathways that lead to increased sodium currents; such as occurs for PGE2 via EP receptors and protein kinase (PK) A on another TTX-R sodium channel Na(v) 1.8 (Gold *et al.*, 1998).

Na(v) 1.8 is a sensory neuron specific channel that underlies slowly activating and inactivating TTX-R currents (Akopian *et al.*, 1996; Akopian *et al.*, 1999). Na(v) 1.8 is expressed by DRG and trigeminal nociceptive neurons (Djouhri *et al.*, 2003) and has been shown to accumulate within the nerve terminals of the skin (Zimmermann *et al.*, 2007; Persson *et al.*, 2010). All TTX-S currents acting in nociceptive neurons have relatively hyperpolarized steady-state activation and inactivation characteristics. Thus at the potentials around the threshold, a major fraction of TTX-S channels undergo fast inactivation. Activation-inactivation voltage dependence of Na(v) 1.8 channels is shifted rightward, producing a substantial window current that peaks around the threshold (Cummins and Waxman, 1997). Consequently, the Na(v) 1.8 mediated current contributes most of the sodium current for the upstroke of the action potential (Renganathan *et al.*, 2001; Blair and Bean, 2002). The application of TTX in micromolar concentration to nociceptive neurons does not abolish action potential, as it does for central neurons (Renganathan *et al.*, 2001). Due to depolarized voltage dependence of inactivation and its rapid repriming (recovery from inactivation), Na(v) 1.8 can sustain long depolarization and therefore underlie the repetitive firing of action potential (Renganathan *et al.*, 2001; Blair and Bean, 2002).

Postmytotic ablation of Na(v) 1.8 expressing fibres using diphtheria toxin shows that these neurons are essential for mechanical and cold evoked acute pain, and for inflammatory pain but not for neuropathic pain (Abrahamsen *et al.*, 2008). Unique resistance of the slow inactivation machinery of Na(v) 1.8 channel to cold temperatures, underlies the availability of this channel as a stand alone transmitter of noxious cold (Zimmermann *et al.*, 2007).

Recent findings emphasize the role of TTX-R sodium channels in the direct response of nociceptors to inflammatory cytokines. The two prototypic proinflammatory cytokines interleukin -1β (IL-1β) and tumour necrosis factor α (TNFα) are rapidly released by immune cells during inflammation (Verri *et al.*, 2006). These cytokines contribute to recruitment and activation of immune cells that enhance the inflammation. They also contribute to the establishment of peripheral sensitization via an induction of nerve growth factor (NGF) (Safieh-Garabedian *et al.*, 1995) and a production of PGE2, secondary to induction of cyclooxygenase-2 in immune and other local non-neuronal cells (Maier *et al.*, 1990). Such changes take, however, some time for increased transcription, protein synthesis, mediator release and action, and yet, inflammatory pain generally has a minimal time lag.The rapidness of onset of inflammatory pain implies that proinflammatory mediators have rapid, transcription -independent action on nociceptors. Several lines of evidence indicates that both TNFα and IL-1β (by activation of p38 MAPK) increases TTX-R sodium current (Jin and Gereau, 2006; Binshtok *et al.*, 2008b). IL-1β by relieving resting slow inactivation of TTX-R channels, rapidly, and directly activates nociceptors sufficiently to generate firing of action potentials, even in the absence of exogenous noxious stimuli. Thus, nociceptors in addition to detection of noxious stimuli can also directly signal the presence of ongoing inflammation (Binshtok *et al.*, 2008b).

Although action potentials in nociceptors is based upon the TTX-R sodium channels, the most intriguing finding in the field in recent years is the paramount importance of the TTX-sensitive Na(v) 1.7 channels for pain (Lampert *et al.*, 2010). A mutation in SCN9A, the gene that encodes the Na(v) 1.7 channels, has been shown to cause severe pain-related phenotypes in humans varying from extreme pain syndromes (Yang *et al.*, 2004; Fertleman *et al.*, 2006) to congenital insensitivity to pain (Cox *et al.*, 2006). Extensive studies of the Na(v) 1.7 channelopathies that underlie painful neuropathies demonstrate how changes in channel kinetics result in substantial alterations of nociceptive excitability (Dib-Hajj *et al.*, 2007).

The Na(v) 1.7 channels are preferentially expressed in DRG and sympathetic ganglion neurons (Sangameswaran *et al.*, 1996; Djouhri *et al.*, 2003). Activation of this channel produces fast activating and inactivating TTX-S currents (Klugbauer *et al.*, 1995). Although these properties are typical for TTX-S sensitive channels, there are several distinctive features of Na(v) 1.7 channels that confer upon Na(v) 1.7 the unique role in detection of noxious stimuli. One of these features of Na(v) 1.7 is atypically slow rate of entry into inactivation from the closed state (Cummins *et al.*, 1998; Herzog *et al.*, 2003). As a result, Na(v) 1.7 will respond to small slow depolarization by producing substantial ramp current (Cummins *et al.*, 1998). Physiologically speaking the Na(v) 1.7-mediated ramp current amplifies transducer or generator potentials. Thus, Na(v) 1.7 serves as a threshold channel that defines the responsiveness of the nociceptive neurons to noxious stimuli. In addition to its crucial role in detection of acute stimuli, there are several lines of evidence that emphasize the role of Na(v) 1.7 in the development of inflammatory and neuropathic pain, both in animals and in humans (Dib-Hajj *et al.*, 2010b). In humans, suffering from painful neuromas, Na(v) 1.7 has been shown to accumulate within the axons. Activated p38 and ERK1/2 MAPK are also upregulated, implying that MAPK-mediated modulation of Na(v) 1.7 might underlie the ectopic firing from the site of neuroma (Black *et al.*, 2008; Stamboulian *et al.*, 2010). Activated p38 MAPK has been shown to increase the levels of Na(v) 1.7 in the models of diabetic neuropathy (Chattopadhyay *et al.*, 2008). On the other hand knocking out of Na(v) 1.7 in Na(v) 1.8 expressing neurons did not impair neuropathic pain but reduces inflammatory pain (Nassar *et al.*, 2004). The role of Na(v) 1.7 in inflammatory pain is well established and described in numerous publications (see Dib-Hajj *et al.*, 2010a for review). For example, genetic manipulations of the level of expression of Na(v) 1.7 in primary afferents shows that decrease or ablation of Na(v) 1.7 protein affects the ability of the animals to develop thermal hyperalgesia following CFA-induced inflammation (Yeomans *et al.*, 2005).

The Na(v) 1.3 is another TTX-S sodium channel subtype. Mainly it is expressed during embryonic development (Waxman *et al.*, 1994) but could be also found in adult animals following axotomy and inflammation (Dib-Hajj *et al.*, 1999). Na(v) 1.3 recovers rapidly from fast inactivation (fast re-priming rate) and therefore might account for the high frequency bursts of action potentials – a typical sigh of chronic pain (Momin and Wood, 2008).

The restricted expression of sodium channels Na(v)1.3, Na(v) 1.7, Na(v)1.8, and Na(v)1.9, their involvement in chronic pain and the direct link of Na(v)1.7 to pain states in humans make them ideal targets for research to develop more effective drugs with less side effects. However, only a few subtype selective sodium channel blockers have been reported (Priest, 2009; Zhang *et al.*, 2010), and none have been shown to produce local analgesia.

We have suggested a different strategy to selectively target pain (Binshtok et al., 2007). This strategy is based, first on the location of the binding site of local anaesthetics on the inside of the pore of sodium channels (Ragsdale *et al.*, 1994, 1996; Yarov-Yarovoy *et al.*, 2002; McNulty *et al.*, 2007; Sheets and Hanck, 2007; Ahern *et al.*, 2008; Muroi and Chanda, 2009), and second, on the membrane impermeability of the charged local anaesthetic QX-314. The permanently charged QX-314 blocks sodium channels only when applied from the inside, but not the outside of neuronal membranes (Frazer and M, 1968; Strichartz, 1973). This feature of QX-314 could be exploited to block only selected neurons if there was some way to allow it to enter specific neurons but not others. A possible strategy to do this is to use naturally-expressed large-pore ion channels as entry ports for QX-314 (or similar permanently charged sodium channel blockers) into neurons. The candidate channel we chose to investigate first was transient receptor potential (TRP) vanilloid 1(TRPV1), a member of the large TRP channel super family (Clapham *et al.*, 2001a).

IV. Charge and Target! Targeted Delivery of Membrane Impermeant Sodium Channel Blockers into Nociceptive Neurons to Selectively Block Pain

Targeted delivery of therapeutic compounds to selective cell types is of great clinical importance and can minimize undesired side effects. Development of drug delivery systems is crucial for targeting. We have suggested that nociceptors are equipped with the natural drug delivery systems.These are high threshold large pore cation non-selective channels expressed selectively by nociceptive neurons and serve as transducers of noxious stimuli.

A. Transduction: How do You Say "Pain" in Heattish?

One of the fundamental questions in physiology is how the outside world is perceived by our senses. In other words, how the exogenous chemical and physical stimuli are translated or transduced into the language of the nervous system electrical signals? Seminal discovery of the TRP ion channel led to a substantial breakthrough in our comprehension of the mechanisms of sensory perception. A landmark article by Minke *et al* in 1992 (Hardie and Minke, 1992), where he demonstrated that the *TRP* gene encodes a calcium permeable channel that "senses" light, providing a foundation to the barrage of more recent discoveries emphasizing the role of TRP channels as the main sensory detectors. Numerous publications in the leading journals demonstrated that TRP channels "see" lights and "hear" sounds, "feel" touch, "tastes" and smells (Damann *et al.*, 2008). They also warn us about actual or potential tissue damage (Wang and Woolf, 2005). TRPs become "hot" target-molecules for treatment of pain, itch, anxiety, and respiratory pathologies. Recent discoveries propose that TRP channels can also serve as a natural "drug-delivery" system for the selective application of therapeutic agents to specific cell types without affecting other (Binshtok *et al.*, 2007).

At the beginning of the 20th century none of those ion channels were known, and the concept of how they should work was least developed and hardly believed (Perl, 2007). It took a century before the "... considerable evidence that the skin is provided with a set of nerve endings whose specific office is to be amenable to stimuli that do the skin injury, stimuli that in continuing to act would injure it still further" (Sherrington, 1903) got the molecular proofmark. At the end of the millennium, finally the first nociceptive transducer, called TRPV1, was characterized (Caterina *et al.*, 1997). During the following years more and more channels were added to the list. The TRP-channel- family grew in members but also other channels such as acid sensing ion channels (ASIC), P2X-receptors and potassium and ligand-gated ion channels were found and shown to be responsible for transducing noxious stimuli (Woolf and Ma, 2007). Researchers tried to connect the ability to sense a certain form of stimulus to certain ion-channels assuming that only one channel was committed to one modality. After some years of work we had to realize that it was not as easy as we thought. For example, at first it was believed that TRPV1 alone was responsible for sensing heat-pain (over 42 °C) (Caterina *et al.*, 2000), but in fact it was found that a lot of other TRP-channels (TRPV1-4) had similar structural properties and therefore the ability to transduce thermal sensitivity in the warm-hot range, and so the whole concept had to be re-thought (Dhaka *et al.*, 2006). To complicate things once more, despite the fact that one single modality or form of stimulus seems to be perceived and defined by different transducers, those transducers themselves also seem to be activated by a lot of different stimuli other then temperatures (Macpherson *et al.*, 2005; Xu *et al.*, 2006). Moreover, it is even possible that single TRP-channels could be forming heteromultimers together (Liapi and Wood, 2005) whereas the properties of these constructs concerning transduction are not clearly defined yet. The next question is how these different families of nociceptors are defined and why they are so important for the understanding of pain detection. In this chapter we focus on these "pain" transducer molecules that could potentially serve as therapeutic targets and also may provide "natural" drug delivery systems to selectively target pain fibers.

B. Transient Receptor Potential (TRP) Channels: the Route of Pain or Path for Pain release

One of the most important and by far largest groups or noxious-stimulus detector molecules belongs to theTRP channel family (Julius and Basbaum, 2001). TRP-channels were discovered in 1977 in the *Drosophila melanogaster* fly because of a mutation in a *TRP*-gene that caused photoreceptors to show a transient instead of sustained response when exposed to continuous intense light (Minke, 1977). The first human TRP-channel (TRPC1) was described in 1995 (Wes *et al.*, 1995), the first cloning of a nociceptive TRP-channel was performed by David Julius's group in 1997 (Caterina *et al.*, 1997). Further research demonstrated that in addition to their role as detectors of common noxious stimuli like heat, cold, and low pH TRP-channels also taste sweet, bitter, and umami (Zhang *et al.*, 2003). Moreover TRP channels bring us the exotic tastes of red hot chili, wasabi, and garlic (Patapoutian *et al.*, 2009). Six different TRP channel families with around 28 members exist, all of whom have a similar structure as non-selective-cation-permeable pores built of six transmembrane segments assembled as homo or hetero tetramers (Clapham *et al.*, 2001b).

The TRPC (canonical) subfamily posses excitatory cation non-selective cationic channels that are activated by the stimulation of G-protein-coupled receptors (GPCRs) or receptor-tyrosine kinases (Clapham, 2003). TRPC1 and 5 can be found in the CNS (Greka *et al.*, 2003), where TRPC5 has an essential function in innate fear (Riccio *et al.*, 2009). TRPC2 was proven to be involved in sensing pheromones in rodents (Stowers *et al.*, 2002) without having any function in humans. TRPC4 is a part of the vasoregulatory mechanisms (Freichel *et al.*, 2001), and also TRPC3, 6 and 7, which seem to share nearly 75 percent identical amino-acid-sequence, seem to be integrated in the process of vasoregulation in smooth and cardiac muscle cells (Trebak *et al.*, 2003).

There are eight members belonging to the TRPM (melastatin) subfamily. While TRPM1 forms a crucial part in the signal transduction pathway in retinal cells (Morgans *et al.*, 2010), TRPM2 seems to play a role in sensing oxidant stress (Hara *et al.*, 2002) and TRPM3 has been shown to be responsible for Ca^{2+} uptake in the kidney (Grimm *et al.*, 2003). TRPM4 and TRPM5 are the only monovalent-selective ion channels of the whole TRP family. While TRPM4 is responsible for sensing mechanotransduction in vasculature (Yin and Kuebler, 2010), TRPM5 can be found in nearly every cell expressing taste receptors, belonging to of the pathway controlling taste sensations like sweet, umami, and bitter (Perez *et al.*, 2002). TRPM6 and 7 are special by virtue of functional kinase domains that seem to play a role in Mg^{2+} homeostasis (Nadler *et al.*, 2001). Finally TRPM8 was found in 2002 (McKemy *et al.*, 2002; Peier *et al.*, 2002), to be activated by physical cooling and cooling-agents like menthol. Further investigation in TRPM8 knockout-mice showed that this TRP-channel is the major sensor of innocuous and noxious cold in mammalians (Bautista *et al.*, 2007; Colburn *et al.*, 2007).

The TRPP (polycystin) subfamily consists of three TRP-channels (TRPP2, 3, and 5) which are synonyms for the polycystic kidney disease proteins PKD2, PKD2L1, and PKD2L2 respectively. Mutations in TRPP1 which is not integrated into this TRP-channel subfamily but only seems to have a TRP-like domain and in TRPP2, lead to autosomal polycystic kidney disease (Wu *et al.*, 1998). Another function of TRPP2 and 3 seems to be mechanosensation in the primary cilium of kidney cells (Nauli *et al.*, 2003). TRPML1, 2, and 3 form the small TRP sub-family called mucolipins which seem to play a role in mucolipidosis (Sun *et al.*, 2000) and pigmentation defects in rodents (Di Palma *et al.*, 2002).

Named after a "hot"-pepper derived vanilloid compound, usually known as capsaicin, the TRPV sub-family includes six TRP-channels. TRPV1, 2, 3, and 4 all are responsible for sensing warmth but in different ranges. TRPV2 which shares up to 50 percent structural correlation with TRPV1, – senses noxious heat at over 52 °C (Caterina *et al.*, 1999), TRPV3 at temperatures of over 31 °C (Xu *et al.*, 2002), and TRPV4 at around 25 °C (Guler *et al.*, 2002). In addition, it was suggested that TRPV3 forms heteromultimers with TRPV1 because their distribution along neurons seems similar and overlapping (Smith *et al.*, 2002). TRPV5 and 6 mostly arise in transporting epithelia in the kidney and in the intestine, being the most Ca^{2+}-selective (permeability ratio $P_{Ca}/P_{Na} > 100$) TRP-channels and therefore might suggest that they are responsible for Ca^{2+} uptake (den Dekker *et al.*, 2003).

C. Pain TRPs

1. *TRPV 1*

TRPV1, the first "pain" TRP-channel ever to be characterized, is a cation non-selective channel with high permeability to Ca^{2+}. TRPV1 consists of six transmembrane domains and assemblies as homo or hetero-tetramers (Moiseenkova-Bell and Wensel, 2009). The channel is opened by the active ingredient of hot chili capsaicin, noxious heat (>43 °C), decreased pH and lipids such as anandomide -that also activates cannabinoid type 1 receptor (Palazzo *et al.*, 2010). There is a long list of other natural substances from tarantula toxins (Bohlen *et al.*, 2010) to clove (Park *et al.*, 2009; Yang et al., 2003) and camphor (Xu *et al.*, 2005) that can activate this channel and, therefore, produce burning pain sensation. The channel function is modulated by phosphatidylinositol-4, 5-bisphosphate (PIP2), while the jury is still out about the direction of this modulation. Initially, PIP2 was believed to exert an inhibitory effect on the activation of TRPV1 (Caterina *et al.*, 1997). However, recent experiments have shown instead a strong activation (Stein *et al.*, 2006). Such modulation is likely to be physiologically important, since many G protein coupled receptors can regulate PIP2.

There are evidence that TRPV1 channels have intrinsic voltage-dependence (Ahern and Premkumar, 2002; Premkumar *et al.*, 2002; Voets *et al.*, 2004; Matta and Ahern, 2007), and when activated by capsaicin, outward rectification of the currents is due in part to voltage-dependent closing of channels at strongly negative voltages. At least for cloned heterologously-expressed channels, TRPV1 can be opened in the absence of ligands by strong non-physiological depolarization (Voets *et al.*, 2004). The temperature-induced shift of the TRPV1-activation curve was suggested as a possible mechanism of heat-induced opening of TRPV1. The exact molecular mechanism that underlies the opening of TRPV1 channels remains unknown. Recently, a mechanism of heat-induced activation of the TRPV1 receptor was suggested by Patwardhan *et al.*, (Patwardhan *et al.*, 2010). The researchers demonstrated that heating metabolizes membrane' linoleic acid into 9- and 13-hydroxyoctadecadienoic acid (9- and 13-HODE). These metabolites are able to directly activate TRPV1 channels and therefore they resemble new endogenous agonists of the TRPV1 receptor. TRPV1 knockout mice show shortfalls in heat nociception demonstrating that TRPV1 is a part of the apparatus of sensing acute thermal noxious stimuli (Caterina *et al.*, 2000). Because of the diminished or rather total absence of reactions of these knockout-mice to capsaicin, it could also be shown that TRPV1 was the only receptor in humans being responsible for its detection (Park *et al.*, 2006).

The channel is mostly found in small- and medium-diameter nociceptive sensory neurons which are likely to give rise to C-fibers (Tominaga *et al.*, 1998), while approximately 50 percent of all DRG and TG neurons express TRPV1.

Expression analyzes of pulpal primary afferent neurons demonstrate that they also express TRPV1 channels. Thus, tooth pain, evoked by temperature stimuli is likely to be mediated via the activation of these receptors (Park *et al.*, 2006). Ro *et al.* showed that trigeminal afferents innervating masseter muscle also express TRPV1 receptors. Activation of these receptors by intramuscular injection of TRPV1 agonists mimics signs of craniofacial muscle nociception (Ro *et al.*, 2009).

The activity of TPRV1 is modulated, among other things, by phosphorylation and dephosphorylation. Dephosphorylation is the main action leading to a reduction of the channel's activities (Docherty *et al.*, 1996) while phosphorylation, via kinases like PKA and PKC, increase it (Michael and Priestley, 1999; Ahern and Premkumar, 2002). Various proinflammatory mediators activate these protein kinases upstream (Meents *et al.*, 2010). These mediators, via the activation of PKC and PKA, act on TRPV1 channels to either open them (as for bradykinin effect on TRPA1 via B2 (Bautista *et al.*, 2006b)); increase in their expression (as for action of NGF on TRPV1) (Ji *et al.*, 2002; Zhang *et al.*, 2005) or sensitize TRPV1 channels by a reduction of their threshold, such that they are active at the physiological temperatures (as for PGI_2 and PGE_2) (Moriyama *et al.*, 2005). This PGI_2 and PGE_2-mediated activation of the TRPV1 channels at the normal body temperatures "drives" nociceptors and thereby leads to spontaneous pain after surgery (Banik and Brennan, 2009) or inflammation (Moriyama *et al.*, 2005). In addition to prostaglandins, NGF activated phosphatidylinositol-3-kinase (PI3K) has been also shown to effect PKCε and PKA-mediated enhancement of TRPV1 activation (Bonnington and McNaughton, 2003). PKCε, which is downstream of PI3K, as well as PKA, produces phosphorylation of serines 502 and 800 and thereby lowers the activation threshold of TRPV1 channels. Using different signaling mechanisms, NGF (via activation of tyrosine kinase receptor A (TrkA)) also mediates translocation of TRPV1 channels into the membrane of the nociceptive neurons (Zhang *et al.*, 2005). This insertion involves activation of tyrosine kinase from the Src family that phosphorylates tyrosine residue Y200 (Zhang *et al.*, 2005). Interestingly, recent evidence indicates that the increase in TRPV1 levels changes following post-transcriptional mechanisms rather than due to changes in gene expression ((Puntambekar *et al.*, 2005) see also (Meents *et al.*, 2010)) Considering the fact that TRPV1 lacks a known binding domain for PKA association, well documented PKA-induced modulation of TRPV1 channel (Bhave *et al.*, 2002; Mohapatra and Nau, 2003) must act via a scaffolding protein (Schnizler *et al.*, 2008). A-kinase-anchoring-proteins (AKAPs), are known mediators of PKA signaling (Bregman *et al.*, 1989) and have been shown to interact with TRPV1 channels (Colledge *et al.*, 2000).

The up-regulation of TRPV1 channels at the peripheral nervous system in neuropathic pain conditions takes place not only in C- fibers but also in the myelinated A-fibers. Several lines of evidence demonstrate that nerve injury produce up-regulation of TRPV1 channels in spinal terminals of non-injured neurons (Hudson *et al.*, 2001). All of the above suggest that the changes in TRPV1 expression pattern following injury, in addition to possible mechanism for thermal hyperalgesia, may also account for changes underlying mechanical allodynia.

Considering the role of the TRPV1 channel in inflammatory and neuropathic pain and its selective distribution in pain afferents, it is very reasonable to assume that selective blockade of TRPV1 will be beneficial for the relief of chronic pain. Several selective antagonists of TRPV1 channels were recently developed. BCTC (N- (4-tertiarybutylphenyl)-4-3-chloropyridin-2-yl) (tetrahydropyrazine-1(2H)-carboxamide) that was synthesized in 2003, showed prominent pain relief in mechanical and thermal hyperalgesia two weeks after partial sciatic nerve injury when used in the rat models of chronic pain (Pomonis *et al.*, 2003).

Another potent and selective antagonist of human and rat TRPV1 receptors, the 1-isoquinol in-5- yl-3- (4- trifluoromethyl -benzyl) urea- A -425619 was efficient in models of inflammatory, postoperative pain and neuropathic pain (Honore *et al.*, 2005). The effect was restrained to pain fibers since treated animals did not show any motor deficit.

These promising results and lack of the side effects in the animal models paved the road for clinical trials for SB-705498 which reached phase II trial (Chizh *et al.*, 2007). Others antagonists, such as AMG-517 also got tested in a Phase II trial but led to substantial and long-lasting hyperthermia with increase of body core temperatures to 40 °C (Gavva *et al.*, 2008), leading to the drawback of these substances. This disappointing phenomenon opens new horizons for the comprehension of additional functions of TRPV1 channels beyond transduction of noxious heat. These findings lead to the barrage of articles emphasizing the role of tonically activated TRPV1 channels in the regulation of body temperature. A systematic study performed by Steiner *et al.* (Steiner *et al.*, 2007) showed that tonic non thermal activation of TRPV1 channels in the abdominal viscera by yet unidentified factors inhibits skin vasoconstriction and thermogenesis, thus having a suppressive effect on body temperature.

The TRPV1 channels are also expressed in central neurons. In the hippocampus, activation of TRPV1 channels by anandamide tunes synaptic inputs and leads to long term depression in dentate gyrus (Gibson *et al.*, 2008; Chavez *et al.*, 2010).

Development of more selective TRPV1 anatgonists that cannot penetrate the blood brain barrier (BBB) might prevent central side effects. More detailed comprehension of the expression pattern and effects of thermal and non-thermal activation of TRPV1 channels is essential for efficient and selective pain relief.

Recently, the pore of the TRPV1 channel has been utilized as a delivery system for membrane impermeant sodium channel blockers into nociceptive neurons that consequently produce pain selective analgesia (Binshtok *et al.*, 2007). The idea of this novel approach originated from the observation made by David Corey's group (Meyers *et al.*, 2003). Meyers and colleagues showed that in HEK cells expressing cloned TRPV1 receptors, the application of capsaicin could induce intracellular staining of the neurons by FM1-43, a dye of molecular weight of 452. As mentioned above, TRPV1 molecules form ion channels that are permeable to cations, including calcium, and have little selectivity among Na, K, and Cs (Caterina *et al.*, 1997). Hellwig and colleagues (Hellwig *et al.*, 2004) showed that there is some measurable permeability of the large cations tetraethyl ammonium (MW 130) and N-methyl-D-glucamine (NMDG, MW 195), which are impermeant in classic nonselective cation channels such as nicotinic acetylcholine receptors and NMDA receptors. Several large polyamines such as spermine (charge +4, MW 202) and spermidine (charge +3, MW 145) are also permeant through TRPV1 channels (Ahern *et al.*, 2006).

It is still unclear what the size limit is for molecules that can permeate through TRPV1 receptors. An indication of a possible upper limit on permeation of cations through TRPV1 channels is provided by AG489, a cationic acylpolyamine molecule of MW 490 from the venom of the spider *Agelenopsis aperta* (Kitaguchi and Swartz, 2005). This polyamine is an extremely potent blocker of TRPV1 channels when present externally, with a Kd near 0.3 micromole at −40 mV. The block is strongly voltage-dependent, with little block at +40 mV compared to −40 mV, suggesting entry into the channel and a pore-blocking mechanism. Recent work by Chung *et al.* showed that the permeability of TRPV1 channel isn't a constant value, since the pore of TRPV1 channel itself could dilate by about 20 percent following prolonged or intensive activation (Chung *et al.*, 2008b). Thus the cation non-selective large pore of TRPV1 channel might serve as a perfect gate for charged and therefore membrane impermeant compounds, to enter the cytoplasm. Furthermore, since in the peripheral nervous system TRPV1 channels are expressed only by nociceptive neurons TRPV1 channels could be used for targeted drug delivery of charged compounds selectively into nociceptors and not into low threshold sensory and motor neurons.

2. *TRPA 1*

Originally called ankyrin transmembrane protein 1 (ANKTM1) because of its more than a dozen ankyrin repeats in its N terminus, the gene of TRPA1was first described in 1999 (Jaquemar *et al.*, 1999). TRPA1 almost always co-located with TRPV1 (Story *et al.*, 2003; Bautista *et al.*, 2005). In trigeminal ganglion, TRPA1 containing neurons co-stained both for the marker of peptinergic neurons Substance P (about 27%) and for the marker of nonpeptinergic neurons IB4 (about 45%) (Kim *et al.*, 2010b).

With the exception of capsaicin, TRPA1 can be activated by a lot of different, mostly pungent chemicals like isothiocyanates, cinnamaldehyde, and allicin, making food taste interesting by bringing flavors of horseradish, mustard, cinnamon, and garlic (Bandell *et al.*, 2004; Jordt *et al.*, 2004). These chemicals act on TRPA1 via covalent modification of cysteines (Macpherson *et al.*, 2007a). Regardless of their shape, compounds activating TRPA1 all seem to have the same chemical properties which is why it is their chemical reactivity and not their specificity to a binding site that makes them affect the channel (Hinman *et al.*, 2006). Following this idea, other agents with a similar nature have been shown to act on TRPA1. The substances such as acrolein (Bautista *et al.*, 2006a; Macpherson *et al.*, 2007b), an irritant mostly found in cigarette smoke, formaldehyde (McNamara *et al.*, 2007), and the endogenous 4- hydroxynonenal (4-HNE) (Trevisani *et al.*, 2007) directly activate the TRPA1 channel. The latter is by far the most interesting as it mostly arises out of the process of lipid-peroxidation. TRPA1 knock-out mice are insensitive to mustard-oil and allicin -proving that TRPA1 is the only receptor for these compounds, and have strong deficits in somatosensory chemosensation (Bautista *et al.*, 2006b). All of the above does not only confirm the role of this channel as a receptor for sensing noxious stimuli, but also underlines its crucial function as a major sensor of chemical damage.

A recent study demonstrates that the oral pungency caused by oleocanthal, the extract of extra-virgin olive oil - is also mediated via the activation of TRPA1 receptors selectively in the oral cavity (Peyrot des Gachons *et al.*, 2011). Interestingly, snakes use TRPA1 receptors which are expressed in the neurons that innervate the pit organ, to create the infrared image of their prey (Gracheva *et al.*, 2010). In addition to all that, Zurborg *et al.* also showed that TRPA1 can be activated by Ca^{2+} (Zurborg *et al.*, 2007). Concerning this last fact, it is possible that TRPA1 also acts as an amplifier for the intracellular Ca^{2+}, thereby converging signals from other channels such as TRPV1. On the other hand, increase of intracellular Ca^{2+} leads to a desensitization of TRPA1 (Akopian *et al.*, 2007). Surprisingly, local (Leffler *et al.*, 2008) and general anesthetics (Matta *et al.*, 2008; Satoh and Yamakage, 2009) are able to activate TRPV1 and TRPA1channels.

Consideration of the facts that the application of bradykinin sensitize TRPV1 to heat (Cesare and McNaughton, 1996), and that TRPV1 and TRPA1 are almost exclusively expressed together, Bautista and colleagues (Bautista *et al.*, 2006b) provided the evidence that there is a functional coupling between these two receptors in response to the bradykinin pathway.

Several lines of evidence indicate that TRPA1 channels are activated by noxious cold (Story *et al.*, 2003; Jordt *et al.*, 2004; Zurborg *et al.*, 2007). However the jury is still out about the role of TRPA1 in cold sensation since other studies demonstrated a higher percentage of TRPA1 expressing neurons in rat TG do react onto mustard oil but not to cold stimuli (Nagata *et al.*, 2005). Interestingly, similarly to TRPV1 (Chung *et al.*, 2008a), the pore of the TRPA1 channel undergoes substantial dilation (Chen *et al.*, 2009). In their elegant study, Chen and colleagues showed that the permeability of the TRPA1 pore (P_{NMDG}/P_{NA}) could be increased ~4.4-fold compared to baseline and that the opening of TRPA1 provided a pathway for Yo-Pro an otherwise membrane impermeant fluorescent divalent cation with molecular weight of 376 Da to enter the neurons.

3. *TRPM8 Receptors*

The TRP melastatin 8 (TRPV8) was discovered and characterized in 2002 as a sensor for cooling and menthol (McKemy *et al.*, 2002; Peier *et al.*, 2002). The TRPM8 is expressed by small and medium TG and DRG neurons and is activated in-vitro by the temperature drop below 26 °C and over the range of both noxious and innoxious cold temperatures (McKemy *et al.*, 2002; Peier *et al.*, 2002). Colburn and colleagues demonstrated that TRPM8 is required for the developments of injury-induced hypersensitivity to cold (Colburn *et al.*, 2007). Interestingly cold-induced analgesia is also mediated via TRPM8 receptors (Dhaka *et al.*, 2007). Recent development of genetically encoded axonal tracer green florescent protein (GFP), that labels TRPM8 axons in-vivo, clarified the role of these puzzling receptors in cold nociception (Takashima *et al.*, 2007). TRPM8 is expressed in both myelinated (Aδ) fibers and non-myelinated C fibers. Surprisingly, about 40% of TRPM8 expressing TG neurons and 60% of DRG neurons did not express neither neurofilament NF200 (the marker for the myelinated fibers), or peripherin (an intermediate filament expressed exclusively in non-myelinated neurons), implying that there is a segregated population of small sensory neurons that currently could only be characterized by the expression of TRPM8. There is a large fraction of TRPM8-expressing neurons that also express TRPV1 channels and also stains for CGRP, implying their nociceptive nature (Park *et al.*, 2006; Hjerling-Leffler *et al.*, 2007). The variety of cold modalities mediated by TRPM8-expressing neurons could be explained by the diversity of fibers that contain the TRPM8. To prove that TRPM8 are expressed on different types of small fibers a model with clear morphological differences in innervation patterns of these fibers is needed. The tooth provides on optimal model since cold-sensitive Aδ and C fibers have innervated distinctive areas of the molar. Aδ fibers end superficially and innervate dentin whereas C fibers innervates pulp (Byers and Narhi, 2002). From this model its clear now that TRPM8 are expressed both in the Aδ fibers and C-fibers (Byers and Narhi, 2002). The fact that TRPM8 are expressed in morphologically and functionally distinct fibers could explain their multiple cold sensor function.

4. *P2X-receptors*

In addition to exogenous factors that evoke pain by direct activation of TRP channels, the initial pain from tissue damage may result from the release of endogenous cytoplasmic components that also acts on nociceptors. Some of these factors will modulate properties of TRP channels (Patwardhan *et al.*, 2010); some will directly activate sodium channels to produce pain hypersensitivity (Binshtok *et al.*, 2008b). Other endogenous factors, such as ATP, activate nociceptors directly by acting on specific ligand gated ion channels, purinioceptors and thereby directly contribute to nociception. There are two distinctive groups within the family of purinioceptors, namely P1-receptors (called A1, A2A, A2B, and A3), that are activated by adenosine and P2-receptors that are activated by ATP but also ADP (Burnstock *et al.*, 1978). The latter group can again be divided into two sub-groups, the metabotropic G-protein-coupled P2Y-receptors, and P2X-receptors (Lustig *et al.*, 1993; Webb *et al.*, 1993). There are seven subtypes of P2X-receptors all of which are ionotropic and in this function form pores that span the cell-membrane. These pores change their conformation from closed to open state when motivated by ATP, overall resembling sodium channels (ENaCs) in shape and configuration (North, 2002). Because of the fact of the nearly ubiquitous spread of ATP and its degradation products throughout the body, P2X receptors are involved in various physiological processes and pain is one of them (Burnstock, 1999). P2X-receptors were found to act in spinal projections of nociceptive neurons (Kim *et al.*, 2008) but also in the periphery, responsible for transducing noxious-stimuli. First evidence for the role of P2X receptors in nociception is that P2X3 receptors is nearly exclusively expressed by a small subset of nociceptive fibers (Chen *et al.*, 1995; Lewis *et al.*, 1995). Seminal work by Cook *et al* using tooth pulp innervating afferents, demonstrated that P2X3 mediates nociception (Cook *et al.*, 1997). Activation of P2X3 and P2X2/3 receptors has been shown to be sufficient to elicit nocifensive behavior, following stimulation of tooth pulp (Adachi *et al.*, 2010). Substance P, via neurokinin-1 receptor, produces sensitization of P2X3 receptors which contributes to inflammatory pain hypersensitivity (Park *et al.*, 2010). Another neuropeptide that is released during migraine, Calcitonine Gene Related Protein CGRP upregulates expression of P2X3 receptors in TG neurons (Fabbretti *et al.*, 2006). This mechanism might contribute to pain sensitization during the states of migraine. Moreover, enhancement of P2X receptor activity in the trigeminal nucleus mediates trigeminal pain in the genetic model of familial hemiplegic migraine (Nair *et al.*, 2010). Deep tissue inflammation in craniofacial area modulates the expression of P2X3 receptors in TG neurons and may contribute to inflammatory hyperalgesia (Ambalavanar *et al.*, 2005). P2X3 receptors have been shown to mediate heat hyperalgesia in a unilateral infraorbital nerve ligation model, a rat model of trigeminal neuropathic pain (Shinoda *et al.*, 2007). In P2X3 the knockout- mice, mechanical allodynia was greatly reduced in a model of neuropathic pain (Cockayne *et al.*, 2000; Souslova *et al.*, 2000).

The selective expression of TRPV1, TRPA1, TRPM8, and P2X3 channels in nociceptive neurons, together with the relatively large pores of TRPV1, TRPA1, and P2X3 and dynamic pores size of TRPV1 and TRPA1 makes them a perfect gate for the selective entry of charged sodium channel blockers into nociceptors.

We examined whether we can achieve nociceptive selective blockade by targeting membrane impermeant sodium channel blocker into nociceptors via the pore of TRPV1 channels using a combination of QX-314 and capsaicin, a TRPV1 agonist and the pungent ingredient in chilli peppers (Binshtok *et al.*, 2007). We found that QX-314, when administered alone to DRG neurons, was without effect on $Na_{(V)}$, as expected. In contrast, co-application of QX-314 with capsaicin dramatically inhibited the sodium current (by ~90%), consistent with the idea that QX-314 enters the neurons through TRPV1 channels and blocks from inside. This action completely abolished the ability to generate action potentials and was seen only in small TRPV1 expressing DRG neurons, with large non-capsaicin-responsive neurons unaffected (Binshtok *et al.*, 2007). The effect was also seen in TRPV1 expressing TG neurons, where it was also shown that the blockade of sodium current and action potentials is irreversible after washing capsaicin and QX-314, consistent with the notion that QX-314 is trapped inside the neurons after the TRPV1 channels close (Kim *et al.*, 2010a).

In vivo experiments suggested that TRPV1-mediated entry of QX-314 could be used to produce nociceptor selective block of excitability and axonal conduction. Local injection in rodents of QX-314 alone was, as expected, was without effect (Binshtok *et al.*, 2007; Binshtok *et al.*, 2009). Injection of capsaicin alone subcutaneously elicited a nociceptive reaction that lasted about ~15 minutes (Binshtok *et al.*, 2007) and a similar reaction was elicited by perineural injection (Binshtok *et al.*, 2009), reflecting the presence of TRPV1 expression on the axons of nociceptors in peripheral nerves (Hoffmann *et al.*, 2008). However, when QX-314 was co-applied with capsaicin, either subcutaneously or perineurally, there was a long lasting block of heat and mechanical pain, with no block in motor function (Binshtok *et al.*, 2007). Subsequent experiments on the jaw opening reflex confirmed the specificity of the combination for nociceptor fibres in sensory nerves, and demonstrated the blockade of dental pain (Kim *et al.*, 2010a).

We interpreted these data as showing that we could indeed exploit TRPV1 as a "drug-delivery portal" mechanism to target QX-314 into neurons at sufficient concentrations to block sodium currents and action potentials, with the differential expression of TRPV1 providing specificity for the delivery of the drug only into nociceptors.

This approach could be used clinically to produce long lasting regional analgesia while preserving motor and autonomic function. In addition to the application of this technology for surgery and childbirth, this technique could also be used to diminish postoperative and cancer pain, as well as inflammatory and neuropathic pain. Further research is needed to adapt this approach for the clinical use.

Moreover, this approach represents a novel concept of the targeted delivery of impermeant compounds and can be used not only to block activity but also modulate intracellular signal transduction and metabolism pathways in pain-sensing neurons a well as cancer or any other TRP-expressing cells, while minimizing effects on other types of cells.

V. Concluding Remarks

A detailed understanding of processes that underlie the detection and transmission of nociceptive information is required for the development of efficient and selective pain therapies. In this chapter we reviewed the current knowledge regarding the peripheral aspects of pain perception. Nociceptive neurons express a wide repertoire of proteins that detect and transmit high threshold noxious stimuli. By virtue of their selective expression by the nociceptors, these proteins constitute the perfect targets for selective pain blockade. Large non-selective pores of high threshold nociceptive transducer channels can serve as a natural delivery system for targeted application of various blockers of electrical activity as well as modulators of intracellular signal transduction and metabolic pathways to pain-sensing neurons as well as or any other TRP-expressing cells, while minimizing unwanted effects on the other non-TRP expressing cells.

References

Abrahamsen, B., Zhao, J., Asante, C.O., Cendan, C.M., Marsh, S., Martinez-Barbera, J.P., Nassar, M. A., Dickenson, A.H., and Wood, J.N. (2008). The cell and molecular basis of mechanical, cold, and inflammatory pain. *Science* **321**, 702–705.

Adachi, K., Shimizu, K., Hu, J.W., Suzuki, I., Sakagami, H., Koshikawa, N., Sessle, B.J., Shinoda, M., Miyamoto, M., Honda, K., and Iwata, K. (2010). Purinergic receptors are involved in tooth-pulp evoked nocifensive behavior and brainstem neuronal activity. *Molecular pain* **6**, 59.

Ahern, C.A., Eastwood, A.L., Dougherty, D.A., and Horn, R. (2008). Electrostatic contributions of aromatic residues in the local anesthetic receptor of voltage-gated sodium channels. *Circ. Res.* **102**, 86–94.

Ahern, G.P., and Premkumar, L.S. (2002). Voltage-dependent priming of rat vanilloid receptor: effects of agonist and protein kinase C activation. *The Journal of Physiology* **545**, 441–451.

Ahern, G.P., Wang, X., and Miyares, R.L. (2006). Polyamines are potent ligands for the capsaicin receptor TRPV1. *The Journal of biological chemistry* **281**, 8991–8995.

Akopian, A.N., Sivilotti, L., and Wood, J.N. (1996). A tetrodotoxin-resistant voltage-gated sodium channel expressed by sensory neurons. *Nature* **379**, 257–262.

Akopian, A.N., Ruparel, N.B., Jeske, N., and Hargreaves, K.M. (2007). Transient receptor potential TRPA1 channel desensitization in sensory neurons is agonist dependent and regulated by TRPV1-directed internalization. *The Journal of physiology* **583**, 175–193.

Akopian, A.N., Souslova, V., England, S., Okuse, K., Ogata, N., Ure, J., Smith, A., Kerr, B.J., McMahon, S.B., Boyce, S., Hill, R., Stanfa, L.C., Dickenson, A.H., and Wood, J.N. (1999). The tetrodotoxin-resistant sodium channel SNS has a specialized function in pain pathways. *Nature neuroscience* **2**, 541–548.

Amaya, F., Wang, H., Costigan, M., Allchorne, A.J., Hatcher, J.P., Egerton, J., Stean, T., Morisset, V., Grose, D., Gunthorpe, M.J., Chessell, I.P., Tate, S., Green, P.J., and Woolf, C.J. (2006). The voltage-gated sodium channel Na(v)1.9 is an effector of peripheral inflammatory pain hypersensitivity. *J. Neurosci.* **26**, 12852–12860.

Ambalavanar, R., Moritani, M., and Dessem, D. (2005). Trigeminal P2X3 receptor expression differs from dorsal root ganglion and is modulated by deep tissue inflammation. *Pain* **117**, 280–291.

Baker, M.D. (2005). Protein kinase C mediates up-regulation of tetrodotoxin-resistant, persistent Na+ current in rat and mouse sensory neurones. *J. Physiol.* **567**, 851–867.

Baker, M.D., Chandra, S.Y., Ding, Y., Waxman, S.G., and Wood, J.N. (2003). GTP-induced tetrodotoxin-resistant Na+ current regulates excitability in mouse and rat small diameter sensory neurones. *J. Physiol.* **548**, 373–382.

Bandell, M., Story, G.M., Hwang, S.W., Viswanath, V., Eid, S.R., Petrus, M.J., Earley, T.J., and Patapoutian, A. (2004). Noxious cold ion channel TRPA1 is activated by pungent compounds and bradykinin. *Neuron* **41**, 849–857.

Banik, R.K., and Brennan, T.J. (2009). Trpv1 mediates spontaneous firing and heat sensitization of cutaneous primary afferents after plantar incision. *Pain* **141**, 41–51.

Basbaum, A.I., Bautista, D.M., Scherrer, G., and Julius, D. (2009). Cellular and molecular mechanisms of pain. *Cell* **139**, 267–284.

Bautista, D.M., Siemens, J., Glazer, J.M., Tsuruda, P.R., Basbaum, A.I., Stucky, C.L., Jordt, S.E., and Julius, D. (2007). The menthol receptor TRPM8 is the principal detector of environmental cold. *Nature* **448**, 204–208.

Bautista, D. M., Movahed, P., Hinman, A., Axelsson, H. E., Sterner, O., Hogestatt, E. D., Julius, D., Jordt, S. E., and Zygmunt P. M. (2005). Pungent products from garlic activate the sensory ion channel TRPA1. Proceedings of the National Academy of Sciences of the United States of America. **102**, 12248–12252.

Bautista, D.M., Jordt, S.E., Nikai, T., Tsuruda, P.R., Read, A.J., Poblete, J., Yamoah, E.N., Basbaum, A.I., and Julius, D. (2006a). TRPA1Mediates the Inflammatory Actions of Environmental Irritants and Proalgesic Agents. *Cell*1269–1282

Bautista, D.M., Jordt, S.E., Nikai, T., Tsuruda, P.R., Read, A.J., Poblete, J., Yamoah, E.N., Basbaum, A.I., and Julius, D. (2006b). TRPA1 mediates the inflammatory actions of environmental irritants and proalgesic agents. *Cell* **124**, 1269–1282.

Bhave, G., Zhu, W., Wang, H., Brasier, D.J., Oxford, G.S., and Gereau, RW. (2002). cAMP-dependent protein kinase regulates desensitization of the capsaicin receptor (VR1) by direct phosphorylation. *Neuron* **35**, 721–731.

Binshtok, A.M., Bean, B.P., and Woolf, C.J. (2007). Inhibition of nociceptors by TRPV1-mediated entry of impermeant sodium channel blockers. *Nature* **449**, 607–610.

Binshtok, A.M., Wang, H., Zimmermann, K., Amaya, F., Vardeh, D., Shi, L., Brenner, G.J., Ji, R.R., Bean, B.P., Woolf, C.J., and Samad, T.A. (2008a). Nociceptors are interleukin-1beta sensors. *J. Neurosci.* **28**, 14062–14073.

Binshtok, A.M., Wang, H., Zimmermann, K., Amaya, F., Vardeh, D., Shi, L., Brenner, G.J., Ji, R.R., Bean, B.P., Woolf, C.J., and Samad, T. (2008b). Nociceptors are interleukin-1beta sensors. *The Journal of neuroscience: the official journal of the Society for Neuroscience* **28**, 14062–14073.

Binshtok, A.M., Gerner, P., Oh, S.B., Puopolo, M., Suzuki, S., Roberson, D.P., Herbert, T., Wang, C. F., Kim, D., Chung, G., Mitani, A.A., Wang, G.K., Bean, B.P., and Woolf, C.J. (2009). Coapplication of lidocaine and the permanently charged sodium channel blocker QX-314 produces a long-lasting nociceptive blockade in rodents. *Anesthesiology* **111**, 127–137.

Black, J.A., Nikolajsen, L., Kroner, K., Jensen, T.S., and Waxman, S.G. (2008). Multiple sodium channel isoforms and mitogen-activated protein kinases are present in painful human neuromas. *Annals of neurology* **64**, 644–653.

Blair, N.T., and Bean, B.P. (2002). Roles of tetrodotoxin (TTX)-sensitive Na+ current, TTX-resistant Na+ current, and Ca2+ current in the action potentials of nociceptive sensory neurons. *J. Neurosci.* **22**, 10277–10290.

Bohlen, C.J., Priel, A., Zhou, S., King, D., Siemens, J., and Julius, D. (2010). A bivalent tarantula toxin activates the capsaicin receptor, TRPV1, by targeting the outer pore domain. *Cell* **141**, 834–845.

Bonnington, J.K., and McNaughton, P.A. (2003). Signalling pathways involved in the sensitisation of mouse nociceptive neurones by nerve growth factor. *The Journal of Physiology* **551**, 433–446.

Bourinet, E., Alloui, A., Monteil, A., Barrere, C., Couette, B., Poirot, O., Pages, A., McRory, J., Snutch, T.P., Eschalier, A., and Nargeot, J. (2005). Silencing of the Cav3.2 T-type calcium channel gene in sensory neurons demonstrates its major role in nociception. *Embo J.* **24**, 315–324.

Bregman, D.B., Bhattacharyya, N., and Rubin, C.S. (1989). High affinity binding protein for the regulatory subunit of cAMP-dependent protein kinase II-B. Cloning, characterization, and expression of cDNAs for rat brain P150. *The Journal of biological chemistry* **264**, 4648–4656.

Burnstock, G. (1999). Current status of P2X receptors: distribution and pathophysiological roles. *Proc. West Pharmacol. Soc.* **42**, 119–121.

Burnstock, G., Cocks, T., Crowe, R., and Kasakov, L. (1978). Purinergic innervation of the guinea-pig urinary bladder. *British Journal of Pharmacology* **63**, 125–138.

Byers, M. R., and Narhi, M. V. O. (2002). Nerve supply of pulpodentin complex and responces to injury. In: Dental Pulp (K. M. Hargreaves and H. E.Goodis Eds.), carol Stream, Il: Quintessence Publishing Co., 151–179.

Cardenas, C.G., Del Mar, L.P., and Scroggs, R.S. (1995). Variation in serotonergic inhibition of calcium channel currents in four types of rat sensory neurons differentiated by membrane properties. *Journal of Neurophysiology* **74**, 1870–1879.

Caterina, M.J., Rosen, T.A., Tominaga, M., Brake, A.J., and Julius, D. (1999). A capsaicin-receptor homologue with a high threshold for noxious heat. *Nature* **398**, 436–441.

Caterina, M.J., Schumacher, M.A., Tominaga, M., Rosen, T.A., Levine, J.D., and Julius, D. (1997). The capsaicin receptor: a heat-activated ion channel in the pain pathway. *Nature* **389**, 816–824.

Caterina, M.J., Leffler, A., Malmberg, A.B., Martin, W.J., Trafton, J., Petersen-Zeitz, K.R., Koltzenburg, M., Basbaum, A.I., and Julius, D. (2000). Impaired nociception and pain sensation in mice lacking the capsaicin receptor. *Science* **288**, 306–313.

Catterall, W. A., and Mackie, K. (2007). Local Anesthetics. In: Goodman & Gilman's The pahrmacological basis of therapeutics, 11 Edition (J. G. Hardman and L. E. Limbird, Eds.), McGraw-Hill, 367–385.

Cesare, P., and McNaughton, P. (1996). A novel heat-activated current in nociceptive neurons and its sensitization by bradykinin. Proceedings of the National Academy of Sciences of the United States of America. **93**, 15435–15439.

Chattopadhyay, M., Mata, M., and Fink, D.J. (2008). Continuous delta-opioid receptor activation reduces neuronal voltage-gated sodium channel (NaV1.7) levels through activation of protein kinase C in painful diabetic neuropathy. *The Journal of neuroscience: the official journal of the Society for Neuroscience* **28**, 6652–6658.

Chavez, A.E., Chiu, C.Q., and Castillo, P.E. (2010). TRPV1 activation by endogenous anandamide triggers postsynaptic long-term depression in dentate gyrus. *Nature neuroscience* **13**, 1511–1518.

Chen, C.C., Akopian, A.N., Sivilotti, L., Colquhoun, D., Burnstock, G., and Wood, J.N. (1995). A P2X purinoceptor expressed by a subset of sensory neurons. *Nature* **377**, 428–431.

Chen, J., Kim, D., Bianchi, B.R., Cavanaugh, E.J., Faltynek, C.R., Kym, P.R., and Reilly, R.M. (2009). Pore dilation occurs in TRPA1 but not in TRPM8 channels. *Molecular pain* **5**, 3.

Chen, W.K., Liu, I.Y., Chang, Y.T., Chen, Y.C., Chen, C.C., Yen, C.T., and Shin, H.S. (2010). Ca(v) 3.2 T-type Ca2+ channel-dependent activation of ERK in paraventricular thalamus modulates acid-induced chronic muscle pain. *The Journal of neuroscience: the official journal of the Society for Neuroscience* **30**, 10360–10368.

Chizh, B.A., O'Donnell, M.B., Napolitano, A., Wang, J., Brooke, A.C., Aylott, M.C., Bullman, J.N., Gray, E.J., Lai, R.Y., Williams, P.M., and Appleby, J.M. (2007). The effects of the TRPV1 antagonist SB-705498 on TRPV1 receptor-mediated activity and inflammatory hyperalgesia in humans. *Pain* **132**, 132–141.

Choi, S., Na, H.S., Kim, J., Lee, J., Lee, S., Kim, D., Park, J., Chen, C.C., Campbell, K.P., and Shin, H. S. (2007). Attenuated pain responses in mice lacking Ca(V)3.2 T-type channels. *Genes Brain Behav.* **6**, 425–431.

Chung, M.K., Güler, A.D., and Caterina, M.J. (2008a). TRPV1 shows dynamic ionic selectivity during agonist stimulation. *Nature neuroscience* **11**, 555–564.

Chung, M.K., Guler, A.D., and Caterina, M.J. (2008b). TRPV1 shows dynamic ionic selectivity during agonist stimulation. *Nat Neurosci.* **11**, 555–564.

Clapham, D.E. (2003). TRP channels as cellular sensors. *Nature* **426**, 517–524.

Clapham, D.E., Runnels, L.W., and Strübing, C. (2001a). The TRP ion channel family. *Nature reviews Neuroscience* **2**, 387–396.

Clapham, D.E., Runnels, L.W., and Strabing, C. (2001b). The TRP ion channel family. *Nature reviews Neuroscience* **2**, 387–396.

Cockayne, D.A., Hamilton, S.G., Zhu, Q.M., Dunn, P.M., Zhong, Y., Novakovic, S., Malmberg, A.B., Cain, G., Berson, A., Kassotakis, L., Hedley, L., Lachnit, W.G., Burnstock, G., McMahon, S.B., and Ford, A.P. (2000). Urinary bladder hyporeflexia and reduced pain-related behaviour in P2X3-deficient mice. *Nature* **407**, 1011–1015.

Colburn, R.W., Lubin, M.L., Stone Jr., D.J., Wang, Y., Lawrence, D., D'Andrea, M.R., Brandt, M.R., Liu, Y., Flores, C.M., and Qin, N. (2007). Attenuated cold sensitivity in TRPM8 null mice. *Neuron* **54**, 379–386.

Colledge, M., Dean, R.A., Scott, G.K., Langeberg, L.K., Huganir, R.L., and Scott, J.D. (2000). Targeting of PKA to glutamate receptors through a MAGUK-AKAP complex. *Neuron* **27**, 107–119.

Cook, S.P., Vulchanova, L., Hargreaves, K.M., Elde, R., and McCleskey, E.W. (1997). Distinct ATP receptors on pain-sensing and stretch-sensing neurons. *Nature* **387**, 505–508.

Copel, C., Osorio, N., Crest, M., Gola, M., Delmas, P., and Clerc, N. (2009). Activation of neurokinin 3 receptor increases Na(v)1.9 current in enteric neurons. *The Journal of Physiology* **587**, 1461–1479.

Coste, B., Crest, M., and Delmas, P. (2007). Pharmacological dissection and distribution of NaN/Nav1.9, T-type Ca2+ currents, and mechanically activated cation currents in different populations of DRG neurons. *The Journal of general physiology* **129**, 57–77.

Cox, J.J., Reimann, F., Nicholas, A.K., Thornton, G., Roberts, E., Springell, K., Karbani, G., Jafri, H., Mannan, J., Raashid, Y., Al-Gazali, L., Hamamy, H., Valente, E.M., Gorman, S., Williams, R., McHale, D.P., Wood, J.N., Gribble, F.M., and Woods, C.G. (2006). An SCN9A channelopathy causes congenital inability to experience pain. *Nature* **444**, 894–898.

Cummins, T.R., and Waxman, S.G. (1997). Downregulation of tetrodotoxin-resistant sodium currents and upregulation of a rapidly repriming tetrodotoxin-sensitive sodium current in small spinal sensory neurons after nerve injury. *The Journal of neuroscience: the official journal of the Society for Neuroscience* **17**, 3503–3514.

Cummins, T.R., Howe, J.R., and Waxman, S.G. (1998). Slow closed-state inactivation: a novel mechanism underlying ramp currents in cells expressing the hNE/PN1 sodium channel. *The Journal of neuroscience: the official journal of the Society for Neuroscience* **18**, 9607–9619.

Cummins, T.R., Dib-Hajj, S.D., Black, J.A., Akopian, A.N., Wood, J.N., and Waxman, S.G. (1999). A novel persistent tetrodotoxin-resistant sodium current in SNS-null and wild-type small primary sensory neurons. *The Journal of neuroscience: the official journal of the Society for Neuroscience* **19**, RC43.

Damann, N., Voets, T., and Nilius, B. (2008). TRPs in our senses. *Current biology: CB* **18**, R880–889.

den Dekker, E., Hoenderop, J.G., Nilius, B., and Bindels, R.J. (2003). The epithelial calcium channels, TRPV5 & TRPV6: from identification towards regulation. *Cell Calcium* **33**, 497–507.

Dhaka, A., Viswanath, V., and Patapoutian, A. (2006). Trp ion channels and temperature sensation. *Annual review of neuroscience* **29**, 135–161.

Dhaka, A., Murray, A.N., Mathur, J., Earley, T.J., Petrus, M.J., and Patapoutian, A. (2007). TRPM8 is required for cold sensation in mice. *Neuron* **54**, 371–378.

Di Palma, F., Belyantseva, I. A., Kim, H. J., Vogt, T. F., Kachar, B., and Noben-Trauth, K. (2002). Mutations in Mcoln3 associated with deafness and pigmentation defects in varitint-waddler (Va) mice. Proceedings of the National Academy of Sciences of the United States of America **99**, 14994–14999.

Dib-Hajj, S., Black, J.A., Cummins, T.R., and Waxman, S.G. (2002). NaN/Nav1.9: a sodium channel with unique properties. *Trends Neurosci.* **25**, 253–259.

Dib-Hajj, S.D., Black, J.A., and Waxman, S.G. (2009a). Voltage-gated sodium channels: therapeutic targets for pain. *Pain medicine (Malden, Mass)* **10**, 1260–1269.

Dib-Hajj, S.D., Cummins, T.R., Black, J.A., and Waxman, S.G. (2007). From genes to pain: Na v 1.7 and human pain disorders. *Trends in neurosciences* **30**, 555–563.

Dib-Hajj, S.D., Cummins, T.R., Black, J.A., and Waxman, S.G. (2010a). Sodium channels in normal and pathological pain. *Annual Review of Neuroscience* **33**, 325–347.

Dib-Hajj, S.D., Cummins, T.R., Black, J.A., and Waxman, S.G. (2010b). Sodium Channels in Normal and Pathological Pain. *Annual Review of Neuroscience*

Dib-Hajj, S.D., Binshtok, A.M., Cummins, T.R., Jarvis, M.F., Samad, T., and Zimmermann, K. (2009b). Voltage-gated sodium channels in pain states: role in pathophysiology and targets for treatment. *Brain research reviews* **60**, 65–83.

Dib-Hajj, S.D., Fjell, J., Cummins, T.R., Zheng, Z., Fried, K., LaMotte, R., Black, J.A., and Waxman, S.G. (1999). Plasticity of sodium channel expression in DRG neurons in the chronic constriction injury model of neuropathic pain. *Pain* **83**, 591–600.

Djouhri, L., Fang, X., Okuse, K., Wood, J.N., Berry, C.M., and Lawson, S.N. (2003). The TTX-resistant sodium channel Nav1.8 (SNS/PN3): expression and correlation with membrane properties in rat nociceptive primary afferent neurons. *The Journal of Physiology* **550**, 739–752.

Docherty, R.J., Yeats, J.C., Bevan, S., and Boddeke, H.W. (1996). Inhibition of calcineurin inhibits the desensitization of capsaicin-evoked currents in cultured dorsal root ganglion neurones from adult rats. *Pflügers Archiv: European journal of physiology* **431**, 828–837.

Dogrul, A., Gardell, L.R., Ossipov, M.H., Tulunay, F.C., Lai, J., and Porreca, F. (2003). Reversal of experimental neuropathic pain by T-type calcium channel blockers. *Pain* **105**, 159–168.

Everill, B., and Kocsis, J.D. (1999). Reduction in potassium currents in identified cutaneous afferent dorsal root ganglion neurons after axotomy. *Journal of Neurophysiology* **82**, 700–708.

Everill, B., Rizzo, M.A., and Kocsis, J.D. (1998). Morphologically identified cutaneous afferent DRG neurons express three different potassium currents in varying proportions. *Journal of Neurophysiology* **79**, 1814–1824.

Fabbretti, E., D'Arco, M., Fabbro, A., Simonetti, M., Nistri, A., and Giniatullin, R. (2006). Delayed upregulation of ATP P2X3 receptors of trigeminal sensory neurons by calcitonin gene-related peptide. *The Journal of neuroscience: the official journal of the Society for Neuroscience* **26**, 6163–6171.

Fertleman, C.R., Baker, M.D., Parker, K.A., Moffatt, S., Elmslie, F.V., Abrahamsen, B., Ostman, J., Klugbauer, N., Wood, J.N., Gardiner, R.M., and Rees, M. (2006). SCN9A mutations in paroxysmal extreme pain disorder: allelic variants underlie distinct channel defects and phenotypes. *Neuron* **52**, 767–774.

Frazer, D.T., M Y (1968). The site of action and active form of local anesthetics. Experiments with quaternary compounds. *The Journal of pharmacology and experimental therapeutics.*

Frazier, D.T., Narahashi, T., and Yamada, M. (1970). The site of action and active form of local anesthetics. II. Experiments with quaternary compounds. *J. Pharmacol. Exp. Ther.* **171**, 45–51.

Fredrickson, M.J., Krishnan, S., and Chen, C.Y. (2010). Postoperative analgesia for shoulder surgery: a critical appraisal and review of current techniques. *Anaesthesia* **65**, 608–624.

Freichel, M., Suh, S.H., Pfeifer, A., Schweig, U., Trost, C., Weissgerber, P., Biel, M., Philipp, S., Freise, D., Droogmans, G., Hofmann, F., Flockerzi, V., and Nilius, B. (2001). Lack of an endothelial store-operated Ca2+ current impairs agonist-dependent vasorelaxation in TRP4–/–mice. *Nature cell biology* **3**, 121–127.

Gavva, N.R et al., (2008). Pharmacological blockade of the vanilloid receptor TRPV1 elicits marked hyperthermia in humans. *Pain* **136**, 202–210.

Gibson, H.E., Edwards, J.G., Page, R.S., Van Hook, M.J., and Kauer, J.A. (2008). TRPV1 channels mediate long-term depression at synapses on hippocampal interneurons. *Neuron* **57**, 746–759.

Gold, M.S., Levine, J.D., and Correa, A.M. (1998). Modulation of TTX-R INa by PKC and PKA and their role in PGE2-induced sensitization of rat sensory neurons in vitro. *J. Neurosci.* **18**, 10345–10355.

Gracheva, E.O., Ingolia, N.T., Kelly, Y.M., Cordero-Morales, J.F., Hollopeter, G., Chesler, A.T., Sanchez, E.E., Perez, J.C., Weissman, J.S., and Julius, D. (2010). Molecular basis of infrared detection by snakes. *Nature* **464**, 1006–1011.

Greka, A., Navarro, B., Oancea, E., Duggan, A., and Clapham, D.E. (2003). TRPC5 is a regulator of hippocampal neurite length and growth cone morphology. *Nature neuroscience* **6**, 837–845.

Grimm, C., Kraft, R., Sauerbruch, S., Schultz, G., and Harteneck, C. (2003). Molecular and functional characterization of the melastatin-related cation channel TRPM3. *The Journal of biological chemistry* **278**, 21493–21501.

Guler, A.D., Lee, H., Iida, T., Shimizu, I., Tominaga, M., and Caterina, M. (2002). Heat-evoked activation of the ion channel, TRPV4. *The Journal of neuroscience: the official journal of the Society for Neuroscience* **22**, 6408–6414.

Hara, Y., Wakamori, M., Ishii, M., Maeno, E., Nishida, M., Yoshida, T., Yamada, H., Shimizu, S., Mori, E., Kudoh, J., Shimizu, N., Kurose, H., Okada, Y., Imoto, K., and Mori, Y. (2002). LTRPC2 Ca2+-permeable channel activated by changes in redox status confers susceptibility to cell death. *Molecular cell* **9**, 163–173.

Hardie, R.C., and Minke, B. (1992). The trp gene is essential for a light-activated Ca2+ channel in Drosophila photoreceptors. *Neuron* **8**, 643–651.

Hawkins, J.L. (2010). Epidural analgesia for labor and delivery. *N. Engl. J. Med.* **362**, 1503–1510.

Heavner, J.E. (2007). Local anesthetics. *Current Opinion in Anaesthesiology*336–342

Hellwig, N., Plant, T.D., Janson, W., Schafer, M., Schultz, G., and Schaefer, M. (2004). TRPV1 acts as proton channel to induce acidification in nociceptive neurons. *J. Biol. Chem.* **279**, 34553–34561.

Herzog, R.I., Cummins, T.R., and Waxman, S.G. (2001). Persistent TTX-resistant Na+ current affects resting potential and response to depolarization in simulated spinal sensory neurons. *J. Neurophysiol.* **86**, 1351–1364.

Herzog, R.I., Cummins, T.R., Ghassemi, F., Dib-Hajj, S.D., and Waxman, S.G. (2003). Distinct repriming and closed-state inactivation kinetics of Nav1.6 and Nav1.7 sodium channels in mouse spinal sensory neurons. *J. Physiol.* **551**, 741–750.

Hille, B. (1977a). Local anesthetics: hydrophilic and hydrophobic pathways for the drug-receptor reaction. *J. Gen. Physiol.* **69**, 497–515.

Hille, B. (1977b). The pH-dependent rate of action of local anesthetics on the node of Ranvier. *J. Gen. Physiol.* **69**, 475–496.

Hinman, A., Chuang, H. H., Bautista, D. M., and Julius, D. (2006). TRP channel activation by reversible covalent modification. Proceedings of the National Academy of Sciences of the United States of America. **103**, 19564–19568.

Hjerling-Leffler, J., Alqatari, M., Ernfors, P., and Koltzenburg, M. (2007). Emergence of functional sensory subtypes as defined by transient receptor potential channel expression. *The Journal of neuroscience: the official journal of the Society for Neuroscience* **27**, 2435–2443.

Hoffmann, T., Sauer, S.K., Horch, R.E., and Reeh, P.W. (2008). Sensory transduction in peripheral nerve axons elicits ectopic action potentials. *J. Neurosci.* **28**, 6281–6284.

Hogan, M.V., Grant, R.E., and Lee Jr., L. (2009). Analgesia for total hip and knee arthroplasty: a review of lumbar plexus, femoral, and sciatic nerve blocks. *Am. J. Orthop. (Belle Mead NJ)* **38**, E129–133.

Honore, P., Wismer, C.T., Mikusa, J., Zhu, C.Z., Zhong, C., Gauvin, D.M., Gomtsyan, A.E.1., Kouhen, R., Lee, C.H., Marsh, K., Sullivan, J.P., Faltynek, C.R., and Jarvis, M.F. (2005). A-425619 [1-isoquinolin-5-yl-3-(4-trifluoromethyl-benzyl)-urea], a novel transient receptor potential type V1 receptor antagonist, relieves pathophysiological pain associated with inflammation and tissue injury in rats. *The Journal of pharmacology and experimental therapeutics* **314**, 410–421.

Hucho, T., and Levine, J.D. (2007). Signaling pathways in sensitization: toward a nociceptor cell biology. *Neuron* **55**, 365–376.

Hudson, L.J., Bevan, S., Wotherspoon, G., Gentry, C., Fox, A., and Winter, J. (2001). VR1 protein expression increases in undamaged DRG neurons after partial nerve injury. *The European journal of neuroscience* **13**, 2105–2114.

Indo, Y., Tsuruta, M., Hayashida, Y., Karim, M.A., Ohta, K., Kawano, T., Mitsubuchi, H., Tonoki, H., Awaya, Y., and Matsuda, I. (1996). Mutations in the TRKA/NGF receptor gene in patients with congenital insensitivity to pain with anhidrosis. *Nat. Genet.* **13**, 485–488.

Jagodic, M.M., Pathirathna, S., Nelson, M.T., Mancuso, S., Joksovic, P.M., Rosenberg, E.R., Bayliss, D.A., Jevtovic-Todorovic, V., and Todorovic, S.M. (2007). Cell-specific alterations of T-type calcium current in painful diabetic neuropathy enhance excitability of sensory neurons. *The Journal of neuroscience: the official journal of the Society for Neuroscience* **27**, 3305–3316.

Jagodic, M.M., Pathirathna, S., Joksovic, P.M., Lee, W., Nelson, M.T., Naik, A.K., Su, P., Jevtovic-Todorovic, V., and Todorovic, S.M. (2008). Upregulation of the T-type calcium current in small rat sensory neurons after chronic constrictive injury of the sciatic nerve. *Journal of Neurophysiology* **99**, 3151–3156.

Jaquemar, D., Schenker, T., and Trueb, B. (1999). An ankyrin-like protein with transmembrane domains is specifically lost after oncogenic transformation of human fibroblasts. *The Journal of biological chemistry* **274**, 7325–7333.

Ji, R.R., Samad, T.A., Jin, S.X., Schmoll, R., and Woolf, C.J. (2002). p38 MAPK activation by NGF in primary sensory neurons after inflammation increases TRPV1 levels and maintains heat hyperalgesia. *Neuron* **36**, 57–68.

Jin, X., and Gereau, RW. (2006). Acute p38-mediated modulation of tetrodotoxin-resistant sodium channels in mouse sensory neurons by tumor necrosis factor-alpha. *J. Neurosci.* **26**, 246–255.

Jordt, S.E., Bautista, D.M., Chuang, H.H., McKemy, D.D., Zygmunt, P.M., Hogestatt, E.D., Meng, I. D., and Julius, D. (2004). Mustard oils and cannabinoids excite sensory nerve fibres through the TRP channel ANKTM1. *Nature* **427**, 260–265.

Julius, D., and Basbaum, A.I. (2001). Molecular mechanisms of nociception. *Nature* **413**, 203–210.

Jyvasjarvi, E., and Kniffki, K.D. (1987). Cold stimulation of teeth: a comparison between the responses of cat intradental A delta and C fibres and human sensation. *The Journal of Physiology* **391**, 193–207.

Kim, D.S., Choi, J.O., Rim, H.D., and Cho, H.J. (2002). Downregulation of voltage-gated potassium channel a gene expression in dorsal root ganglia following chronic constriction injury of the rat sciatic nerve. *Molecular Brain Research* **105**, 146–152.

Kim, H.Y., Kim, K., Li, H.Y., Chung, G., Park, C.K., Kim, J.S., Jung, S.J., Lee, M.K., Ahn, D.K., Hwang, S.J., Kang, Y., Binshtok, A.M., Bean, B.P., Woolf, C.J., and Oh, S.B. (2010a). Selectively targeting pain in the trigeminal system. *Pain* **150**, 29–40.

Kim, Y.S., Son, J.Y., Kim, T.H., Paik, S.K., Dai, Y., Noguchi, K., Ahn, D.K., and Bae, Y.C. (2010b). Expression of transient receptor potential ankyrin 1 (TRPA1) in the rat trigeminal sensory afferents and spinal dorsal horn. *The Journal of Comparative Neurology* **518**, 687–698.

Kim, Y.S., Paik, S.K., Cho, Y.S., Shin, H.S., Bae, J.Y., Moritani, M., Yoshida, A., Ahn, D.K., Valtschanoff, J., Hwang, S.J., Moon, C., and Bae, Y.C. (2008). Expression of P2X3 receptor in the trigeminal sensory nuclei of the rat. *The Journal of Comparative Neurology* **506**, 627–639.

Kitagawa, J., Takeda, M., Suzuki, I., Kadoi, J., Tsuboi, Y., Honda, K., Matsumoto, S., Nakagawa, H., Tanabe, A., and Iwata, K. (2006). Mechanisms involved in modulation of trigeminal primary afferent activity in rats with peripheral mononeuropathy. *The European journal of neuroscience* **24**, 1976–1986.

Kitaguchi, T., and Swartz, K.J. (2005). An inhibitor of TRPV1 channels isolated from funnel Web spider venom. *Biochemistry* **44**, 15544–15549.

Klugbauer, N., Lacinova, L., Flockerzi, V., and Hofmann, F. (1995). Structure and functional expression of a new member of the tetrodotoxin-sensitive voltage-activated sodium channel family from human neuroendocrine cells. *Embo J.* **14**, 1084–1090.

Koller, C. (1884). On the use of cocaine for producing anaesthesia on the eye. *Lancet* **2**, 990.

Lampert, A., O'Reilly, A.O., Reeh, P., and Leffler, A. (2010). Sodium channelopathies and pain. *Pflügers Archiv: European journal of physiology* **460**, 249–263.

Leffler, A., Fischer, M.J., Rehner, D., Kienel, S., Kistner, K., Sauer, S.K., Gavva, N.R., Reeh, P.W., and Nau, C. (2008). The vanilloid receptor TRPV1 is activated and sensitized by local anesthetics in rodent sensory neurons. *J. Clin. Invest.* **118**, 763–776.

Lewis, C., Neidhart, S., Holy, C., North, R.A., Buell, G., and Surprenant, A. (1995). Coexpression of P2X2 and P2X3 receptor subunits can account for ATP-gated currents in sensory neurons. *Nature* **377**, 432–435.

Liapi, A., and Wood, J.N. (2005). Extensive co-localization and heteromultimer formation of the vanilloid receptor-like protein TRPV2 and the capsaicin receptor TRPV1 in the adult rat cerebral cortex. *The European journal of neuroscience* **22**, 825–834.

Loeser, J.D., and Treede, R.D. (2008). The Kyoto protocol of IASP Basic Pain Terminology. *Pain* **137**, 473–477.

Lustig, K. D., Shiau, A. K., Brake, A. J., and Julius, D. (1993). Expression cloning of an ATP receptor from mouse neuroblastoma cells. Proceedings of the National Academy of Sciences of the United States of America. **90**, 5113–5117.

Macpherson, L.J., Geierstanger, B.H., Viswanath, V., Bandell, M., Eid, S.R., Hwang, S., and Patapoutian, A. (2005). The pungency of garlic: activation of TRPA1 and TRPV1 in response to allicin. *Current biology: CB* **15**, 929–934.

Macpherson, L.J., Dubin, A.E., Evans, M.J., Marr, F., Schultz, P.G., Cravatt, B.F., and Patapoutian, A. (2007a). Noxious compounds activate TRPA1 ion channels through covalent modification of cysteines. *Nature* **445**, 541–545.

Macpherson, L.J., Xiao, B., Kwan, K.Y., Petrus, M.J., Dubin, A.E., Hwang, S., Cravatt, B., Corey, D. P., and Patapoutian, A. (2007b). An ion channel essential for sensing chemical damage. *The Journal of neuroscience: the official journal of the Society for Neuroscience* **27**, 11412–11415.

Maier, J.A., Hla, T., and Maciag, T. (1990). Cyclooxygenase is an immediate-early gene induced by interleukin-1 in human endothelial cells. *J. Biol. Chem.* **265**, 10805–10808.

Maingret, F., Coste, B., Padilla, F., Clerc, N., Crest, M., Korogod, S.M., and Delmas, P. (2008). Inflammatory mediators increase Nav1.9 current and excitability in nociceptors through a coincident detection mechanism. *J. Gen. Physiol.* **131**, 211–225.

Matta, J.A., and Ahern, G.P. (2007). Voltage is a partial activator of rat thermosensitive TRP channels. *The Journal of Physiology* **585**, 469–482.

Matta, J. A., Cornett, P. M., Miyares, R. L., Abe, K., Sahibzada, N., and Ahern, G. P. (2008). General anesthetics activate a nociceptive ion channel to enhance pain and inflammation. Proceedings of the National Academy of Sciences of the United States of America **105**, 8784–8789.

McKemy, D.D., Neuhausser, W.M., and Julius, D. (2002). Identification of a cold receptor reveals a general role for TRP channels in thermosensation. *Nature* **416**, 52–58.

McNamara, C. R., Mandel-Brehm, J., Bautista, D. M., Siemens, J., Deranian, K. L., Zhao, M., Hayward, N. J., Chong, J. A., Julius, D., Moran, M. M., and Fanger, C. M. (2007). TRPA1 mediates formalin-induced pain. Proceedings of the National Academy of Sciences of the United States of America. **104**, 13525–13530.

McNulty, M.M., Edgerton, G.B., Shah, R.D., Hanck, D.A., Fozzard, H.A., and Lipkind, G.M. (2007). Charge at the lidocaine binding site residue Phe-1759 affects permeation in human cardiac voltage-gated sodium channels. *J. Physiol.* **581**, 741–755.

Meents, J.E., Neeb, L., and Reuter, U. (2010). TRPV1 in migraine pathophysiology. *Trends in molecular medicine* **16**, 153–159.

Meyer, R. A., Ringkamp, M., Campbell, J. N., and Raja, S. N. (2008). Peripheral Mechanisms of Cutaneous Nociception. In: Wall and Melzak's Texbook of Pain (McMahon SB, Koltzenburg M, eds), Philadelphia: Elsevier, 3–34.

Meyers, J.., MacDonald, R.B., Duggan, A., Lenzi, D., Standaert, D.G., Corwin, J.T., and Corey, D.P. (2003). Lighting up the senses: FM1-43 loading of sensory cells through nonselective ion channels. *J. Neurosci.* **23**, 4054–4065.

Michael, G.J., and Priestley, J.V. (1999). Differential expression of the mRNA for the vanilloid receptor subtype 1 in cells of the adult rat dorsal root and nodose ganglia and its down-regulation by axotomy. *The Journal of neuroscience: the official journal of the Society for Neuroscience* **19**, 1844–1854.

Minke, B. (1977). Drosophila mutant with a transducer defect. *Biophys. Struct. Mech.* **3**, 59–64.

Mohapatra, D.P., and Nau, C. (2003). Desensitization of capsaicin-activated currents in the vanilloid receptor TRPV1 is decreased by the cyclic AMP-dependent protein kinase pathway. *The Journal of biological chemistry* **278**, 50080–50090.

Moiseenkova-Bell, V.Y., and Wensel, T.G. (2009). Hot on the trail of TRP channel structure. *The Journal of general physiology* **133**, 239–244.

Momin, A., and Wood, J.N. (2008). Sensory neuron voltage-gated sodium channels as analgesic drug targets. *Current opinion in neurobiology* **18**, 383–388.

Morgans, C.W., Brown, R.L., and Duvoisin, R.M. (2010). TRPM1: the endpoint of the mGluR6 signal transduction cascade in retinal ON-bipolar cells. *Bioessays* **32**, 609–614.

Moriyama, T., Higashi, T., Togashi, K., Iida, T., Segi, E., Sugimoto, Y., Tominaga, T., Narumiya, S., and Tominaga, M. (2005). Sensitization of TRPV1 by EP1 and IP reveals peripheral nociceptive mechanism of prostaglandins. *Mol. Pain.* **1**, 3.

Muroi, Y., and Chanda, B. (2009). Local anesthetics disrupt energetic coupling between the voltage-sensing segments of a sodium channel. *J. Gen. Physiol.* **133**, 1–15.

Murray, J.M., Derbyshire, S., and Shields, M.O. (2010). Lower limb blocks. *Anaesthesia* **65**(Suppl 1); 57–66.

Nadler, M.J., Hermosura, M.C., Inabe, K., Perraud, A.L., Zhu, Q., Stokes, A.J., Kurosaki, T., Kinet, J. P., Penner, R., Scharenberg, A.M., and Fleig, A. (2001). LTRPC7 is a Mg.ATP-regulated divalent cation channel required for cell viability. *Nature* **411**, 590–595.

Nagata, K., Duggan, A., Kumar, G., and Garcia-Anoveros, J. (2005). Nociceptor and hair cell transducer properties of TRPA1, a channel for pain and hearing. *The Journal of neuroscience: the official journal of the Society for Neuroscience* **25**, 4052–4061.

Nair, A., Simonetti, M., Birsa, N., Ferrari, M.D., van den Maagdenberg, A.M., Giniatullin, R., Nistri, A., and Fabbretti, E. (2010). Familial hemiplegic migraine Ca(v)2.1 channel mutation R192Q enhances ATP-gated P2X3 receptor activity of mouse sensory ganglion neurons mediating trigeminal pain. *Molecular pain* **6**, 48.

Nakagawa, K., Takeda, M., Tsuboi, Y., Kondo, M., Kitagawa, J., Matsumoto, S., Kobayashi, A., Sessle, B.J., Shinoda, M., and Iwata, K. (2010). Alteration of primary afferent activity following inferior alveolar nerve transection in rats. *Molecular pain* **6**, 9.

Nassar, M. A., Stirling, L. C., Forlani, G., Baker, M. D., Matthews, E. A., Dickenson, A. H., and Wood, J. N. (2004). Nociceptor-specific gene deletion reveals a major role for Nav1.7 (PN1) in acute and inflammatory pain. Proceedings of the National Academy of Sciences of the United States of America. **101**, 12706–12711.

Nauli, S.M., Alenghat, F.J., Luo, Y., Williams, E., Vassilev, P., Li, X., Elia, A.E., Lu, W., Brown, E.M., Quinn, S.J., Ingber, D.E., and Zhou, J. (2003). Polycystins 1 and 2 mediate mechanosensation in the primary cilium of kidney cells. *Nat. Genet.* **33**, 129–137.

Nelson, M.T., Joksovic, P.M., Perez-Reyes, E., and Todorovic, S.M. (2005). The endogenous redox agent L-cysteine induces T-type Ca2+ channel-dependent sensitization of a novel subpopulation of rat peripheral nociceptors. *The Journal of neuroscience: the official journal of the Society for Neuroscience* **25**, 8766–8775.

Nelson, M.T., Woo, J., Kang, H.W., Vitko, I., Barrett, P.Q., Perez-Reyes, E., Lee, J.H., Shin, H.S., and Todorovic, S.M. (2007). Reducing agents sensitize C-type nociceptors by relieving high-affinity zinc inhibition of T-type calcium channels. *The Journal of neuroscience: the official journal of the Society for Neuroscience* **27**, 8250–8260.

North, R.A. (2002). Molecular physiology of P2X receptors. *Physiological reviews* **82**, 1013–1067.

Ostman, J.A.R., Nassar, M.A., Wood, J.N., and Baker, M.D. (2008). GTP up-regulated persistent Na+ current and enhanced nociceptor excitability require NaV1.9. *The Journal of physiology* **586**, 1077–1087.

Palazzo, E., Luongo, L., de Novellis, V., Berrino, L., Rossi, F., and Maione, S. (2010). Moving towards supraspinal TRPV1 receptors for chronic pain relief. *Molecular pain* **6**, 66.

Park, C.K., Kim, M.S., Fang, Z., Li, H.Y., Jung, S.J., Choi, S.Y., Lee, S.J., Park, K., Kim, J.S., and Oh, S.B. (2006). Functional expression of thermo-transient receptor potential channels in dental primary afferent neurons: implication for tooth pain. *The Journal of biological chemistry* **281**, 17304–17311.

Park, C.K., Kim, K., Jung, S.J., Kim, M.J., Ahn, D.K., Hong, S.D., Kim, J.S., and Oh, S.B. (2009). Molecular mechanism for local anesthetic action of eugenol in the rat trigeminal system. *Pain* **144**, 84–94.

Park, C.K., Bae, J.H., Kim, H.Y., Jo, H.J., Kim, Y.H., Jung, S.J., Kim, J.S., and Oh, S.B. (2010). Substance P sensitizes P2X3 in nociceptive trigeminal neurons. *Journal of dental research* **89**, 1154–1159.

Park, S.Y., Choi, J.Y., Kim, R.U., Lee, Y.S., Cho, H.J., and Kim, D.S. (2003). Downregulation of voltage-gated potassium channel alpha gene expression by axotomy and neurotrophins in rat dorsal root ganglia. *Mol. Cells.* **16**, 256–259.

Patapoutian, A., Tate, S., and Woolf, C.J. (2009). Transient receptor potential channels: targeting pain at the source. *Nature reviews Drug discovery* **8**, 55–68.

Patwardhan, A.M., Akopian, A.N., Ruparel, N.B., Diogenes, A., Weintraub, S.T., Uhlson, C., Murphy, R.C., and Hargreaves, K.M. (2010). Heat generates oxidized linoleic acid metabolites that activate TRPV1 and produce pain in rodents. *JCI*

Peier, A.M., Moqrich, A., Hergarden, A.C., Reeve, A.J., Andersson, D.A., Story, G.M., Earley, T.J., Dragoni, I., McIntyre, P., Bevan, S., and Patapoutian, A. (2002). A TRP channel that senses cold stimuli and menthol. *Cell* **108**, 705–715.

Perez, C.A., Huang, L., Rong, M., Kozak,J.A., Preuss, A.K., Zhang, H., Max, M., and Margolskee, R. F. (2002). A transient receptor potential channel expressed in taste receptor cells. *Nature neuroscience* **5**, 1169–1176.

Perl, E.R. (2007). Ideas about pain, a historical view. *Nature reviews Neuroscience* **8**, 71–80.

Persson, A.K., Black, J.A., Gasser, A., Cheng, X., Fischer, T.Z., and Waxman, S.G. (2010). Sodium-calcium exchanger and multiple sodium channel isoforms in intra-epidermal nerve terminals. *Molecular pain* **6**, 84.

Peyrot des Gachons, C., Uchida, K., Bryant, B., Shima, A., Sperry, J.B., Dankulich-Nagrudny, L., Tominaga, M., Smith 3rd, A.B., Beauchamp, G.K., and Breslin, P.A. (2011). Unusual pungency from extra-virgin olive oil is attributable to restricted spatial expression of the receptor of oleocanthal. *The Journal of neuroscience: the official journal of the Society for Neuroscience* **31**, 999–1009.

Pomonis, J.D., Harrison, J.E., Mark, L., Bristol, D.R., Valenzano, K.J., and Walker, K. (2003). N-(4-Tertiarybutylphenyl)-4-(3-cholorphyridin-2-yl)tetrahydropyrazine -1(2H)-carbox-amide (BCTC), a novel, orally effective vanilloid receptor 1 antagonist with analgesic properties: II. in vivo characterization in rat models of inflammatory and neuropathic pain. *The Journal of pharmacology and experimental therapeutics* **306**, 387–393.

Premkumar, L.S., Agarwal, S., and Steffen, D. (2002). Single-channel properties of native and cloned rat vanilloid receptors. *The Journal of Physiology* **545**, 107–117.

Priest, B.T. (2009). Future potential and status of selective sodium channel blockers for the treatment of pain. *Curr. Opin. Drug. Discov. Devel.* **12**, 682–692.

Priest, B.T., Murphy, B.A., Lindia, J.A., Diaz, C., Abbadie, C., Ritter, A.M., Liberator, P., Iyer, L.M., Kash, S.F., Kohler, M.G., Kaczorowski, G.J., Macintyre, E., and Martin, W.J. (2005). Contribution of the tetrodotoxin-resistant voltage-gated sodium channel Na. *PNAS*

Puntambekar, P., Mukherjea, D., Jajoo, S., and Ramkumar, V. (2005). Essential role of Rac1/NADPH oxidase in nerve growth factor induction of TRPV1 expression. *Journal of neurochemistry* **95**, 1689–1703.

Ragsdale, D.S., McPhee, J.C., Scheuer, T., and Catterall, W.A. (1994). Molecular determinants of state-dependent block of Na+ channels by local anesthetics. *Science* **265**, 1724–1728.

Ragsdale, D.S., McPhee, J.C., Scheuer, T., and Catterall, W.A. (1996). Common molecular determinants of local anesthetic, antiarrhythmic, and anticonvulsant block of voltage-gated Na+ channels. *Proc. Natl. Acad. Sci. U S A* **93**, 9270–9275.

Renganathan, M., Cummins, T.R., and Waxman, S.G. (2001). Contribution of Na(v)1.8 sodium channels to action potential electrogenesis in DRG neurons. *J. Neurophysiol.* **86**, 629–640.

Riccio, A., Li, Y., Moon, J., Kim, K.S., Smith, K.S., Rudolph, U., Gapon, S., Yao, G.L., Tsvetkov, E., Rodig, S.J., Van't Veer, A., Meloni, E.G., Carlezon Jr., W.A., Bolshakov, V.Y., and Clapham, D.E. (2009). Essential role for TRPC5 in amygdala function and fear-related behavior. *Cell* **137**, 761–772.

Ro, J.Y., Lee, J.S., and Zhang, Y. (2009). Activation of TRPV1 and TRPA1 leads to muscle nociception and mechanical hyperalgesia. *Pain* **144**, 270–277.

Ruetsch, Y.A., Boni, T., and Borgeat, A. (2001). From cocaine to ropivacaine: the history of local anesthetic drugs. *Curr. Top Med. Chem.* **1**, 175–182.

Safieh-Garabedian, B., Poole, S., Allchorne, A., Winter, J., and Woolf, C.J. (1995). Contribution of interleukin-1 beta to the inflammation-induced increase in nerve growth factor levels and inflammatory hyperalgesia. *Br. J. Pharmacol.* **115**, 1265–1275.

Sangameswaran, L., Delgado, S.G., Fish, L.M., Koch, B.D., Jakeman, L.B., Stewart, G.R., Sze, P., Hunter, J.C., Eglen, R.M., and Herman, R.C. (1996). Structure and function of a novel voltage-gated, tetrodotoxin-resistant sodium channel specific to sensory neurons. *The Journal of biological chemistry* **271**, 5953–5956.

Satoh, J., and Yamakage, M. (2009). Desflurane induces airway contraction mainly by activating transient receptor potential A1 of sensory C-fibers. *Journal of anesthesia* **23**, 620–623.

Schmidt, R., Schmelz, M., Forster, C., Ringkamp, M., Torebjork, E., and Handwerker, H. (1995). Novel classes of responsive and unresponsive C nociceptors in human skin. *J. Neurosci.* **15**, 333–341.

Schnizler, K., Shutov, L.P., Van Kanegan, M.J., Merrill, M.A., Nichols, B., McKnight, G.S., Strack, S., Hell, J.W., and Usachev, Y.M. (2008). Protein kinase A anchoring via AKAP150 is essential for TRPV1 modulation by forskolin and prostaglandin E2 in mouse sensory neurons. *The Journal of neuroscience: the official journal of the Society for Neuroscience* **28**, 4904–4917.

Schwarz, W., Palade, P.T., and Hille, B. (1977). Local anesthetics. Effect of pH on use-dependent block of sodium channels in frog muscle. *Biophys. J.* **20**, 343–368.

Scott, N.B. (2010). Wound infiltration for surgery. *Anaesthesia* **65**(1 Suppl); 67–75.

Sheets, M.F., and Hanck, D.A. (2007). Outward stabilization of the S4 segments in domains III and IV enhances lidocaine block of sodium channels. *J. Physiol.* **582**, 317–334.

Sherrington, C.S. (1903). Qualitative difference of spinal reflex corresponding with qualitative difference of cutaneous stimulus. *The Journal of Physiology* **30**, 39–46.

Shinoda, M., Kawashima, K., Ozaki, N., Asai, H., Nagamine, K., and Sugiura, Y. (2007). P2X3 receptor mediates heat hyperalgesia in a rat model of trigeminal neuropathic pain. *The journal of pain: official journal of the American Pain Society* **8**, 588–597.

Smith, G.D., Gunthorpe, M.J., Kelsell, R.E., Hayes, P.D., Reilly, P., Facer, P., Wright, J.E., Jerman, J. C., Walhin, J.P., Ooi, L., Egerton, J., Charles, K.J., Smart, D., Randall, A.D., Anand, P., and Davis, J.B. (2002). TRPV3 is a temperature-sensitive vanilloid receptor-like protein. *Nature* **418**, 186–190.

Souslova, V., Cesare, P., Ding, Y., Akopian, A.N., Stanfa, L., Suzuki, R., Carpenter, K., Dickenson, A., Boyce, S., Hill, R., Nebenuis-Oosthuizen, D., Smith, A.J., Kidd, E.J., and Wood, J.N. (2000). Warm-coding deficits and aberrant inflammatory pain in mice lacking P2X3 receptors. *Nature* **407**, 1015–1017.

Stamboulian, S., Choi, J.S., Ahn, H.S., Chang, Y.W., Tyrrell, L., Black, J.A., Waxman, S.G., and Dib-Hajj, S.D. (2010). ERK1/2 mitogen-activated protein kinase phosphorylates sodium channel Na(v) 1.7 and alters its gating properties. *The Journal of neuroscience: the official journal of the Society for Neuroscience* **30**, 1637–1647.

Stein, A.T., Ufret-Vincenty, C.A., Hua, L., Santana, L.F., and Gordon, S.E. (2006). Phosphoinositide 3-kinase binds to TRPV1 and mediates NGF-stimulated TRPV1 trafficking to the plasma membrane. *The Journal of general physiology* **128**, 509–522.

Steiner, A.A., Turek, V.F., Almeida, M.C., Burmeister, J.J., Oliveira, D.L., Roberts, J.L., Bannon, A. W., Norman, M.H., Louis, J.C., Treanor, J.J., Gavva, N.R., and Romanovsky, A.A. (2007). Nonthermal activation of transient receptor potential vanilloid-1 channels in abdominal viscera tonically inhibits autonomic cold-defense effectors. *The Journal of neuroscience: the official journal of the Society for Neuroscience* **27**, 7459–7468.

Story, G.M., Peier, A.M., Reeve, A.J., Eid, S.R., Mosbacher, J., Hricik, T.R., Earley, T.J., Hergarden, A.C., Andersson, D.A., Hwang, S.W., McIntyre, P., Jegla, T., Bevan, S., and Patapoutian, A. (2003). ANKTM1, a TRP-like channel expressed in nociceptive neurons, is activated by cold temperatures. *Cell* **112**, 819–829.

Stowers, L., Holy, T.E., Meister, M., Dulac, C., and Koentges, G. (2002). Loss of sex discrimination and male-male aggression in mice deficient for TRP2. *Science* **295**, 1493–1500.

Strichartz, G.R. (1973). The inhibition of sodium currents in myelinated nerve by quaternary derivatives of lidocaine. *J. Gen. Physiol.* **62**, 37–57.

Sun, M., Goldin, E., Stahl, S., Falardeau, J.L., Kennedy, J.C., Acierno Jr., J.S., Bove, C., Kaneski, C.R., Nagle, J., Bromley, M.C., Colman, M., Schiffmann, R., and Slaugenhaupt, S.A. (2000). Mucolipidosis type IV is caused by mutations in a gene encoding a novel transient receptor potential channel. *Hum. Mol. Genet.* **9**, 2471–2478.

Takashima, Y., Daniels, R.L., Knowlton, W., Teng, J., Liman, E.R., and McKemy, D.D. (2007). Diversity in the neural circuitry of cold sensing revealed by genetic axonal labeling of transient receptor potential melastatin 8 neurons. *The Journal of neuroscience: the official journal of the Society for Neuroscience* **27**, 14147–14157.

Takeda, M., Kitagawa, J., Takahashi, M., and Matsumoto, S. (2008). Activation of interleukin-1beta receptor suppresses the voltage-gated potassium currents in the small-diameter trigeminal ganglion neurons following peripheral inflammation. *Pain*

Takeda, M., Tsuboi, Y., Kitagawa, J., Nakagawa, K., Iwata, K., and Matsumoto, S. (2011). Potassium channels as a potential therapeutic target for trigeminal neuropathic and inflammatory pain. *Molecular pain* **7**, 5.

Takeda, M., Tanimoto, T., Ikeda, M., Nasu, M., Kadoi, J., Yoshida, S., and Matsumoto, S. (2006). Enhanced excitability of rat trigeminal root ganglion neurons via decrease in A-type potassium currents following temporomandibular joint inflammation. *Neuroscience* **138**, 621–630.

Talley, E.M., Cribbs, L.L., Lee, J.H., Daud, A., Perez-Reyes, E., and Bayliss, D.A. (1999). Differential distribution of three members of a gene family encoding low voltage-activated (T-type) calcium channels. *The Journal of neuroscience: the official journal of the Society for Neuroscience* **19**, 1895–1911.

Taylor, R.E. (1959). Effect of procaine on electrical properties of squid axon membrane. *Am. J. Physiol.* **196**, 1071–1078.

Todorovic, S.M., and Jevtovic-Todorovic, V. (2006). The role of T-type calcium channels in peripheral and central pain processing. *CNS Neurol. Disord. Drug. Targets* **5**, 639–653.

Todorovic, S.M., and Jevtovic-Todorovic, V. (2011). T-type voltage-gated calcium channels as targets for the development of novel pain therapies. *British Journal of Pharmacology*

Todorovic, S.M., Jevtovic-Todorovic, V., Meyenburg, A., Mennerick, S., Perez-Reyes, E., Romano, C., Olney, J.W., and Zorumski, C.F. (2001). Redox modulation of T-type calcium channels in rat peripheral nociceptors. *Neuron* **31**, 75–85.

Tominaga, M., Caterina, M.J., Malmberg, A.B., Rosen, T.A., Gilbert, H., Skinner, K., Raumann, B. E., Basbaum, A.I., and Julius, D. (1998). The cloned capsaicin receptor integrates multiple pain-producing stimuli. *Neuron* **21**, 531–543.

Trebak, M., St., J.B.G., McKay, R.R., Birnbaumer, L., and Putney Jr., J.W. (2003). Signaling mechanism for receptor-activated canonical transient receptor potential 3 (TRPC3) channels. *The Journal of biological chemistry* **278**, 16244–16252.

Trevisani, M., Siemens, J., Materazzi, S., Bautista, D. M., Nassini, R., Campi, B., Imamachi, N., Andre, E., Patacchini, R., Cottrell, G. S., Gatti, R., Basbaum, A. I., Bunnett, N. W., Julius, D., and Geppetti, P. (2007). 4-Hydroxynonenal, an endogenous aldehyde, causes pain and neurogenic inflammation through activation of the irritant receptor TRPA1. Proceedings of the National Academy of Sciences of the United States of America. **104**, 13519–13524.

Tsuboi, Y., Takeda, M., Tanimoto, T., Ikeda, M., Matsumoto, S., Kitagawa, J., Teramoto, K., Simizu, K., Yamazaki, Y., Shima, A., Ren, K., and Iwata, K. (2004). Alteration of the second branch of the trigeminal nerve activity following inferior alveolar nerve transection in rats. *Pain* **111**, 323–334.

Verri, W.A., Cunha, T.M., Parada, C.A., Poole, S., Cunha, F.Q., and Ferreira, Sr. (2006). Hypernociceptive role of cytokines and chemokines: targets for analgesic drug development? *Pharmacology & therapeutics* **112**, 116–138.

Voets, T., Droogmans, G., Wissenbach, U., Janssens, A., Flockerzi, V., and Nilius, B. (2004). The principle of temperature-dependent gating in cold - and heat-sensitive TRP channels. *Nature* **430**, 748–754.

Wang, H., and Woolf, C.J. (2005). Pain TRPs. *Neuron* **46**, 9–12.

Waxman, S.G., Kocsis, J.D., and Black, J.A. (1994). Type III sodium channel mRNA is expressed in embryonic but not adult spinal sensory neurons, and is reexpressed following axotomy. *Journal of Neurophysiology* **72**, 466–470.

Webb, T.., Bateson, A.N., and Barnard, E.A. (1993). Isolation and characterization of a novel family of G protein-coupled receptors. *Biochem. Soc. Trans.* **21**, 199S.

Wes, P. D., Chevesich, J., Jeromin, A., Rosenberg, C., Stetten, G., and Montell, C. (1995). TRPC1, a human homolog of a Drosophila store-operated channel. Proceedings of the National Academy of Sciences of the United States of America. **92**, 9652–9656.

Woolf, C.J., and Ma, Q. (2007). Nociceptors–noxious stimulus detectors. *Neuron* **55**, 353–364.

Wu, G., Hayashi, T., Park, J.H., Dixit, M., Reynolds, D.M., Li, L., Maeda, Y., Cai, Y., Coca-Prados, M., and Somlo, S. (1998). Identification of PKD2L, a human PKD2-related gene: tissue-specific expression and mapping to chromosome 10q25. *Genomics* **54**, 564–568.

Xu, H., Blair, N.T., and Clapham, D.E. (2005). Camphor activates and strongly desensitizes the transient receptor potential vanilloid subtype 1 channel in a vanilloid-independent mechanism. *The Journal of neuroscience: the official journal of the Society for Neuroscience* **25**, 8924–8937.

Xu, H., Delling, M., Jun, J.C., and Clapham, D.E. (2006). Oregano, thyme and clove-derived flavors and skin sensitizers activate specific TRP channels. *Nature neuroscience* **9**, 628–635.

Xu, H., Ramsey, I.S., Kotecha, S.A., Moran, M.M., Chong, J.A., Lawson, D., Ge, P., Lilly, J., Silos-Santiago, I., Xie, Y., DiStefano, P.S., Curtis, R., and Clapham, D.E. (2002). TRPV3 is a calcium-permeable temperature-sensitive cation channel. *Nature* **418**, 181–186.

Yang, B.H., Piao, Z.G., Kim, Y.B., Lee, C.H., Lee, J.K., Park, K., Kim, J.S., and Oh, S.B. (2003). Activation of vanilloid receptor 1 (VR1) by eugenol. *J. Dent. Res.* **82**, 781–785.

Yang, Y., Wang, Y., Li, S., Xu, Z., Li, H., Ma, L., Fan, J., Bu, D., Liu, B., Fan, Z., Wu, G., Jin, J., Ding, B., Zhu, X., and Shen, Y. (2004). Mutations in SCN9A, encoding a sodium channel alpha subunit, in patients with primary erythermalgia. *Journal of Medical Genetics* **41**, 171–174.

Yarov-Yarovoy, V., McPhee, J.C., Idsvoog, D., Pate, C., Scheuer, T., and Catterall, W.A. (2002). Role of amino acid residues in transmembrane segments IS6 and IIS6 of the Na+ channel alpha subunit in voltage-dependent gating and drug block. *J. Biol. Chem.* **277**, 35393–35401.

Yentis, S.M., and Vlassakov, K.V. (1999). Vassily von Anrep, forgotten pioneer of regional anesthesia. *Anesthesiology* **90**, 890–895.

Yeomans, D.C., Levinson, S.R., Peters, M.C., Koszowski, A.G., Tzabazis, A.Z., Gilly, W.F., and Wilson, S.P. (2005). Decrease in inflammatory hyperalgesia by herpes vector-mediated knockdown of Nav1.7 sodium channels in primary afferents. *Hum. Gene. Ther.* **16**, 271–277.

Yin, J., and Kuebler, W.M. (2010). Mechanotransduction by TRP channels: general concepts and specific role in the vasculature. *Cell Biochem. Biophys.* **56**, 1–18.

Yoshida, S., and Matsumoto, S. (2005). Effects of alpha-dendrotoxin on K+ currents and action potentials in tetrodotoxin-resistant adult rat trigeminal ganglion neurons. *The Journal of pharmacology and experimental therapeutics* **314**, 437–445.

Zamponi, G.W., Lewis, R.J., Todorovic, S.M., Arneric, S.P., and Snutch, T.P. (2009). Role of voltage-gated calcium channels in ascending pain pathways. *Brain research reviews* **60**, 84–89.

Zhang, X., Huang, J., and McNaughton, P.A. (2005). NGF rapidly increases membrane expression of TRPV1 heat-gated ion channels. *Embo J.* **24**, 4211–4223.

Zhang, X.F., Shieh, C.C., Chapman, M.L., Matulenko, M.A., Hakeem, A.H., Atkinson, R.N., Kort, M.E., Marron, B.E., Joshi, S., Honore, P., Faltynek, C.R., Krafte, D.S., and Jarvis, M.F. (2010). A-887826 is a structurally novel, potent and voltage-dependent Na(v)1.8 sodium channel blocker that attenuates neuropathic tactile allodynia in rats. *Neuropharmacology* **59**, 201–207.

Zhang, Y., Hoon, M.A., Chandrashekar, J., Mueller, K.L., Cook, B., Wu, D., Zuker, C.S., and Ryba, N.J. (2003). Coding of sweet, bitter, and umami tastes: different receptor cells sharing similar signaling pathways. *Cell* **112**, 293–301.

Zimmermann, K., Leffler, A., Babes, A., Cendan, C.M., Carr, R.W., Kobayashi, J-., Nau, C., Wood, J. N., and Reeh, P.W. (2007). Sensory neuron sodium channel Nav1.8 is essential for pain at low temperatures. *Nature* **447**, 855–858.

Zurborg, S., Yurgionas, B., Jira, J. A., Caspani, O., and Heppenstall, P. A. (2007). Direct activation of the ion channel TRPA1 by Ca2+. *Nature neuroscience* **10**, 277–279.

PERIPHERAL AND CENTRAL MECHANISMS OF OROFACIAL INFLAMMATORY PAIN

Barry J. Sessle

Faculties of Dentistry and Medicine, University of Toronto, 124 Edward Street, Toronto, ON M5G 1G6, Canada

I. Introduction

The face, mouth, and jaws manifest some of the most common pains in the body, and epidemiological investigations have documented the high prevalence rates for several acute or chronic orofacial pain conditions (Lipton *et al.*, 1993; LeResche and Drangsholt, 2008). These pain conditions include many involving inflammation of orofacial tissues and range from acute pulpitis (toothache) and mucositis to chronic arthritic conditions affecting the temporomandibular joint (TMJ. This article will focus on the mechanisms in orofacial tissues and in nociceptive pathways in the brain that underlie the development or maintenance of acute and chronic orofacial inflammatory pain.

II. Overview of Trigeminal Primary Afferent Mechanisms

The trigeminal (V) nerve, which is the fifth cranial nerve, provides the principal sensory innervation of the face and mouth (for review, see Dubner *et al.*, 1978;

DOI: 10.1016/B978-0-12-385198-7.00007-2

Sessle, 2005a, 2009). Many trigeminal primary afferent fibers terminate in the orofacial tissues as free nerve endings and function as nociceptors since they are activated by noxious stimuli. These noxious stimuli may include mechanical stimuli such as a pin prick or surgical incision of the facial skin or oral mucosa, extraction of a tooth, bacterial toxins accessing an exposed dental pulp, the products of an inflammatory process in a jaw muscle, TMJ, tooth, cornea, etc., and chemical irritants (e.g. hot pepper, mustard), or excessively hot or cold liquids coming into contact with the oral mucosa. The activation of the nociceptive endings by a noxious stimulus can result in activation of their parent small-diameter, slowly conducting (A-delta and C-fiber) primary afferent fibers which have their primary afferent cell bodies in the trigeminal ganglion. These nociceptive afferent fibers conduct nerve impulses away from their nociceptive endings into the central nervous system (CNS) and provide the brain with sensory-discriminative information about the quality, location, intensity, and duration of the stimulus.

Several chemicals mediators are involved in the activation of the nociceptive endings (e.g. prostaglandins, bradykinins) as a result of their release following the damage or inflammation of the tissue innervated by the nociceptive endings. Orofacial nociceptive afferents are also subject to considerable modulation since, like spinal nociceptive afferents, there is a peripheral substrate by which complex interactions between the neural, immune, cardiovascular, and endocrine systems can take place (for review, see Meyer *et al.*, 2006; Woolf and Ma, 2007; Matthews and Sessle, 2008). These interactions can take place not only at the afferent's peripheral endings in the orofacial tissues, but also at its cell body in the trigeminal ganglion and can be triggered or maintained by inflammation, as outlined below.

III. Effects of Inflammation and Inflammatory Irritants on Various Trigeminal Nociceptive Afferents

Inflammation of peripheral tissues may be associated with the release of chemical mediators from tissue cells such as mast cells, macrophages, and immune cells (e.g. 5-hydroxytrytamine [5-HT], histamine, tumor necrosis factor [TNF] alpha) or from the nociceptive afferent endings themselves (e.g. substance P) (for review, see Hucho and Levine, 2006; Meyer *et al.*, 2006; Woolf and Ma, 2007). Many of these mediators can act on the nociceptive endings at the site of injury to increase their excitability (Fig. 1). They act by virtue of their action on certain receptors and ion channels of the nociceptive endings, and associated intracellular matrix, signaling, and second messenger systems (e.g. 5-HT; protease-activated;

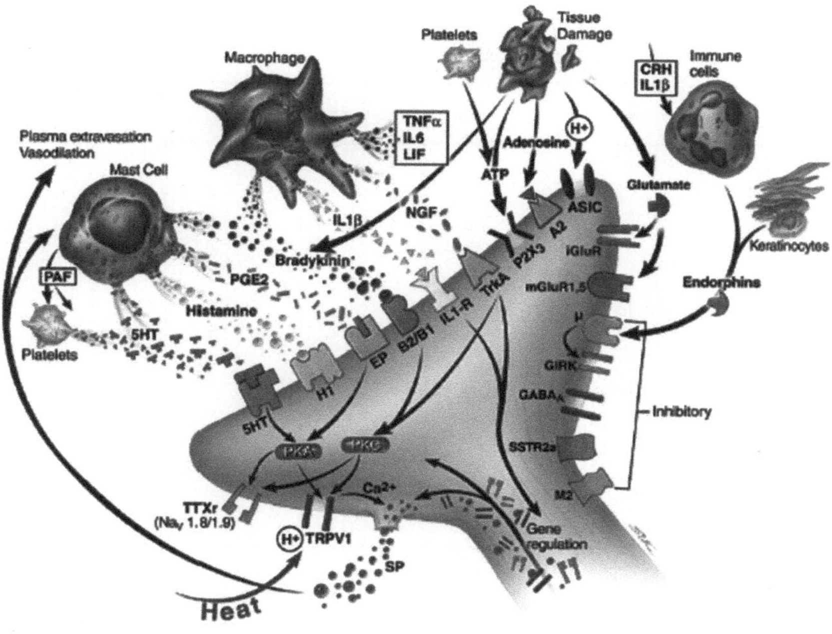

FIG. 1. Peripheral mediators involved in inflammation-related peripheral sensitization following inflammation. Inflammation results in numerous chemicals being released from mast cells, macrophages, immune cells, and injured cells that may alter the sensitivity of peripheral afferent terminals; several of these mediators are shown here. ASIC, acid-sensing ion channel; CRH, corticotrophin-releasing hormone; GIRK, G-protein-copied inward rectifying potassium channel; 5-HT, serotonin; iGluR, ionotropic glutamate receptor; IL-1β, interleukin-1-beta; IL-6, interleukin-6; LIF, leukemia inhibitory factor; M_2, muscarinic receptor; mGluR, metabotropic glutamate receptor; NGF, nerve growth factor; PAF, platelet-activating factor; PGE_2, prostaglandin E_2; PKA, protein kinase A; PKC, protein kinase C; SSTR2A, somatostatin receptor 2A; TNF-α, tumor necrosis factor alpha; TrkA, tyrosine kinase receptor A; TRPV1, transient receptor potential vanilloid 1; TTXr, tetrodotoxin-resistant sodium channel; μ, mu-opioid receptor. (From Meyer *et al.*, 2006).

neurokinin receptors). Inflammatory irritants applied to the tissues also have analogous actions, e.g. capsaicin acts on TRPV1 and mustard oil on TRPA1 ion channels. As a result, the endings may show an enhanced response to subsequent noxious stimuli, and even respond to stimuli that before the tissue damage or inflammation were innocuous, thus reflecting a decreased activation threshold; some may also develop spontaneous activity. Through the spread of the mediators through the tissues, these changes may also occur in other nociceptive endings adjacent to the injury site. This enhanced excitability reflects a so-called peripheral sensitization of the nociceptive endings, and can result in an augmented afferent barrage being conducted along the nociceptive afferents into the CNS. Table I

Table I
Effect of Inflammatory Mediators on Nociceptors and Pain.

Mediator	Effect on nociceptors	Effect on human volunteers
Potassium	Activate	++
Protons	Activate	++
Serotonin	Activate	++
Bradykinin	Activate	+++
Histamine	Activate	+
Tumor necrosis factor α (TNF α)	Sensitize	+
Prostaglandins	Sensitize	±
Leukotrienes	Sensitize	±
Nerve growth factor (NGF)	Sensitize	++
Substance P	Sensitize	±
Interleukin 1 (IL-1)	Sensitize(?)	-
Endotoxin	Sensitize(?)	-
Prolactin	Sensitize	-
Proteases	Activate	-

From Khan *et al.*, 2008

outlines the effects of various inflammatory irritants and mediators on the nociceptive afferent endings.

Thus, by the increased responsiveness to noxious stimuli, decreased activation threshold, spontaneous activity, and involvement of adjacent afferents, peripheral sensitization represents a peripheral nociceptive process that may contribute to the hyperalgesia, allodynia, spontaneous pain and pain spread that are characteristic of most acute or chronic inflammatory pain conditions. Tissue injury or inflammation may also lead to axonal sprouting or abnormal discharges of the nociceptive afferents, representing additional pathophysiological processes in some pain conditions. Also noteworthy is that the nociceptive afferents can undergo phenotypic changes in response to peripheral inflammation, with alterations in the expression of certain receptors or ion channels (e.g., NaV). Transcription of neuropeptides, brain-derived neurotrophic factor (BDNF) and ion channels as well as translation of TRP channels may occur and enhance peripheral (and central) sensitization (Fig. 2), and inflammatory irritants that act upon these receptors or ion channels, can excite or sensitize the afferent endings. Excitatory changes resulting from neural and non-neural processes in the ganglion can also occur in the afferent's ganglion cell body. Inflammation of peripheral tissues, can for example, cause the release of chemical mediators in the ganglion through paracrine processes that affect the afferent's excitability and its discharges conducted

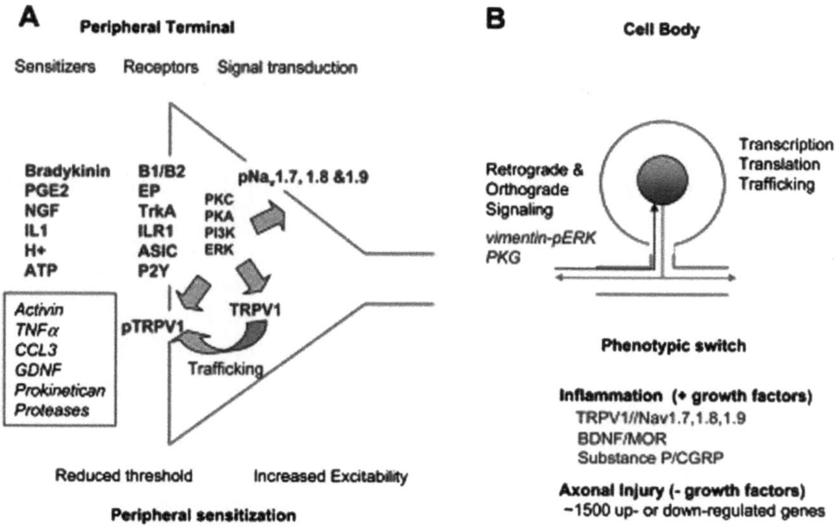

FIG. 2. Chemical mediators, receptors and signal transduction mechanisms involved in peripheral sensitization of peripheral nociceptive ending (A), and phenotypic switches occurring in nociceptor ganglion cell body (B) as a result of inflammation (and axonal injury) by virtue of exposure to retrogradely transported signal molecules or absence of target-derived signals. (From Woolf and Ma, 2007).

into the CNS; non-neural cells (e.g. satellite glial cells) may also play a critical role (see below).

The following outlines inflammation-related effects on the afferents supplying specific orofacial tissues.

The facial skin, cornea, and oral mucosa are supplied by nociceptive afferents that can be activated by inflammatory irritants and their activation can lead to pain (see Belmonte, 2007; Cooper, 2007). For example, capsaicin application to facial skin or cornea acts through TRP receptors to activate nociceptive trigeminal afferents, and elicit nociceptive behavior that includes mechanical allodynia or thermal hyperalgesia (e.g., Diogenes *et al.*, 2006; Honda *et al*, 2008; Akiyama *et al.*, 2010; Okumura *et al.*, 2010), as can Complete Freund's Adjuvant (CFA) or formalin when applied to the perioral skin (e.g., Raboisson and Dallel, 2004; Morgan and Gebhart, 2008; Quintans-Júnior *et al.*, 2010). Peripheral sensitization of trigeminal cutaneous nociceptive afferents can also be produced by some of these inflammatory irritants such as capsaicin, although with others (e.g. mustard oil) it may also produce desensitizing effects (see Lam *et al.*, 2008; 2009a).

The tooth pulp and periodontium are extensively innervated. Little information is available of effects of inflammation on periodontal afferents although "*in vitro*" as well as "*in vivo*" recordings do indicate that periodontal nociceptive afferents can be activated by a variety of mechanical, thermal or chemical stimuli (Mengel *et al*, 1993; Toda *et al*, 2004). In contrast, considerable study has been made of the properties of afferents supplying the tooth pulp which is a common source of pain. The dentine encasing the pulp is also very sensitive despite its relatively sparse innervation, and activation of intradentinal afferents appears to be mainly due to a hydrodynamic mechanism, although the odontoblast (the dentine-forming cell) may play an important role (see Byers and Narhi, 1999; Hu, 2004; Matthews and Sessle, 2008; Magloire *et al.*, 2010). A special feature of the pulp that should be noted is that it has a very low compliance because of its encasement in hard tissues, and this feature is thought to be a factor contributing to the exquisite sensitivity of the tooth in some inflammatory states. Also, the clinical outcome of dental caries reflects an orchestrated process involving bacterial invasion, several inflammatory mediators, immune cells, and other chemical processes within the pulp. These processes may also include growth factors leading to morphological as well as phenotypic changes in the pulp afferent endings, including sprouting, and changes in neuropeptide expression that may be reflected in an increased receptive field size of the afferents (Byers and Narhi, 1999), and so an enhancement of spatial summation that could result in an increase in pain sensitivity.

Many of the peripheral chemical processes, receptors, and ion channels underlying the activation and sensitization of intradental afferents appear to be similar to those identified in other tissues (see above), including intraneural neuropeptides (e.g. substance P, calcitonin gene-related peptide [CGRP]), ATP and TRP receptors, and a number of other chemical mediators (e.g. histamine, 5-HT, opioids, cytokines) released from pulp tissue cells; several of these also contribute to pulp inflammatory, repair, and regenerative processes. Novel approaches to study these mediators or effects of inflammatory irritants have been introduced, and involve pulpal perfusion and microdialysis techniques, including their application to human pulps in situ (Chidiac *et al.*, 2001; Bowles *et al.*, 2003; see Khan and Hargreaves, 2008, 2010), showing for example that compared to normal healthy teeth, an inflamed pulp has increased levels of substance P which can itself modulate the inflammatory process through several mechanisms. Also noteworthy is that while many of the mediators activate and/or sensitize the afferent endings, some appear to have suppressive effects on afferent excitability. For example, opiate receptors occur in the pulp and peripherally applied morphine to an inflamed booth may control dental pain, especially if chronic (Dionne *et al.*, 2001; Jaber *et al.*, 2003).

The endings of many of the nociceptive afferents innervating the masticatory muscles and TMJ may respond to a wide range of peripheral stimuli that cause pain in humans and nociceptive behavior in rodent models of deep orofacial pain, including inflammatory agents such as capsaicin, mustard oil, and CFA (see Gazerani and Arendt-Nielsen, 2005; Sessle, 2006; Cairns, 2007). Capsaicin for example not only activates and sensitizes TMJ nociceptive afferents, but also sometimes desensitizes them (Lam *et al.*, 2009a). Several recent studies utilizing electrophysiological, immunohistochemical, and behavioral approaches have provided evidence for agonists acting peripherally on glutamate, GABA or opiate receptors, just to name a few, as also having modulatory effects on these musculoskeletal craniofacial afferents and their effects in the CNS; sex hormones (e.g., estrogens) also can modulate their activity, and there are documented sex differences in their responsiveness to some of these agonists (e.g., Cairns *et al*, 2001a, 2003; Lam *et al.*, 2005b, 2009a, b; Wang *et al*, 2010; see Lam *et al.*, 2005a; Cairns, 2007). Several other chemicals acting as inflammatory mediators have also been used in human TMJ and masticatory muscles (e.g. see Kopp, 2001; Milam, 2006; Kopp and Alstergren, 2008). These studies have implicated some neuropeptides (e.g. substance P, CGRP), 5-HT, cytokines (e.g. 1L-1β, TNFα) or other inflammatory mediators such as prostaglandins in TMJ or muscle pain conditions associated with inflammation. For example, 5-HT, 1L-1β and prostaglandins are not present in the TMJ synovial fluid of healthy subjects, but are detectable in inflamed TMJ synovial fluid, suggesting they may prove to be useful diagnostic markers or therapeutic targets. The same applies to glutamate levels in the jaw muscles of temporomandibular disorder patients, although glutamate *per se* does not appear to produce a significant inflammatory response (Castrillon *et al.*, 2010).

Cranial vessels and the meninges are supplied by small-diameter afferents that can be activated by noxious stimuli (Strassman *et al.*, 1996; Burstein *et al.*, 2006; Strassman and Levy, 2006; Messlinger, 2009) that may be associated with the subsequent development of vasodilatation related to neurogenic inflammation. They can also be activated or sensitized by the application to these tissues of an "inflammatory soup" containing several inflammatory and algesic chemicals. The activation and modulation of these afferents by inflammation and related peripheral neurochemical processes (e.g., 5-HT) are thought to be important factors in the initiation and control of certain headaches such as migraine.

There is also evidence that non-neural cells, the satellite glial cells that envelop the primary afferent neurons in the trigeminal ganglion, provide not only metabolic and structural support of the neurons but can also modulate their excitability (for review, see Chiang *et al.*, 2011). The inflammatory irritants or inflammation *per se* (or nerve injury) produce orofacial mechano-allodynia and a variety of ganglion changes, such as gene expression and intracellular molecular alterations, and neuropeptide generation in trigeminal ganglion neurons as well as an increase in neuronal excitability (Ambalavanar and Dessem, 2009; Takeda *et al.*, 2009; Vaughn and Gold, 2010). It is also noteworthy that some inflammatory-related events in tissues of one trigeminal division may produce intracellular changes (e.g., ERK, p38MAPK, and phosphatases) in neurons and satellite glial cells in all three divisions of the trigeminal ganglion, and so possibly contribute to peripheral mechanisms, underlying the spread of orofacial pain (Thalakoti *et al.*, 2007. Freeman *et al.*, 2008). Paracrine processes may also be involved since the neuropeptides substance P and CGRP are released from trigeminal ganglion cells following inflammation and affect satellite glial cell activity (Takeda *et al.*, 2009), supporting other evidence of a role for these neuropeptides in modulating satellite glial cell function in the trigeminal ganglion (Vause *et al.*, 2009). There is a recent evidence that gap junctions (Hanani, 2005; Thalakoti *et al.*, 2007; Garrett and Durham, 2008; O'Hara *et al.*, 2008) in addition to paracrine processes may be important in the spread of excitation between the satellite glial cells as well as to trigeminal ganglion neurons. While many details of the processes underlying neuron-glia interactions in the trigeminal ganglion are still unclear, these processes likely are critical in determining the generation of increased or abnormal afferent activity that can influence both neuronal as well as glial function in the CNS nociceptive mechanisms underlying orofacial inflammatory (and neuropathic) pain (see below).

The numerous peripheral chemical mediators, ion channels, receptors, and intracellular processes involved in orofacial nociceptive activation and sensitization related to inflammation are all potential targets for the development of new and more effective therapeutic approaches. Common non-steroidal anti-inflammatory drugs (NSAIDs), as well as many more recently analgesics such as COX-2 inhibitors have their main analgesic and anti-inflammatory actions in peripheral tissues (e.g. on PGE2 synthesis). However, the multiplicity of processes, many of which act in parallel, also means that targetting any one or only a few is unlikely to have a major impact therapeutically. The development of effective agents that act further downstream on the consequences of the increased afferent excitability associated with inflammation, will be likely prove a more useful and fruitful avenue (see Hucho and Levine, 2007).

IV. Overview of Trigeminal Nociceptive Pathways and Organizational Features

The trigeminal primary afferents project to the trigeminal brainstem sensory nuclear complex where they synapse on second-order neurons. The trigeminal brainstem complex can be subdivided into the main or principal sensory nucleus and the spinal tract nucleus, which is comprised of three subnuclei: oralis, interpolaris, and caudalis (Fig. 3). The neurons in each nucleus and subnucleus are arranged in a topographic manner; many are low-threshold mechanoreceptive (LTM) neurons, that provide the brain with spatiotemporal information about orofacial tactile stimuli, others instead code for non-noxious warming or cooling of facial skin or mucosa (for review, see Dubner *et al.*, 1978; Sessle, 2006, 2009). There are also many neurons that respond to noxious stimuli and that represent crucial brainstem elements in orofacial pain, as outlined below.

Although the other subnuclei (interpolaris, oralis) of the trigeminal brainstem complex may contribute to the brainstem mechanisms of orofacial pain (see Sessle,

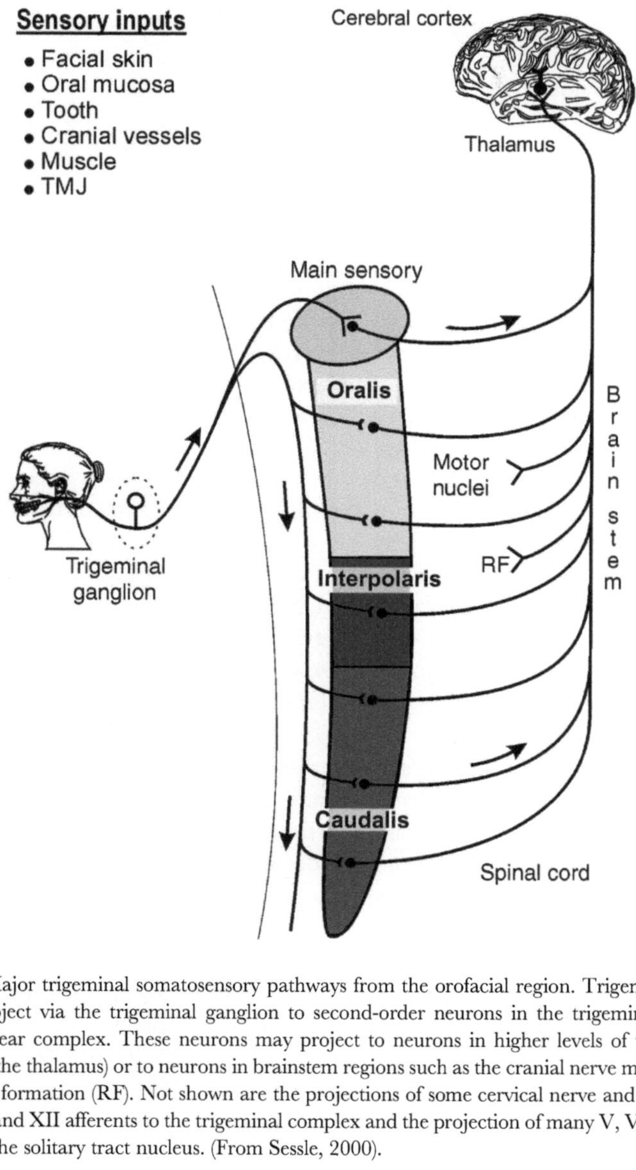

FIG. 3. Major trigeminal somatosensory pathways from the orofacial region. Trigeminal primary afferents project via the trigeminal ganglion to second-order neurons in the trigeminal brainstem sensory nuclear complex. These neurons may project to neurons in higher levels of the brain (for example, in the thalamus) or to neurons in brainstem regions such as the cranial nerve motor nuclei or the reticular formation (RF). Not shown are the projections of some cervical nerve and cranial nerve VII, IX, X, and XII afferents to the trigeminal complex and the projection of many V, VII, IX, and X afferents to the solitary tract nucleus. (From Sessle, 2000).

2006; Woda, 2003; Dostrovsky and Sessle, 2007), subnucleus caudalis has been especially implicated in orofacial nociceptive mechanisms on the basis of clinical, behavioral, anatomical, immunocytochemical, and electrophysiological findings (for review, see Dubner *et al.*, 1978; Dubner and Bennett, 1983; Sessle, 2000, 2005a, b;

Dostrovsky and Sessle, 2007). For example, like the spinal dorsal horn, small-diameter afferents ending in subnucleus caudalis release neuropeptides (e.g. substance P) as well as ATP, and excitatory amino acids such as glutamate that excite nociceptive neurons (nociceptive-specific, NS; and wide dynamic range, WDR). These two types of nociceptive neurons predominate in the superficial and deep laminae of the subnucleus caudalis, and process and relay nociceptive afferent information to higher brain centers (e.g. thalamus) or local (brainstem) centers such as those involved in facial, jaw, and tongue skeletal muscle reflexes, and autonomic reflex responses evoked by noxious orofacial stimuli (Fig. 3). The subnucleus caudalis now is often termed the medullary dorsal horn because of its many similarities with the spinal dorsal horn. There are however several distinguishing characteristics of subnucleus caudalis, including a caudal component merging with the cervical dorsal horn, and a rostral component forming a distinctive transition region with the subnucleus interpolaris; each if these two components has its own unique morphological and functional features that may be differentially involved in contributing to perceptual, endocrine, autonomic, and muscle reflex responses to noxious stimulation of different orofacial tissues (Bereiter *et al.*, 2000; Dubner and Ren, 2004).

Some caudalis nociceptive neurons respond only to the stimulation of a cutaneous or mucosal mechanoreceptive field and, as a consequence, they are thought to play an important role in our ability to localize, detect, and discriminate superficial noxious stimuli. However, most of them can also be activated by peripheral afferent inputs from other tissues, e.g., tooth pulp, TMJ, jaw muscle, or cerebrovasculature (Sessle, 2000, 2005a; Dostrovsky and Sessle, 2007). Such features are thought to provide an important neural substrate for central sensitization (see below) and for the very common clinical findings of poor localization, and referral of pain from deep tissues or from teeth.

Both WDR and NS neurons also occur in several thalamic regions (e.g. ventrobasal thalamus, nucleus submedius, intralaminar nuclei) as well as in the main cortical targets of these thalamic nuclei (e.g. the insula, primary and secondary somatosensory cortices, and cingulate cortex) (Sessle, 2005a; Dostrovsky and Sessle, 2007). Like the ascending spinal nociceptive pathways, nociceptive neurons in the central trigeminal nociceptive system can be modulated by segmental and descending circuits within the CNS that utilize a number of chemical mediators (e.g. opioids, norepinephrine, GABA, glycine, 5-HT) (Sessle, 2000, 2005a, b; Dubner and Ren, 2004; Bereiter, 2007; Dostrovsky and Sessle, 2007). Many of these segmental or descending substrates are inhibitory, and there is evidence that they contribute to the efficacy of several pain-relieving approaches (e.g., acupuncture, deep brain stimulation, analgesic drugs such as morphine, tricyclic antidepressants, and carbamazepine). Some however have facilitatory effects on the trigeminal nociceptive neurons, as outlined below.

The trigeminal nociceptive transmission can be enhanced by peripheral afferent inputs to the CNS as a result of trauma or inflammation of peripheral tissues or nerves that result in a barrage of nociceptive primary afferent input into the CNS. This barrage may lead to prolonged neuroplastic alterations in nociceptive pathways that collectively have been termed central sensitization. Trigeminal central sensitization is reflected in an enhanced excitability of nociceptive neurons that may be manifested as an increase in their spontaneous activity, expansion of their mechanoreceptive field, lowering of their activation threshold, and enhancement of their peripherally evoked nociceptive responses [Sessle, 2000, 2005b]. Such changes are thought to contribute to persistent orofacial pain and respectively to its common characteristics of spontaneous pain, pain spread and referral, allodynia, and hyperalgesia. Trigeminal central sensitization involves several receptor mechanisms, ion channels, and intracellular signaling processes; these include neurokinin and purinergic as well as NMDA and non-NMDA glutamatergic receptor mechanisms (see Sessle, 2000, 2005b; Dubner and Ren, 2004). It is especially evident in subnucleus caudalis but also occurs in subnucleus oralis and higher brain regions such as the ventrobasal thalamus, although subnucleus caudalis has been shown to be responsible for the expression of central sensitization in these structures by way of its projections to both (see below).

It is also noteworthy that in addition to their well-known "housekeeping" roles, glia in the CNS have important and unique roles in modulation of neuronal excitability. Both astroglia and microglia can mediate immune responses and can switch to a much more active ("activated") state by CNS injury and inflammation, as well as by peripheral inflammation (and nerve damage) (see Milligan and Watkins, 2009; Chiang *et al.*, 2011). Both may also interact and influence each other's involvement in exaggerated nociceptive responses to injury or inflammation, such as central sensitization. It is also important to note that disruption of glial function is reported to have no effect on nociceptive behavioral responses to thermal or mechanical stimuli in intact animals, suggesting that glia may not make a significant contribution to normal pain processing, but are instead involved in conditions of pain enhancement (see Milligan and Watkins, 2009).

V. Effects of Inflammation and Inflammatory Irritants on Central Trigeminal Nociceptive Mechanisms

The nociceptive neurons in subnuclei caudalis and oralis and higher centers such as ventrobasal thalamus can be activated not only by noxious mechanical or thermal stimulation of orofacial tissues but also by inflammatory irritants applied to orofacial tissues (e.g. Amano *et al.*, 1986; Broton *et al.*, 1988; Chiang *et al.*, 1998; Burstein *et al.*, 2006; Goadsby, 2006; Zhang *et al*, 2006; Zanotto *et al.*, 2007; Honda *et al*, 2008; Yamazaki *et al*, 2008; Tashiro *et al.*, 2009, 2010; Akiyama *et al.*, 2010; Chun and Ro, 2010; Kaneko *et al.*, 2010). The application of these irritants to TMJ, tooth pulp, facial skin, masticatory muscle, and cerebrovasculature can evoke a sustained activation of many of these neurons. These agents may also induce nociceptive behavior. For example, injection into cutaneous or deep orofacial tissues of inflammatory irritants such as capsaicin or mustard oil (or non-inflammatory agents such as glutamate), can evoke acute pain and other nociceptive behaviors in humans or experimental animals (e.g. Yu *et al.*, 1994; Cairns *et al.*, 1998, 2003; Capra and Ro, 2004; Gazerani *et al*, 2005; Lam *et al.*, 2005b; Ro, 2008; Wang *et al*, 2010). More sustained pain behavior lasting several hours or even longer can also be induced by formalin or carrageenan application to these tissues (e.g. Duale *et al.*, 1996; Eisenberg *et al.*, 1996; Capra and Ro, 2004; Clemente *et al.*, 2004; Teixeira *et al.*, 2010). Even more persistent nociceptive behavior associated with a chronic inflammatory state can be induced by the injection of CFA into the rat's TMJ or masticatory muscle or by manipulations inducing a sustained inflammatory state in musculoskeletal tissues including the teeth (e.g. Dubner and Ren, 2004; Ro, 2005; Yamazaki *et al.*, 2008; Tsuboi *et al.*, 2011).

In the subnucleus caudalis, various of these peripheral manipulations are associated with the induction of c-Fos expression which is thought to reflect increased neuronal activity (e.g. Wakisaki *et al.*, 1992; Coimbra and Coimbra, 1994; Hathaway *et al.*, 1995; Gojyo *et al.*, 2002; Locher-Claus *et al.*, 2005; Stabile *et al.*, 2009). Electrophysiological changes reflecting central sensitization also occur, e.g. mustard oil or capsaicin application to the TMJ, masticatory muscle or tooth pulp (e.g. Hu *et al*, 1992; Yu *et al.*, 1993; Chiang *et al.*, 1998; Lam *et al.*, 2009b) produces a lowering of the threshold for activation of caudalis NS and WDR neurons by peripheral orofacial stimuli, an increase of neuronal responses to graded noxious stimuli, and an increase in neuronal cutaneous and deep receptive field size (Fig. 4). In contrast, mustard oil application to facial skin is much less effective in inducing these neuronal changes (Yu *et al.*, 1993; Dubner and Ren, 2004). Sex differences were noted above in the responsiveness of some nociceptive trigeminal afferents, and may also occur in the effectiveness of noxious stimuli in exciting caudalis nociceptive neurons, and possibly in inducing central sensitization in them (see Lam *et al.*, 2005a; Bereiter, 2007). The changes in receptive field and response properties of the caudalis nociceptive neurons reflect a neuroplasticity of central trigeminal nociceptive processes that can be produced by orofacial inflammation or inflammatory irritants, and provide a neural substrate that may contribute to the pain spread or referral, and the allodynia and hyperalgesia that may result from the inflammation of orofacial tissues.

Central sensitization of caudalis nociceptive neurons may occur within minutes and last for several minutes after an inflammatory irritant is administered to craniofacial tissues, but it may last for days in the case of a chronic inflammation (or nerve injury) (see Burstein *et al.*, 2000; Sessle, 2000, 2005a,b; Capra and Ro, 2004; Dubner and Ren, 2004). In addition, it has been shown that the caudalis central sensitization induced by mustard oil or capsaicin (or glutamate) application may be

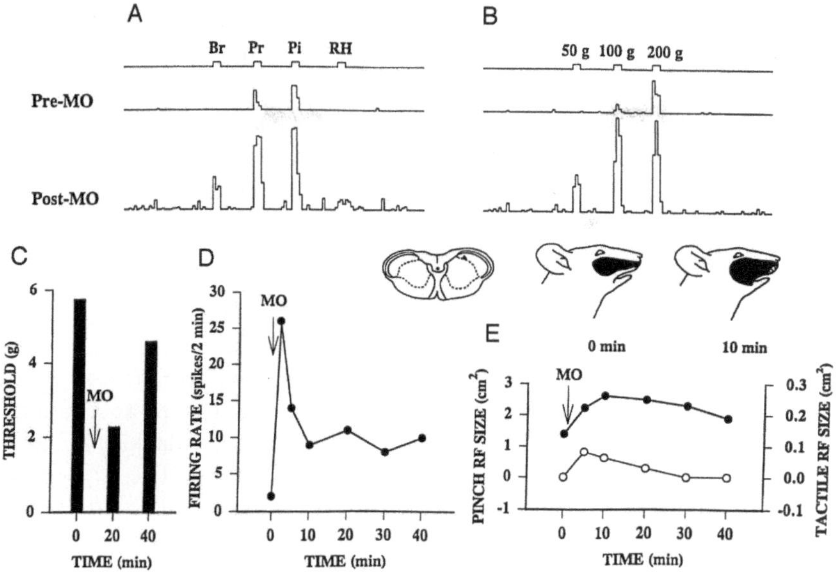

FIG. 4. Example of a caudalis nociceptive-specific (NS) neuron showing changes in spontaneous activity and mechanoreceptive field (RF) and response properties after mustard oil (MO) application to the maxillary molar pulp. A: neuronal responses to mechanical and thermal stimuli applied to the cutaneous RF. Top trace: marker of brush (Br), pressure (Pr), pinch (Pi) and radiant heat (RH). Middle trace: neuronal responses in control conditions (i.e., Pre-MO, before MO application). Bottom trace: neuronal responses to same stimuli 20 min after MO application (i.e., Post-MO, after MO application). B: neuronal responses to graded mechanical stimuli (50, 100, and 200 g). Each stimulus lasts for 3 s, and the **y**-axis scale (omitted) is the same for middle and bottom traces in A and B. Binwidth is 1 s. Note that MO application resulted in this NS neuron taking on features of a WDR neuron, by becoming responsive to light brushing of the facial skin; it also became responsive to radiant heating of its cutaneous RF and much more responsive to graded pinch stimuli. C: profound decrease in mechanical threshold at 20 min and a partial recovery at 40 min after MO application; 0-min value represents the baseline value before MO application; arrow represents the time when MO was applied to the molar pulp. D: MO induced a brief burst of discharges followed by a higher firing rate than the baseline level (0 min). E: MO induced an expansion of cutaneous pinch RF as well as a temporary appearance of tactile RF. ●: values of pinch RF size; ○: values of tactile RF size. Values at 0 min represent the RF size before MO application. Insets: histologically retrieved recording site and RF sizes before (0 min) and 10 min after MO application (i.e., solid area represents pinch RF and shaded area represents a novel tactile RF that also responded to pinch stimulus after MO application). (From Chiang *et al.*, 1998).

accompanied by increased electromyographic (EMG) activity in both jaw-opening and jaw-closing muscles, that is dependent on the functional integrity of caudalis, e.g. it can be abolished by blockade of caudalis or mimicked by activation of caudalis (Yu *et al.*, 1994; Cairns *et al.*, 1998, 2001b; Sunakawa *et al.*, 1999; Tsai *et al.*, 1999; Yao *et al.*, 2009).

The nociceptive behavior evoked by inflammatory irritants and the mustard oil-evoked increases in jaw muscle EMG activity, c-Fos expression and caudalis nociceptive neuronal excitability involve NMDA and non-NMDA glutamatergic receptors as well as several second messenger systems such as NO and kinases, that may also show for example increased expression (e.g. Bereiter and Bereiter, 1996; Cairns *et al.*, 1998; Chiang *et al.*, 1998; Yu *et al.*, 1996; Honda *et al.*, 2008; Noma *et al.*, 2008; see Sessle, 2000; Dubner and Ren, 2004; Capra and Ro, 2004; Bereiter, 2007; Ro, 2008). Furthermore, purinergic receptor mechanisms play a role, since trigeminal central sensitization induced for example by mustard oil applied to a tooth pulp can be mimicked by the caudalis application of P2X receptor subtype agonists, and blocked by the application of P2X subtype antagonists to subnucleus caudalis (Hu *et al.*, 2002; Chiang *et al.*, 2005). Moreover, caudalis central sensitization and enhanced jaw or neck EMG activity can be reflexly induced by the application of P2X agonists to tissues such as tooth pulp, TMJ, or dura, and the reflex effects can be reduced by application to these peripheral tissues or to caudalis of P2X antagonists (Adachi *et al.*, 2010; Watanabe *et al.*, 2010; Yao *et al.*, 2010; Cherkas *et al.*, 2011). The P2X-related neuronal and EMG effects of inflammatory irritants applied to craniofacial tissues are in keeping with evidence that $P2X_3$ receptors on the central terminals of nociceptive primary afferents modulate the release of glutamate and thereby influence the development of caudalis central sensitization (Gu, 2003; Jennings *et al.*, 2006, 2011). As noted below, P2X mechanisms involving glia may also play a role in the central sensitization.

Another important process contributing to trigeminal central sensitization involves alterations to inhibitory mechanisms. There is evidence in humans that some chronic pain conditions (e.g. temporomandibular disorders) reflect a heightened central excitatory state, resulting from a decrease in central inhibitory control mechanisms (Maixner *et al.*, 1998; Sarlani *et al.*, 2004; King *et al.*, 2009). Animal studies using CFA-induced TMJ or muscle inflammation have shown that central sensitization (as reflected in enhanced c-Fos expression) evident in the rostral parts of caudalis at its junction with subnucleus interpolaris, is associated with alterations in descending modulatory influences (see Dubner and Ren, 2004). Not only may descending inhibition (e.g. from rostral ventromedial medulla) be reduced, but also descending facilitation from some structures (e.g. nucleus gigantocellularis, and rostral ventromedial medulla) may be enhanced, and both sets of alterations appear to contribute to the hyperalgesia associated with peripheral inflammation (see Sessle, 2000; Dubner and Ren, 2004; Bereiter, 2007; Shimizu *et al.*, 2009) and involve several chemical mediators and receptors as well as glial cells (also see below). These mediators and receptor processes include 5-HT, NMDA, GABA, IL-Iβ, and opioids, For example, consistent with observations of the involvement of endogenous opioids in trigeminal nociceptive mechanisms (see above), central mu and kappa opioid depressive effects may be involved also in central sensitization since the caudalis central sensitization, the associated enhanced jaw muscle EMG activity and other nociceptive behaviors produced by inflammatory irritant application to the tooth pulp or TMJ are limited, by the recruitment of central opioid inhibitory mechanisms (Yu *et al.*, 1994; Sunakawa *et al.*, 1999; Tambeli *et al.*, 2001; Tashiro *et al.*, 2009; Fischer *et al.*, 2009). Also, there may be sex differences in the opioid-related modulatory effects (Bereiter *et al.*, 2000; Flores *et al.*, 2003; Bereiter, 2007).

It was noted above that trigeminal central sensitization is not limited to subnucleus caudalis, but can also be induced in the NS and WDR neurons in subnucleus oralis by inflammatory irritant application to the tooth pulp, jaw muscle, or facial skin (e.g. Hu *et al.*, 1992; Raboisson *et al.*, 1995; Park *et al.*, 2001). Nonetheless, the development of central sensitization induced in oralis nociceptive neurons seems to be at least partly linked with the function of subnucleus caudalis. Caudalis (especially via its substantia gelatinosa) can modulate oralis through NMDA and purinergic receptor mechanisms within caudalis itself, since NMDA or P2X receptor antagonist-induced blockade of caudalis interferes with oralis central sensitization (Woda *et al.*, 2001; Hu *et al.*, 2002). Subnucleus caudalis also appears to play a key role in the expression of central sensitization at higher levels of the trigeminal system. Application of the inflammatory irritant mustard oil, for example, to the rat tooth pulp induces thalamic central sensitization reflected in a lowered activation threshold, receptive field expansion and enhanced responses to noxious stimulation of nociceptive neurons, in the ventrobasal and mediodorsal nucleus of the thalamus (Kaneko *et al.*, 2005, 2010; Zhang *et al.*, 2006; Kawamura *et al.*, 2010). The ventrobasal thalamic central sensitization is dependent on the functional integrity of subnucleus caudalis since it can be abolished if subnucleus caudalis is blocked (but not if subnucleus oralis is blocked) (Park *et al.*, 2006). These findings complement the documentation (see above) of the vital role played by caudalis in the development of oralis central sensitization and in the accompanying enhancement of jaw muscle activity, and suggest that caudalis is crucial for the development of central sensitization in the trigeminal nociceptive system, since if the development of central sensitization in caudalis can be prevented, then central sensitization may not be expressed in other parts of the system to which caudalis relays.

There is also recent evidence that disruption of trigeminal brainstem glial cell function interferes with the development and maintenance of central sensitization in caudalis nociceptive neurons (for review, see Chiang *et al.*, 2011). In the case of microglia, there is now considerable evidence that microglia in the spinal dorsal horn becomes activated in spinal models of chronic inflammatory pain. Once activated, microglia produce and release cytokines and various inflammatory mediators and other agents that interact with other microglia and with astroglia and neurons (see Hanisch and Kettenmann, 2007; Abbadie *et al.*, 2009; Gao and Ji, 2010). In trigeminal inflammatory pain models, up-regulation of the microglial marker OX42 may occur in subnucleus caudalis for up to 21 days following formalin injection into the perioral region (Yeo *et al.*, 2001). The OX42 also may appear as early as 1 day after experimental tooth movement-induced masseter muscle allodynia, and is followed by increased expression of astroglia marker (GFAP); administration of the microglial inhibitor minocycline can attenuate both the allodynia and the GFAP expression (Liu *et al.*, 2009). Microglial involvement in trigeminal nociceptive mechanisms may however be much more rapid than is evident from such labelling studies. The caudalis central sensitization that can be detected within 20 minutes following mustard oil application to a rat or mouse molar tooth pulp can be pre-emptively blocked by prior medullary application of an inhibitor of microglial p38MAPK (Xie *et al.*, 2007) or minocycline (Chiang *et al.*, 2010b). It is especially noteworthy that the effects of the microglial inhibitors in this acute pulp inflammatory pain model do not affect the baseline nociceptive properties of the nociceptive neurons, but are limited to their hyperexcitable state that is reflected in central sensitization, which is consistent with the behavioral effects of glial suppression (see above). Furthermore, additional studies using this model (Chiang *et al.*, 2005; Itoh *et al.*, 2009) suggest an important role in central sensitization not only of $P2X_3$ (see above) but also of other P2X receptor subtypes ($P2X_4$, $P2X_7$) in caudalis that are located primarily on microglia. Activation of $P2X_7$ receptors may promote microglia to produce and release excessive amounts of ATP and pro-inflammatory cytokines, as well as trigger astroglia to release cytokines, chemokines, and glutamate, and lead to persistent neuronal changes (see Miller *et al.*, 2009; Milligan and Watkins, 2009; Surprenant and North, 2009).

In addition to their release of chemical mediators and their modulation by microglia (see above), astroglia express several neurotransmitter receptors (e.g. NMDA and metabotropic glutamatergic, TrkB, purinergic, neurokinin, cytokine receptors). These glial cells can modulate the uptake of K^+ and glutamate, the uptake and release of glucose-derived transmitters (glutamate and GABA), and the release of gliotransmitters such as glutamate, ATP, and BDNF (see Hertz and Zickles, 2004; Kang *et al.*, 2008; Parpura and Dorec, 2010) and thereby modulate the activity of nearby neurons and glial cells. These astroglial processes include the "glutamate-glutamine shuttle" (see Hertz and Zielke, 2004; Chiang *et al.*, 2011) which is a crucial astroglial mechanism involved in central sensitization (Fig. 5). These processes play a crucial role in the acute tooth pulp inflammatory pain model noted above, since medullary administration of the astroglial inhibitor fluoroacetate or shuttle inhibitors MSO or MeAIB or gap junction blockers such as carbanoxolone can pre-emptively block the development of caudalis central sensitization, induced by mustard oil application to the molar tooth pulp (Chiang *et al.*, 2007, 2008, 2010a) (Fig. 6). Astroglia inhibitors also suppress the mustard oil-induced medullary release of glutamate (Chiang *et al.*, 2010c). These findings are consistent with documentation that tooth pulp injury induces changes in caudalis astroglia (Canzobre and Ríos, 2010) and also suggest that astroglial gap junctions and hemi-channels may be involved in the excitation of neurons and other cells in subnucleus caudalis. Like the effects of microglial inhibitors (see above), these

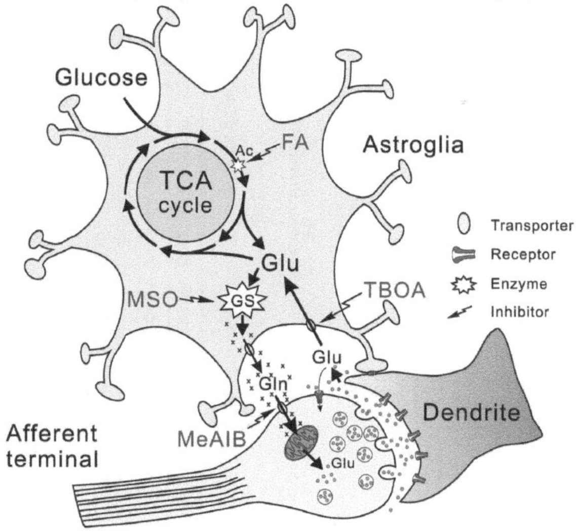

FIG. 5. Astroglial glutamate-glutamine shuttle. Astroglia take up extracellular glutamate released from the primary afferent central terminals (and GABA) through astrocytic transporters (GLT-1, GLAST), and then the glutamate is converted by glutamine synthetase (GS) into glutamine (an important precursor for glutamate and GABA), which is then trafficked through transporters into glutamatergic neuronal terminals to replenish the glutamate transmitter pool. This process, the "*glutamate-glutamine shuttle*" (or cycle), is crucial in nociceptive neuronal central sensitization and is specific to astroglia. Fluoroacetate (FA) is a specific blocker of aconitase (Ac) which is critically involved in the astroglial metabolic tricarboxylic acid (TCA) cycle. Methionine sulfoximine (MSO) is a specific blocker of glutamine synthetase (GS) that converts glutamate (Glu) into glutamine (Gln). Threobeta-benzyloxyasparate (TBOA) is a selective blocker of GLT-1 and GLAST transporters. Methylamino-isobutyric acid (MeAIB) is a specific blocker of neuronal glutamine transporter. (From Chiang *et al.*, 2011).

astroglial inhibitors do not affect the baseline nociceptive properties of caudalis neurons but are limited to their hyperexcitable state, consistent with the behavioral literature noted above. Figure 7 illustrates some of these features in normal nociceptive processing and in orofacial inflammatory pain states.

Likewise, in chronic orofacial inflammatory pain models, medullary administration of astroglia inhibitor 7 days after the induction of a chronic pulpitis can temporarily relieve the mechanical behavioral hypersensitivity and the maintained caudalis central sensitization, that are features of this model of chronic inflammatory dental pain (Miyamoto *et al.*, 2010; Tsuboi *et al.*, 2011). Studies using a chronic muscle inflammatory model showed that astroglial GFAP and IL-1β expressions are increased in rostral subnucleus caudalis from 30 min to 7 days after CFA injection into the masseter muscle (Guo *et al.*, 2007) and that localized caudalis microinjections of astroglial inhibitors reduce the associated masseter hyperalgesia

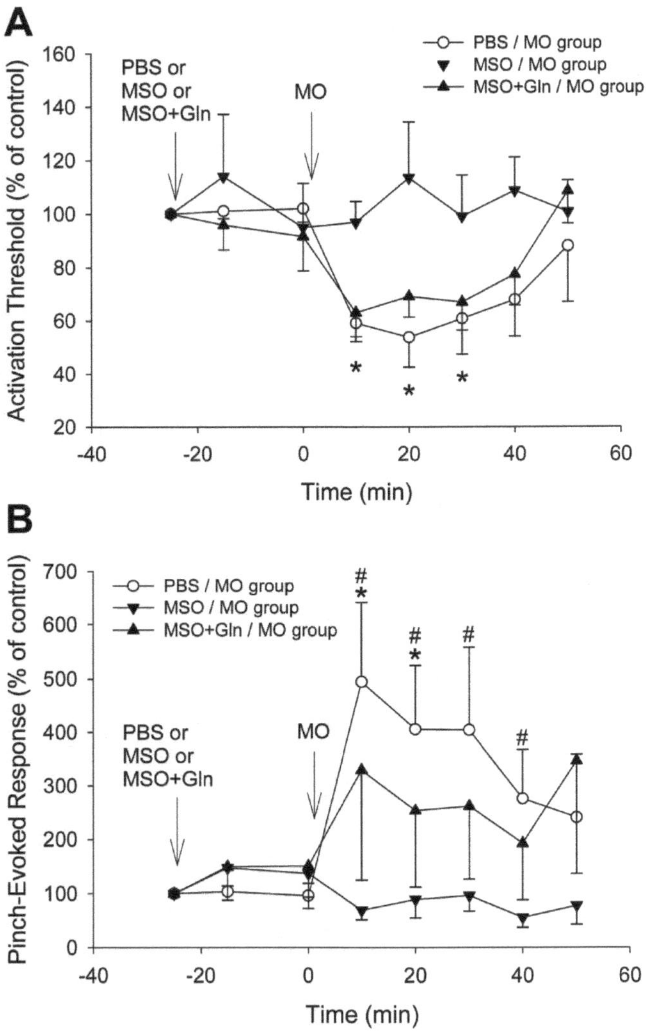

FIG. 6. Intrathecal superfusion of methionine sulfoximine (MSO) blocked the mustard oil (MO)-induced central sensitization and glutamate release in subnucleus caudalis; superfusion by phosphate-buffered saline (PBS, as control) instead of MSO was ineffective. Time course of neuroplastic changes in nociceptive-specific (NS) neurons' mechanical activation threshold (A) and responses to mechanical stimulation (B) reflecting central sensitization induced by application to the rat tooth pulp of MO. Significant differences occurred between the PBS/MO or MSO+Gln/MO and MSO/MO groups ($P<0.001$ or $P<0.02$, respectively, 2-way ANOVA; #$P<0.05$, Bonferroni t-test). Note that superfusion of MSO blocked the MO-induced neuroplastic changes in NS neurons, while simultaneous superfusion of glutamine (Gln) could restore the MO-induced neuroplastic changes. In A and B, arrows indicate the application time (at 0 min) of chemicals or PBS, and error bars represent SEM. (Modified from Chiang *et al.*, 2007).

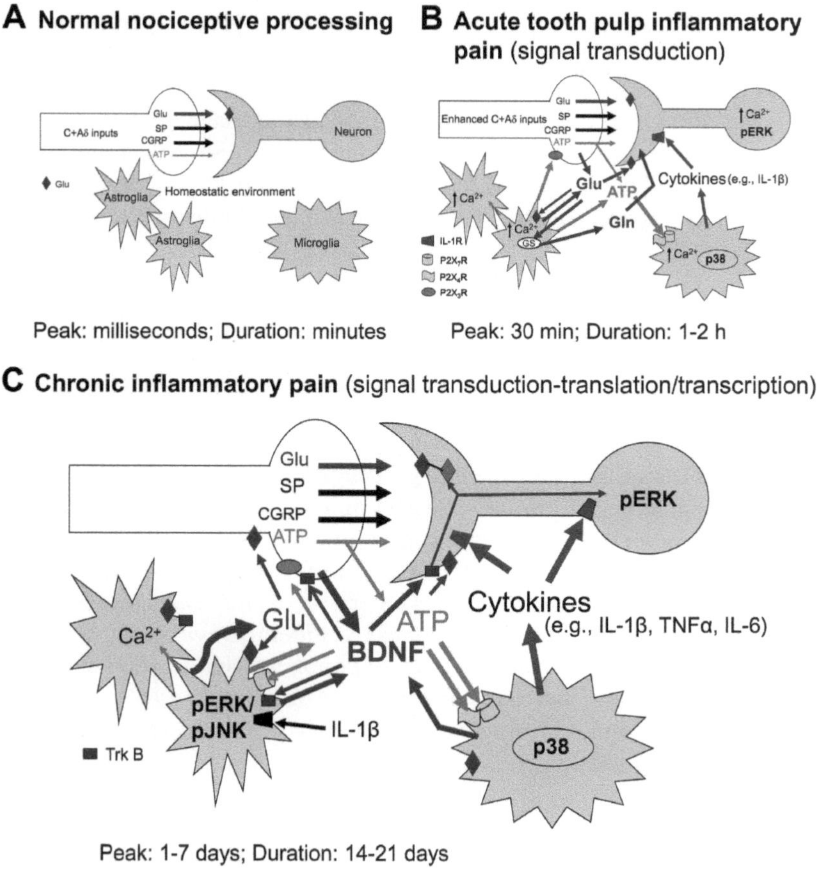

FIG. 7. Diagrams showing normal nociceptive processing in trigeminal subnucleus caudalis (A) and caudalis neuron-glia interactions in acute tooth pulp inflammatory pain (B) and chronic inflammatory pain (C) conditions. Different colors represent different pathways of individual mediators; the different thickness of arrows/fonts represents their importance in individual cases. For figure clarity, some receptors have not been linked with appropriate agonists or mediators and peptidergic (substance P, CGRP) mechanisms are omitted. (Adapted from Chiang *et al.*, 2011). (For interpretation of the references to color in this figure legend, the reader is referred to the Web version of the chapter.).

manifested in this model (Shimizu *et al.*, 2009). Further investigation into the role of glial cells in trigeminal central sensitization, associated with orofacial inflammation promises to provide important insights into how pain develops and may become sustained in orofacial inflammatory states.

These various observations pointing to the integral role that central sensitization plays in acute and chronic orofacial inflammatory pain states and the critical involvement of several chemical mediators and glial cell processes have improved our understanding of the central mechanisms underlying these states. Further study of these processes and the underlying intracellular and intercellar mechanisms involved, as well the introduction of investigations aimed at clarifying the genetic and environmental determinants of these mechanisms, holds out promise of providing insights into neural and non-neural targets for the development of new therapeutic approaches to control orofacial inflammatory pain.

VI. Summary

This article has reviewed current understanding of the peripheral and central mechanisms underlying acute and chronic orofacial inflammatory pain conditions. These conditions may be associated not only with the activation of trigeminal nociceptive primary afferents and neurons in the trigeminal nociceptive pathways in the CNS, but may also produce a sustained hyperexcitability (sensitization) of these neural elements that may contribute to the allodynia, hyperalgesia, spontaneous pain, and pain spread or referral, that are characteristic of many of these conditions. There is considerable evidence that a variety of chemical mediators are involved in these peripheral sensitization and central sensitization processes, and emerging evidence is pointing also to the crucial involvement of non-neural processes (e.g. associated with glial cells) in these inflammatory pain conditions.

References

Abbadie, C., Bhangoo, S., De Koninck, Y., Malcangio, M., Melik-Parsadaniantz, S. and White, F.A. (2009). Chemokines and pain mechanisms. *Brain Res. Rev.* **60**, 125–134.

Adachi, K., Shimizu, K., Hu, J.W., Suzuki, I., Sakagami, H., Koshikawa, N., Sessle, B.J., Shinoda, M., Miyamoto, M., Honda, K., and Iwata, K. (2010). Purinergic receptors are involved in tooth-pulp evoked nocifensive behavior and brainstem neuronal activity. *Molecular Pain***6**, 59 (pp.) in press.

Akiyama, T., Carstens, M.I. and Carstens, E. (2010). Facial injections of pruritogens and algogens excite partly overlapping populations of primary and second-order trigeminal neurons in mice. *J. Neurophysiol.* **104**, 2442–2450.

Amano, N., Hu, J.W. and Sessle, B.J. (1986). Responses of neurons in feline trigeminal subnucleus caudalis (medullary dorsal horn) to cutaneous, intraoral and muscle afferent stimuli. *J. Neurophysiol.* **55**, 227–243.

Ambalavanar, R. and Dessem, D. (2009). Emerging peripheral receptor targets for deep-tissue craniofacial pain therapies. *J. Dent, Res.* **88**, 201–211.

Belmonte, C. (2007). Ocular nociceptors. In: Schmidt, R.F., Willis, W.D. (Eds.), *Encyclopedia of Pain*. Springer, Heidelberg, Germany, pp. 1504–1507 Section 10.

Bereiter, D.A. (2007). Trigeminal brainstem nuclear complex. Immunohistochemistry and neurochemistry. In: Schmidt, R.F., Willis, W.D. (Eds.), *Encyclopedia of Pain.* Springer, Heidelberg, Germany, pp. 2541–2543 Section 10.

Bereiter, D.A. and Bereiter, D.F. (1996). N-methyl-D-aspartate and non-N-methyl-D-aspartate receptor antagonism reduces fos-like immunoreactivity in central trigeminal neurons after corneal stimulation in the rat. *Neurosci.* **73**, 249–258.

Bereiter, D.A., Hiraba, H. and Hu, J.W. (2000). Trigeminal subnucleus caudalis beyond homologies with the spinal dorsal horn. *Pain* **88**, 221–224.

Bowles, W.R., Flores, C.M., Jackson, D.L. and Hargreaves, K.M. (2003). beta 2-Adrenoceptor regulation of CGRP release from capsaicin-sensitive neurons. *J. Dent. Res.* **82**, 308–311.

Broton, J.G., Hu, J.W. and Sessle, B.J. (1988). Effects of temporomandibular joint stimulation on nociceptive and nonnociceptive neurons of the cat's trigeminal subnucleus caudalis (medullary dorsal horn). *J. Neurophysiol.* **59**, 1575–1589.

Burstein, R., Levy, D., Jakubowski, M. and Woolf, C.J. (2006). Peripheral and central sensitization related to headaches. In: Olesen, J., goadsby, P.J., Ramadan, N.B., Tfelt-HansenF P, Tfelt-HansenF P., WelchF K.M.A, WelchF K.M.A. (Eds.), *The Headaches, 3rd edition. Lippincott Williams & Wilkins, Philadelphia, pp. 121–129.*

Burstein, R., Yarnitsky, D., Goor-Aryeh, I., Ransil, B.J. and Bajwa, Z.H. (2000). An association between migraine and cutaneous allodynia. *Ann. Neurol.* **47**, 614–624.

Byers, M.R. and Narhi, M.V.O. (1999). Dental injury models: experimental tools for understanding neuroinflammatory interactions and polymodal nociceptor functions. *Crit. Rev. Oral Biol. Med.* **10**, 4–39.

Cairns, B. (2007). Nociceptors in the orofacial region: Temporomandibular joint and masseter muscle. In: Schmidt, R.F., Willis, W.D. (Eds.), *Encyclopedia of Pain.* Springer-Verlag, Heidelberg, pp. 1410–1427.

Cairns, B.E., Sessle, B.J. and Hu, J.W. (1998). Evidence that excitatory amino acid receptors within the temporomandibular joint region are involved in the reflex activation of the jaw muscles. *J. Neurosci.* **18**, 8056–8064.

Cairns, B.E., Hu, J.W., Arendt-Nielsen, L., Sessle, B.J. and Svensson, P. (2001a). Sex-related differences in human pain perception and rat afferent discharge evoked by injection of glutamate into the masseter muscle. *J. Neurophysiol* **86**, 782–791.

Cairns, B.E., Sessle, B.J. and Hu, J.W. (2001b). Temporomandibular-evoked jaw muscle reflex: role of brainstem NMDA and non-NMDA receptors. *NeuroReport* **12**, 1875–1878.

Cairns, B.E., Svensson, P., Wang, K., Hupfeld, S., Graven-Nielsen, T., Sessle, B.J., Berde, C.B., and Arendt-Nielsen, L. (2003). Activation of peripheral NMDA receptors contributes to human pain and rat afferent discharges evoked by injection of glutamate into the masseter muscle. *J. Neurophysiol.* **90**, 2098–2105.

Canzobre, M.C. and Ríos, H. (2010). Pulpar tooth injury induces plastic changes in S100B positive astroglial cells in the trigeminal subnucleus caudalis. *Neurosci. Lett.* **470**, 71–75.

Capra, N.F. and Ro, J.Y. (2004). Human and animal experimental models of acute and chronic muscle pain: intramuscular algesic injection. *Pain* **110**, 3–7.

Castrillon, E., Ernberg, M., Cairns, B.E., Wang, K., Sessle, B.J., Arendt-Nielsen, L. and Svensson, P. (2010). Interstitial glutamate concentration is elevated in the masseter muscle of myofascial temporomandibular disorder patients. *J. Orofacial. Pain* **24**, 350–360.

Cherkas, P., Dostrovsky, J.O. and Sessle, B.J. (2011). Activation of peripheral P2X receptors is sufficient to induce central sensitization in rat medullary dorsal horn nociceptive neurons. submitted

Chidiac, J.J., Hawwa, N., Baliki, M., Safieh-Garabedian, B., Rifai, K., Jabbur, S.J. and Saade, N.E. (2001). A perfusion technique for the determination of pro-inflammatory mediators induced by intradental application of irritants. *J. Pharmacol. Toxicol. Methods* **46**, 125–130.

Chiang, C.Y., Park, S.J., Kwan, C.L., Hu, J.W. and Sessle, B.J. (1998). NMDA receptor mechanisms contribute to neuroplasticity induced in caudalis nociceptive neurons by tooth pulp stimulation. *J. Neurophysiol.* **80**, 2621–2631.

Chiang, C.Y., Zhang, S., Xie, Y.F., Hu, J.W., Dostrovsky, J.O., Salter, M.W. and Sessle, B.J. (2005). Endogenous ATP involvement in mustard oil-induced central sensitization in trigeminal subnucleus caudalis (medullary dorsal horn). *J. Neurophysiol.* **94**, 1751–1760.

Chiang, C.Y., Wang, J., Xie, Y.F., Zhang, S., Hu, J.W., Dostrovsky, J.O. and Sessle, B.J. (2007). Astroglial glutamate-glutamine shuttle is involved in central sensitization of nociceptive neurons in rat medullary dorsal horn. *J. Neurosci.* **27**, 9068–9076.

Chiang, C.Y., Li, Z., Dostrovsky, J.O., Hu, J.W. and Sessle, B.J. (2008). Glutamine uptake contributes to central sensitization in the medullary dorsal horn. *Neuroreport* **19**, 1151–1154.

Chiang, C.Y., Dostrovsky, J.O., Iwata, K., and Sessle, B.J. (2011). Role of glia in orofacial pain. *The Neuroscientist*, **17**, 303–320.

Chiang, C.Y., Li, Z., Dostrovsky, J.O. and Sessle, B.J. (2010a). Central sensitization in medullary dorsal horn involves gap junctions and hemichannels. *Neuroreport* **21**, 233–237.

Chiang, C.Y., Itoh, K., Dostrovsky, J.O. and Sessle, B.J. (2010b). Minocycline attenuates central sensitization in medullary dorsal horn in rats. *Pain Res. Manage* **15**(2); 103.

Chiang, C., Itoh, K., Li, Z., Cherkas, P.S., Kumar, N., Beggs, S., Dostrovsky, J.O., Salter, M.W., Coderre, T.J. and Sessle, B.J. (2010d). Central sensitization in the rat medullary dorsal horn is dependent on glial cell function. *Abstracts of IASP World Congress on Pain* Montreal, August 2010.

Chun, Y.H. and Ro, J.Y. (2010). Electrophysiological characterization of the rat trigeminal caudalis (Vc) neurons following intramuscular injection of capsaicin. *Neurosci. Lett.* **469**, 289–293.

Clemente, J.T., Parada, C.A., Veiga, M.C., Gear, R.W. and Tambeli, C.H. (2004). Sexual dimorphism in the antinociception mediated by kappa opioid receptors in the rat temporomandibular joint. *Neurosci. Lett.* **372**, 250–255.

Coimbra, F. and Coimbra, A. (1994). Dental noxious input reaches the subnucleus caudalis of the trigeminal complex in the rat, as shown by c-fos expression upon thermal or mechanical stimulation. *Neurosci. Lett.* **173**, 201–204.

Cooper, B. (2007). Nociceptors in the orofacial region: Skin/mucosa. In: Schmidt, R.F., Willis, W.D. (Eds.), *Encyclopedia of Pain.* Springer-Verlag, Heidelberg.

Diogenes, A., Patwardhan, A., Ruparel, N., Goffin, A., Akopian, A. and Hargreaves, K.M. (2006). Prolactin modulates TRPV1 in female rat trigeminal sensory neurons. *J. Neurosci.* **26**, 8126–8136.

Dionne, R.A., Lepinski, A.M., Gordon, S.M., Jaber, L., Brahim, J.S. and Hargreaves, K.M. (2001). Analgesic effects of peripherally administered opioids in clinical models of acute and chronic inflammation. *Clin Pharmacol Ther.* **70**(1); 66–73.

Dostrovsky, J.O., and Sessle, B.J. (2007). Nociceptive processing in the brainstem. In "*Encyclopedia of Pain*" (R. F. Schmidt and W. D. Willis, Eds.), Section 10, Springer, Heidelberg, Germany, 1370–1373.

Duale, C., Luccarini, P., Cadet, R. and Woda, A. (1996). Effects of morphine microinjections into the trigeminal sensory complex on the formalin test in the rat. *Exp. Neurol.* **142**, 331–339.

Dubner, R. and Bennett, G.J. (1983). Spinal and trigeminal mechanisms of nociception. *Ann. Rev, Neurosci.* **6**, 381–418.

Dubner, R. and Ren, K. (2004). Brainstem mechanisms of persistent pain following injury. *J. Orofac. Pain* **18**, 299–305.

Dubner, R., Sessle, B.J. and Storey, A.T. (1978). *The Neural Basis of Oral and Facial Function.* Plenum Press, New York 483.

Eisenberg, E., Vos, B.P. and Strassman, A.M. (1996). The peripheral antinociceptive effect of morphine in a rat model of facial pain. *Neurosci.* **72**, 519–525.

Fischer, L., Arthuri, M.T., Torres-Chávez, K.E. and Tambeli, C.H. (2009). Contribution of endogenous opioids to gonadal hormones-induced temporomandibular joint antinociception. *Behav. Neurosi.* **123**, 1129–1140.

Freeman, S.E., Patil, V.V. and Durham, P.L. (2008). Nitric oxide-proton stimulation of trigeminal ganglion neurons increases mitogen-activated protein kinase and phosphatase expression in neurons and satellite glial cells. *Neurosci.* **157**, 542–555.

Flores, C.A., Shughrue, P., Petersen, S.L. and Mokha, S.S. (2003). Sex-related differences in the distribution of opioid receptor-like 1 receptor mRNA and colocalization with estrogen receptor mRNA in neurons of the spinal trigeminal nucleus caudalis in the rat. *Neurosci.* **118**, 769–778.

Gao, Y.J. and Ji, R.R. (2010). Chemokines, neuronal-glial interactions, and central processing of neuropathic pain. *Pharmacol. Ther.* **126**, 56–68.

Garrett, F.G. and Durham, P.L. (2008). Differential expression of connexins in trigeminal ganglion neurons and satellite glial cells in response to chronic or acute joint inflammation. *Neuron Glia Biol.* **4**, 295–306.

Gazerani, P. and Arendt-Nielsen, L. (2005). The impact of ethnic differences in response to capsaicin-induced trigeminal sensitization. *Pain* **117**, 223–229.

Goadsby, P. J. (2006). Headache: clinical and basic science advances relevant to practice. In "Proceedings of the 11th World Congress on Pain" (H. Flor, E. Kalso and J. O. Dostrovsky, Eds.). IASP Press, Seattle, 633–649.

Gojyo, F., Sugiyo, S., Kuroda, R., Kawabata, A., Varathan, V., Shigenaga, Y. and Takemura, M. (2002). Effects of somatosensory cortical stimulation on expression of c-Fos in rat medullary dorsal horn in response to formalin-induced noxious stimulation. *J. Neurosci. Res.* **68**, 479–488.

Gu, J.G. (2003). P2X receptor-mediated modulation of sensory transmission to the spinal cord dorsal horn. *Neuroscientist* **9**, 370–378.

Hanisch, U.K. and Kettenmann, H. (2007). Microglia: active sensor and versatile effector cells in the normal and pathologic brain. *Nat. Neurosci.* **10**, 1387–1394.

Hathaway, C.B., Hu, J.W., and Bereiter, D.A. (1995). Distribution of fos-like immunoreactivity in the caudal brainstem of the rat following noxious chemical stimulation of the temporomandibular joint. *J. Comp. Neurol* **356**, 444–456.

Hertz, L. and Zielke, H.R. (2004). Astrocytic control of glutamatergic activity: astrocytes as stars of the show. *Trends Neurosci.* **27**, 735–743.

Honda, K., Kitagawa, J., Sessle, B.J., Kondo, M., Tsuboi, Y., Yonehara, Y. and Iwata, K. (2008). Mechanisms involved in an increment of multimodal excitability of medullary and upper cervical dorsal horn neurons following cutaneous capsaicin treatment. *Mole. Pain* **4**, 59.

Hu, J.W. (2004). Tooth pulp. In: Miles, T.S., Nauntofte, B., Svensson, P. (Eds.), *Clinical Oral Physiology*. Copenhagen, Quintessence, pp. 141–163.

Hu, B., Chiang, C.Y., Hu, J.W., Dostrovsky, J.O. and Sessle, B.J. (2002). P2X receptors in trigeminal subnucleus caudalis modulate central sensitization in trigeminal subnucleus oralis. *J. Neurophysiol.* **88**, 1614–1624.

Hu, J.W., Sessle, B.J., Raboisson, P., Dallel, R. and Woda, A. (1992). Stimulation of craniofacial muscle afferents induces prolonged facilitatory effects in trigeminal nociceptive brainstem neurones. *Pain* **48**, 53–60.

Hucho, T. and Levine, J.D. (2007). Signaling pathways in sensitization: toward a nociceptor cell biology. *Neuron* **55**, 365–376.

Itoh, K., Chiang, C. Y., Dostrovsky, J. O., and Sessle, B. J. (2009). Medullary application of P2X7 receptor agonist produces central sensitization-like responses in the rat medullary dorsal horn (MDH). Abstracts #01047, IUPS, Kyoto, July.

Jaber, L., Swaim, W.D. and Dionne, R.A. (2003). Immunohistochemical localization of μ-opioid receptors in human dental pulp. *J. Endo.* **29**, 108–110.

Jennings, E.A., Christie, M.J. and Sessle, B.J. (2006). ATP potentiates neurotransmission in the rat trigeminal subnucleus caudalis. *NeuroReport* **17**, 1507–1510.

Jennings, E.A., Williams, M.C., Cho, H., Bardoni, R., Salter, M.W. and Sessle, B.J. (2011). Mechanisms underlying the excitatory actions of adenosine triphosphate (ATP) on neurons in the rat medullary dorsal horn (trigeminal subnucleus caudalis). *J. Neurophysiol* submitted.

Kaneko, M., Kaneko, T., Kaneko, R., Chokechanachaisakul, U., Kawamura, J., Sunakawa, M., Okiji, T., and Suda, H. (2010). The role of N-methyl-D-aspartate receptor subnunits in the rat thalamic mediodorsal nucleus during central sensitization. *Brain Res*, in press.

Kaneko, M., Sunakawa, M., Matsui, Y. and Suda, H. (2005). Responsiveness changes of tooth pulp driven-neurons in thalamic ventral posteromedial and mediodorsal nuclei following experimental pulpitis and naloxone administration in rats. *J. Oral Biosci.* **47**, 135–148.

Kang, J., Kang, N., Lovatt, D., Torres, A., Zhao, Z., Lin, J. and Nedergaard, M. (2008). Connexin 43 hemichannels are permeable to ATP. *J. Neurosci.* **28**, 4702–4711.

Kawamura, J., Kaneko, T., Kaneko, M., Sunakawa, M., Kaneko, R., Chokechanachaisakul, U., Okiji, T. and Suda, H. (2010). Neuron-immune interactions in the sensitized thalamus induced by mustard oil application to rat molar pulp. *J. Dent. Res.* **89**, 1309–1314.

Khan, A. and Hargreaves, K.M. (2010). Animal models of orofacial pain. *Methods Mol. Biol* **617**, 93–104.

Khan, A., Ren, K. and Hargreaves, K.M. (2008). Neurochemical factors in injury and inflammation of orofacial tissues. In: Sessle, B.J., Lavigne, G., Dubner, R., Lund, J.P. (Eds.), *"Orofacial Pain", 2nd Edition. Quintessence, Chicago, pp. 45–52.*

King, C.D., Wong, F., Currie, T., Mauderli, A.P., Fillingim, R.B. and Riley 3rd., J.L. (2009). Deficiency in endogenous modulation of prolonged heat pain in patients with irritable bowel syndrome and temporomandibular disorder. *Pain* **143**, 172–178.

Kopp, S. (2001). Neuroendocrine, immune, and local responses related to temporomandibular disorders. *J. Orofac. Pain* **15**, 9–28.

Kopp, S. and Alstergren, P. (2008). Peripheral aspects of cytokines in musculoskeltetal pain. In: Graven-Nielsen, T., Arendt-Nielsen, L., Mense, S. (Eds.), *Fundamentals of Musculoskeletal Pain.* IASP Press, Seattle, pp. 119–137.

Lam, D.K., Sessle, B.J., Cairns, B.E. and Hu, J.W. (2005a). Neural mechanisms of temporomandibular joint and masticatory muscle pain: a possible role for peripheral glutamate receptor mechanisms. *Pain Res. Manage* **10**, 145–152.

Lam, D.K., Sessle, B.J., Cairns, B.E. and Hu, J.W. (2005b). Peripheral NMDA receptor modulation of jaw muscle electromyographic activity induced by capsaicin injection into the temporomandibular joint of rats. *Brain Res.* **1046**, 68–76.

Lam, D.K., Sessle, B.J. and Hu, J.W. (2008). Surgical incision can alter capsaicin-induced central sensitization in rat brainstem nociceptive neurons. *Neurosci.* **156**, 737–747.

Lam, D.K., Sessle, B.J. and Hu, J.W. (2009a). Glutamate and capsaicin effects on trigeminal nociception I: Activation and peripheral sensitization of deep craniofacial trigeminal nociceptive afferents. *Brain Res.* **1251**, 130–139.

Lam, D.K., Sessle, B.J. and Hu, J.W. (2009b). Glutamate and capsaicin effects on trigeminal nociception. II: Activation and central sensitization in brainstem neurons with deep craniofacial afferent input. *Brain Res.* **1253**, 48–59.

LeResche, L. and Drangsholt, M. (2008). Epidemiology of orofacial pain: prevalence, incidence, and risk factors. In: Sessle, B.J., Lavigne, G., Dubner, R., Lund, J.P. (Eds.), *Orofacial Pain, 2nd Edition. Quintessence, Chicago, pp. 13–18.*

Lipton, J.A., Ship, J.A. and Larach-Robinson, D. (1993). Estimated prevalence and distribution of reported orofacial pain in the United States. *JADA* **124**, 115–121.

Liu, X.D., Wang, J.J., Sun, L., Chen, L.W., Rao, Z.R., Duan, L., Cao, R. and Wang, M.Q. (2009). Involvement of medullary dorsal horn glial cell activation in mediation of masseter mechanical allodynia induced by experimental tooth movement. *Arch. Oral Biol.* **54**, 1143–1150.

Magloire, H., Maurin, J.C., Couble, M.L., Shibukawa, Y., Tsumura, M., Thivichon-Prince, B. and Bleicher, F. (2010). Topical Review. Dental pain and odontoblasts: Facts and hypotheses. *J. Orofac. Pain* **24**, 335–349.

Maixner, W., Fillingim, R., Sigurdsson, A., Kincaid, S. and Silva, S. (1998). Sensitivity of patients with painful temporomandibular disorders to experimentally evoked pain Evidence for altered temporal summation of pain. *Pain* **76**, 71–81.

Matthews, B. and Sessle, B.J. (2008). Peripheral mechanisms of orofacial pain. In: Sessle, B.J., Lavigne, G., Dubner, R., Lund, J.P. (Eds.), *Orofacial Pain, 2nd Edition. Quintessence, Chicago, pp. 27–43.*

Mengel, M.K., Jyväsjärvi, E. and Kniffki, K.D. (1993). Identification and characterization of afferent periodontal A delta fibres in the cat. *J. Physiol.* **464**, 393–405.

Messlinger, K. (2009). Migraine: where and how does the pain originate? *Exp. Brain Res.* **196**, 179–193.

Meyer, R.A., Ringkamp, M., Campbell, J.N. and Raja, S.N. (2006). Peripheral mechanisms of cutaneous nociception. In: McMahon, S.B., Koltzenburg, M. (Eds.), *Wall and Melzack's Textbook of Pain, 5th Edition. Elsevier, Amsterdam, pp. 3–34.*

Milam, S.B. (2006). TMJ osteoarthritis. In: Laskin, D., Greene, C.S., Hylander, W. (Eds.), *TMDs. An Evidence-Based Approach to Diagnosis and Treatment.* Quintessence, Chicago, pp. 105–123.

Miller, R.J., Jung, H., Bhangoo, S.K. and White, F.A. (2009). Cytokine and chemokine regulation of sensory neuron function. *Handb. Exp. Pharmacol.* **194**, 417–449.

Milligan, E.D. and Watkins, L.R. (2009). Pathological and protective roles of glia in chronic pain. *Nat. Rev. Neurosci.* **10**, 23–36.

Miyamoto, M., Varathan, V., Cherkas, P.S., Hu, J.W., Tsuboi, Y., Iwata, K., Dostrovsky, J.O., and Sessle, B.J. (2010). Chronic pulp inflammation is associated with central sensitization and glial cell changes in rat medullary dorsal horn. *Abstr. World Congr. Pain PW* **312**.

Morgan, J.R. and Gebhart, G.F. (2008). Characterization of a model of chronic orofacial hyperalgesia in the rat: Contribution of NaV 1.8. *J. Pain* **9**, 522–531.

Noma, N., Tsuboi, Y., Kondo, M., Matsumoto, M., Sessle, B., Kitagawa, J., Kimiko, S. and Iwata, K. (2008). Organization of pERK-immunoreactive cells in trigeminal spinal nucleus caudalis and upper cervical cord following capsaicin injection into oral and craniofacial regions in rats. *J. Comp. Neurol.* **507**, 1428–1440.

O'Hara, P.T., Vit, J.P., Bhargava, A. and Jasmin, L. (2008). Evidence for a role of connexin 43 in trigeminal pain using RNA interference *in vivo*. *J. Neurophysiol.* **100**, 3064–3073.

Okumura, M., Iwata, K., Yasuda, K., Inoue, K., Shinoda, M., Honda, K., Shibuta, K., Yasuda, M. and Kondo, E. (2010). Alternation of gene expression in trigeminal ganglion neurons following complete Freund's adjuvant or capsaicin injection into the rat face. *J. Mol. Neurosci.* **42**, 200–209.

Park, S.J., Chiang, C.Y., Hu, J.W. and Sessle, B.J. (2001). Neuroplasticity induced by tooth pulp stimulation in trigeminal subnucleus oralis involves NMDA receptor mechanisms. *J. Neurophysiol.* **85**, 1836–1846.

Park, S.J., Zhang, S., Chiang, C.Y., Hu, J.W., Dostrovsky, J.O. and Sessle, B.J. (2006). Central sensitization induced in thalamic nociceptive neurons by tooth pulp stimulation is dependent on the functional integrity of trigeminal brainstem subnucleus caudalis but not subnucleus oralis. *Brain Res.* **1112**, 134–145.

Parpura, V. and Zorec, R. (2010). Gliotransmission: Exocytotic release from astrocytes. *Brain Res. Rev.* **63**, 83–92.

Quintans-Júnior, L.J., Melo, M.S., De Sousa, D.P., Araujo, A.A., Onofre, A.C., Gelain, D.P., Gonçalves, J.C., Araújo, D.A., Almeida, J.R. and Bonjardim, L.R. (2010). Antinociceptive effects of citronellal in formalin-, capsaicin-, and glutamate-induced orofacial nociception in rodents and its action on nerve excitability. *J. Orofac. Pain* **24**, 305–312.

Raboisson, P. and Dallel, R. (2004). The orofacial formalin test. *Neurosci. Biobehav. Rev.* **28**, 219–226.

Raboisson, P., Dallel, R., Clavelou, P., Sessle, B.J. and Woda, A. (1995). Effects of subcutaneous formalin on the activity of trigeminal brain stem nociceptive neurones in the rat. *J. Neurophysiol.* **73**, 496–505.

Ro, J.Y. (2005). Bite force measurement in awake rats: a behavioral model for persistent orofacial muscle pain and hyperalgesia. *J. Orofac. Pain* **15**, 159–167.

Ro, J.Y. (2008). Functional role of peripheral glutamate receptors in craniofacial muscle pain and hyperalgesia. In: Graven-Nielsen, T., Arendt-Nielsen, L., Mense, S. (Eds.), *Fundamentals of Musculoskeletal Pain.* IASP Press, Seattle, pp. 33–45.

Sarlani, E., Grace, E.G., Reynolds, M.A. and Greenspan, J.D. (2004). Evidence for up-regulated central nociceptive processing in patients with masticatory myofascial pain. *J. Orofac. Pain* **18**, 41–55.

Sessle, B.J. (2000). Acute and chronic craniofacial pain: brainstem mechanisms of nociceptive transmission and neuroplasticity, and their clinical correlates. *Crit. Rev. Oral Biol. Med.* **11**, 57–91.

Sessle, B.J. (2005a). Orofacial Pain. In: Merskey, H., Loeser, J.D., Dubner, R. (Eds.), *The Paths of Pain 1975-2005.* IASP Press, Seattle, pp. 131–150.

Sessle, B.J. (2005b). Trigeminal central sensitization. *Rev. Analgesia* **8**, 85–102.

Sessle, B.J. (2006). Sensory and motor neurophysiology related to temporomandibular joint function. In: Laskin, D., Greene, C.G., HylanderF W.,HylanderF W.. (Eds.), *Temporomandibular Disorders. An Evidence-Based Approach to Diagnosis And Treatment.* Quintessence, Chicago, pp. 69–88.

Sessle, B.J. (2009). Sensation from the face. Squire, L. (Ed.), *Encyclopedia of Neuroscience.* **8**, Academic Press, Oxford, pp. 585–592.

Shimizu, K., Guo, W., Wang, H., Lagraize, S.C., Zou, S., Iwata, K., Wei, F., Dubner, R. and Ren, K. (2009). Differential involvement of trigeminal transition zone and laminated subnucleus caudalis in orofacial deep and cutaneous hyperalgesia: the effects of interleukin-10 and glial inhibitors. *Mol. Pain* **5**, 75.

Stabile, A.C., Stuani, M.B., Leite-Panissi, C.R. and Rocha, M.J. (2009). Effects of short-term acetaminophen and celecoxib treatment on orthodontic tooth movement and neuronal activation in rat. *Brain Res. Bull.* **79**, 396–401.

Strassman, A.M. and Levy, D. (2006). Response properties of dural nociceptors in relation to headache. *J. Neurophysiol.* **95**, 1298–1306.

Strassman, A.M., Raymond, S.A. and Burstein, R. (1996). Sensitization of meningeal sensory neurons and the origin of headaches. *Nature* **384**, 560–564.

Sunakawa, M., Chiang, C.Y., Sessle, B.J. and Hu, J.W. (1999). Jaw electromyographic (EMG) activity induced by application of algesic chemicals to the rat tooth pulp. *Pain* **80**, 493–501.

Surprenant, A. and North, R.A. (2009). Signaling at purinergic P2X receptors. *Annu. Rev. Physiol.* **71**, 333–359.

Takeda, M., Takahashi, M. and Matsumoto, S. (2009). Contribution of the activation of satellite glia in sensory ganglia to pathological pain. *Neurosci. Biobehav. Rev.* **33**, 784–792.

Tambeli, C.H., Seo, K., Sessle, B.J. and Hu, J.W. (2001). Central μ opioid receptor mechanisms modulate mustard oil-evoked jaw muscle activity. *Brain Res.* **913**, 90–94.

Tashiro, A., Okamoto, K. and Bereiter, D.A. (2009). Chronic inflammation and estradiol interact through MAPK activation to affect TMJ nociceptive processing by trigeminal caudalis neurons. *Neurosci.* **164**, 1813–1820.

Tashiro, A., Okamoto, K., Chang, Z. and Bereiter, D.A. (2010). Behavioral and neurophysiological correlates of nociception in an animal model of photokeratitis. *Neurosci.* **169**, 455–462.

Teixeira, J.M., Oliveira, M.C., Nociti Jr., F.H., Clemente-Napimoga, J.T., Pelegrini-da-Silva, A., Parada, C.A. and Tambeli, C.H. (2010). Involvement of temporomandibular joint P2X3 and P2X2/3 receptors in carrageenan-induced inflammatory hyperalgesia in rats. *Eur. J. Pharmacol.* **645**, 79–85.

Thalakoti, S., Patil, V.V., Damodaram, S., Vause, C.V., Langford, L.E., Freeman, S.E. and Durham, P.L. (2007). Neuron-glia signaling in trigeminal ganglion: implications for migraine pathology. *Headache* **47**, 1008–1023.

Toda, K., Zeredo, J.L., Fujiyama, R., Okada, Y., Oi, K., Hayashi, Y. and Nasution, F.H. (2004). Characteristics of nociceptors in the periodontium–an *in vitro* study in rats. *Brain Res. Bull.* **62**, 345–349.

Tsai, C.M., Chiang, C.Y., Yu, X.M. and Sessle, B.J. (1999). Involvement of trigeminal subnucleus caudalis (medullary dorsal horn) in craniofacial nociceptive reflex activity. *Pain* **81**, 115–128.

Tsuboi, Y., Iwata, K., Dostrovsky, J.O., Chiang, C.Y., Sessle, B.J. and Hu, J.W. (2011). Modulation of astroglial glutamine synthetase activity affects nociceptive behavior and central sensitization of medullary dorsal horn nociceptive neurons in a rat model of chronic pulpitis. *Eur. J. Neurosci, submitted.*

Vaughn, A.H. and Gold, M.S. (2010). Ionic mechanisms underlying inflammatory mediatorinduced sensitization of dural afferents. *J. Neurosci.* **30**, 7878–7888.

Vause, C.V. and Durham, P.L. (2009). CGRP stimulation of iNOS and NO release from trigeminal ganglion glial cells involves mitogen-activated protein kinase pathways. *J. Neurochem.* **110**, 811–821.

Wakisaki, S., Sasaki, Y., Ichikawa, H. and Matsuo, S. (1992). Increase in c-fos-like immunoreactivity in the trigeminal nucleus complex after dental treatment. *Proc. Finn. Dent. Soc.* **88**(Suppl. 1); 551–556.

Wang, K., Svensson, P., Sessle, B.J., Cairns, B.E. and Arendt-Nielsen, L. (2010). Interactions of glutamate and capsaicin evoked-muscle pain on human jaw motor functions. *Clin. Neurophysiol.* **121**, 950–956.

Watanabe, T., Tsuboi, Y., Sessle, B.J., Iwata, K. and Hu, J.W. (2010). P2X and NMDA receptor involvement in temporomandibular joint-evoked reflex activity in rat jaw muscles. *Brain Res.* **1346**, 83–91.

Woda, A. (2003). Pain in the trigeminal system: from orofacial nociception to neural network modeling. *J. Dent. Res.* **82**, 764–768.

Woda, A., Molat, J.L. and Luccarini, P. (2001). Low doses of N-methyl-D-aspartate antagonists in superficial laminae of medulla oblongata facilitate wind-up of convergent neurones. *Neurosci.* **107**, 317–327.

Woolf, C.J. and Ma, Q. (2007). Nociceptors – noxious stimulus detectors. *Neuron* **55**, 353–364.

Xie, Y.F., Zhang, S., Chiang, C.Y., Hu, J.W., Dostrovsky, J.O. and Sessle, B.J. (2007). Involvement of glia in central sensitization in trigeminal subnucleus caudalis (medullary dorsal horn). *Brain Behav. Immun.* **21**, 634–641.

Yamazaki, Y., Ren, K., Shimada, M. and Iwata, K. (2008). Modulation of paratrigeminal nociceptive neurons following temporomandibular joint inflammation in rats. *Exp. Neurol.* **214**, 209–218.

Yao, D., Yoshida, M. and Sessle, B.J. (2009). *Administration of noxious irritant on dura modulates neck muscle activities evoked by mustard oil application to superior sagittal sinus in the rat. Program No.459.9. Abstract Viewer/ Itinerary Planner.* Society for Neuroscience, Washington DC.

Yao, D., Yoshida, M. and Sessle, B.J. (2010). *Dura-evoked neck muscle activity involves purinergic receptor mechanism. Program No. 780. 13/MM13. Abstract Viewer/Itinerary Planner.* Society for Neuroscience, Washington, DC.

Yu, X.-M., Sessle, B.J. and Hu, J.W. (1993). Differential effects of cutaneous and deep application of inflammatory irritant on mechanoreceptive field properties of trigeminal brain stem nociceptive neurons. *J. Neurophysiol.* **70**, 1704–1707.

Yu, X.M., Sessle, B.J., Vernon, H. and Hu, J.W. (1994). Administration of opiate antagonist naloxone induces recurrence of increased jaw muscle activities related to inflammatory irritant application to rat temporomandibular joint region. *J. Neurophysiol.* **72**, 1430–1433.

Yu, X.M., Sessle, B.J., Haas, D.A., Izzo, A., Vernon, H. and Hu, J.W. (1996). Involvement of NMDA receptor mechanisms in jaw electromyographic activity and plasma extravasation induced by inflammatory irritant application to temporomandibular joint region of rats. *Pain* **68**, 169–178.

Zanotto, K.L., Merrill, A.W., Carstens, M.I. and Carstens, E. (2007). Neurons in superficial trigeminal subnucleus caudalis responsive to oral cooling, menthol, and other irritant stimuli. *J. Neurophysiol.* **97**, 966–978.

Zhang, S., Chiang, C.Y., Xie, Y.F., Lu, Y., Hu, J.W., Dostrovsky, J.O. and Sessle, B.J. (2006). Central sensitization in thalamic nociceptive neurons induced by mustard oil application to rat molar tooth pulp. *Neurosci.* **142**, 833–842.

THE ROLE OF TRIGEMINAL INTERPOLARIS-CAUDALIS TRANSITION ZONE IN PERSISTENT OROFACIAL PAIN

Ke Ren and Ronald Dubner

Department of Neural and Pain Sciences, Dental School; & Program in Neuroscience, University of Maryland, Baltimore, MD 21201-1586, USA

The sensory information from dental and craniofacial regions is first relayed in the spinal trigeminal nuclear complex (spinal trigeminal nucleus), which is further divided rostrocaudally into the subnuclei oralis (Vo), interpolaris (Vi) and caudalis (Vc) (Olszewski, 1950). It is widely accepted that nociceptive input from the cranial orofacial region is initially processed in the Vc (Sessle 2000) that exhibits considerable similarity with spinal dorsal horn and thus termed the medullary dorsal horn (MDH) (Gobel 1981). Despite apparent homology in nociceptive processing, recent observations have identified features of trigeminal pain processing in the MDH that are distinctly different from that of the spinal dorsal horn (Bereiter *et al.*, 2000). Further, studies have pointed out increased excitability and sensitization of trigeminal pain pathways in non-laminar regions of the spinal trigeminal nuclear complex, particularly the trigeminal Vi/Vc transition zone, following injury and noxious stimulation of the dental and craniofacial region. Multiple lines of

INTERNATIONAL REVIEW OF NEUROBIOLOGY, VOL. 97
DOI: 10.1016/B978-0-12-385198-7.00008-4

evidence suggest that the trigeminal Vi/Vc transition zone plays an important role in deep tissue pain processing, integrating nociceptive orofacial input, and the development of persistent orofacial pain.

I. Vi/Vc Neuronal Activation after Orofacial Injury

At the obex level, the ventral portion of the laminated Vc merges with the caudal Vi. Thus, rostral Vc with imperfectly laminated structures appears dorsally with Vi (ventral) at the same coronal plane to form the trigeminal Vi/Vc transition zone (Fig. 1A). The dorsal portion of the Vi/Vc transition zone in the rat mainly involves the rostral end of the laminated Vc and the ventral Vi/Vc mainly includes the caudal Vi. Immunostaining with the anti-calcitonin gene-related peptide (CGRP) antibodies, the superficial laminae of the Vc can be clearly seen in the dorsal lateral portion of the Vi/Vc (Fig. 1A). The ventral pole of the Vi/Vc, the CGRP staining in the Vi appears less well organized, whereas the CGRP-like immunoreactivity (LI) is distributed across the full length of the superficial MDH (Fig. 1B). Somatotopy exists in the trigeminal transition zone. For example, the mandibular structures masseter muscle and temporomandibular joint (TMJ) are represented at the dorsomedial Vi/Vc (Klineberg, 1971; Nishimori *et al.*, 1986; Capra, 1987; Takemura *et al.*, 1987; Pfaller and Arvidsson, 1988; Shigenaga *et al.*, 1988; Arvidsson and Raappana 1989); and corneal afferents terminate in the ventral Vi/Vc (Pozo and Cervero 1993; Hirata *et al.*, 1999).

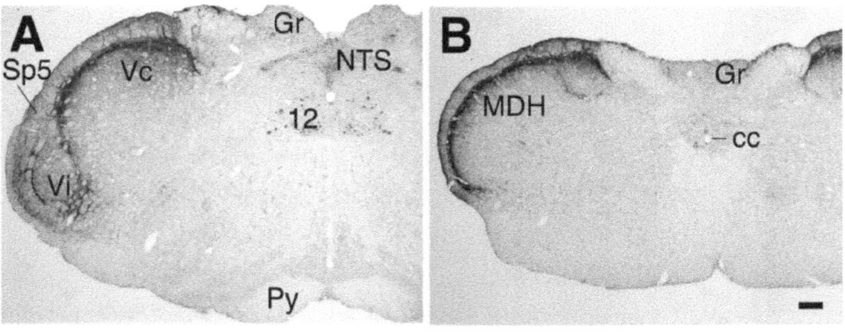

FIG. 1. Digital photomicrograph illustrating the trigeminal Vi/Vc transition zone and laminated subnucleus caudalis (Vc). The sections in A and B were immunostained against anti-CGRP antibodies to illustrate the appearance of the Vi/Vc transition zone (A, about 0.4 mm rostral to the obex) and laminated Vc, or Medullary Dorsal Horn (MDH) (B, about 1.0 mm caudal to the obex). Note the the delineation of the Vi in the ventral Vi/Vc transition zone by calcitonin gene-related peptide staining (A). Scale bar = 0.2 mm. 12, hypoglossal nucleus; cc, central canal; Gr, gracile nucleus; NTS, Nucleus Tractus Solitarius; Py, pyramidal tract; Sp5, spinal trigeminal tract; Vi, subnucleus interpolaris of the spinal trigeminal complex. (Adapted from Wang *et al.*, 2006, with permission from John Willey and Sons, License number: 2514340553127).

An interesting finding in recent years is that neuronal activation, as indicated by Fos protein expression, is consistently observed in the trigeminal Vi/Vc transition zone after a variety of noxious stimuli applied to the dental and craniofacial regions, including dural blood vessel and facial stimulation (Strassman and Vos, 1993, Strassman *et al.*, 1994), corneal stimulation (Bereiter *et al.*, 1994) and intravitreal capsaicin (Chang *et al.*, 2010), noxious stimulation of the tooth (Coimbra and Coimbra, 1994), oral mucous membrane (Sugimoto *et al.*, 1994) and the pulp (Chattipakorn *et al.*, 2002, 2005; Oakden and Boissonade, 1998), chemical stimulation of the rat's tongue (Carstens *et al.*, 1995), mustard oil and adjuvant stimulation of the TMJ (Hathaway *et al.*, 1995; Zhou *et al.* 1999), and masseter muscle inflammation (Imbe *et al.*, 1999; Ro *et al.*, 2003). These studies reveal an interesting pattern of trigeminal nociceptive neuronal activation (Fig. 2). First, stimulation-induced trigeminal Fos protein expression exhibits a bi-modal distribution, with one peak at the caudal Vc/C1,2 and a rostral peak at the Vi/Vc (Strassman and Vos, 1993). Second, while stimulus-induced Fos-LI in the Vc/C1,2, particularly in superficial laminae, is predominantly ipsilateral to the side of stimulation, Fos-LI in

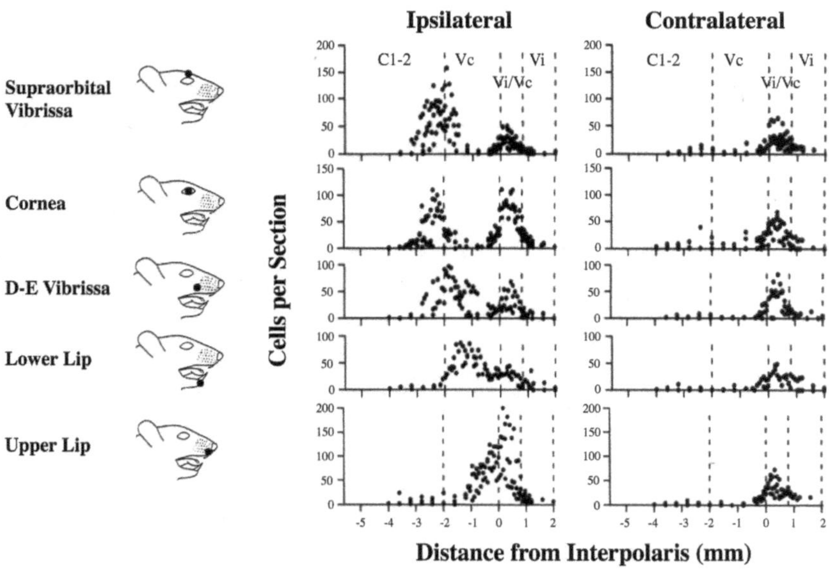

FIG. 2. Rostrocaudal distribution of Fos-immunoreactive neurons in the spinal trigeminal complex after orofacial stimulation. Cartoons on the right show site of stimulation. The number of Fos-positive cells is plotted against the distance from the subnucleus interpolaris. 0 ≈ obex level, positive = rostral, negative = caudal. Note bi-modal distribution of Fos-positive cells along the Vi/Vc and Vc/C1,2 ipsilateral to stimulation and one peak of Fos-positive cells at the Vi/Vc level contralateral to stimulation. (Adapted from Strassman and Vos, 1993, with permission from John Willey and Sons, License number: 2514340716050).

the Vi/Vc transition zone is often expressed bilaterally in the ventral Vi/Vc despite a unilateral injury.

The dual representation of orofacial nociceptive input in the spinal trigeminal complex is consistent with anatomical findings. It is known that sensory inputs from the orofacial region project to two regions of the spinal trigeminal complex, the Vc and caudal Vi (Arvidsson *et al.*, 1992; Capra, and Dessem, 1992). The location of the terminal field in the caudal Vi is constant but the terminal field in the Vc shows somatopic differences. In general, primary afferent fibers from the perioral and perinasal regions, or the most anterior face (tongue, upper lip and snout), terminate most rostrally in the Vc, and fibers from progressively more posterior facial regions (lower lip, cornea, supraorbital vibrassae) terminate at successively lower levels (Shigenaga *et al.*, 1986). Accordingly, primary afferent fibers that convey noxious stimuli from more caudal and lateral regions of the face have progressively more caudal terminations in reference to the obex. The fibers that innervate the circumoral zone terminate near the obex, whereas intermediate and peripheral zones terminate more caudally in the Vc. The anatomical relationship between the orofacial input and central termination explains the Fos expression pattern after noxious stimulation. For example, the terminal field for the lower lip is clearly caudal and separated from the Vi/Vc zone; so are the two distinct Fos peaks (Fig. 2). The primary terminal field for the upper lip is immediately caudal or slightly overlapped with the Vi/Vc zone (Arvidsson *et al.*, 1992). Consistently, the caudal peak of Fos labeling is apparently missing after stimulation of the upper lip, as the Vi/Vc and caudal Fos peaks merge at the obex-Vi/Vc level (Fig. 2) (Strassman and Vos 1993).

What is the significance of neuronal activation at the Vi/Vc level? It has been shown that urethane anesthesia itself can induce Fos at the Vi/Vc, but not at the caudal Vc (Strassman and Vos, 1993). Methohexital (Brevital) anesthesia also induces Fos in the Vi/Vc (Zhou *et al.*, 1999). However, the masseter inflammation-induced Fos in Vi/Vc cannot be explained by the effect of Brevital anesthesia alone (Imbe *et al.*, 1999). Specific neuronal activation at the Vi/Vc transition zone after noxious stimulation, which correlates with behavioral hyperalgesia, suggests a previously unrecognized role of this region in trigeminal pain processing.

II. Functional Input and Output of the Vi/Vc Transition Zone

A. Peripheral Input

By comparing the masseteric inflammation induced Fos-LI to that induced by anesthesia and skin-cut over the masseter muscle, it was found that the bilateral periobex peak of Fos-LI was primarily a response to masseteric inflammation, while the skin-cut mainly induced the caudal ipsilateral peak of Fos-LI (Imbe *et al.*, 1999; Ikeda *et al.*, 2003). These findings suggest that the Vi/Vc transition zone plays an important role in the responses to deep tissue injury. This hypothesis is supported by recent studies discussed below.

Utilizing a double tracing protocol (Capra and Wax, 1989), we studied the central termination of masseter muscle afferents in the trigeminal transition zone, compared with that of the cutaneous afferents (Wang *et al.* 2006). Different neuronal tracers were injected either centrally (FluoroGold; ventral Vi/Vc or MDH) or peripherally (wheat germ agglutinin-conjugated horseradish peroxidase or cholera toxin B; masseter or overlying skin), in the same rat and the convergence of the tracers in the trigeminal ganglion was examined. A population of small- to medium-sized neurons was double-labeled after injections of the tracers into the masseter and Vi/Vc, masseter and MDH, or the skin and MDH. However, only a few double-labeled neurons were occasionally observed after injections of the tracers into the skin and Vi/Vc. These results indicate that while both masseter and cutaneous inputs project to the MDH, masseter afferents provide an additional input to the Vi/Vc. The ventral Vi/Vc also receives direct corneal input (Pozo and Cervero, 1993; Tashiro *et al.*, 2010).

Behavioral pharmacology studies show that injection of an N-methyl-D-aspartate receptor antagonist, AP-5, into the Vi/Vc and MDH attenuated masseter inflammatory hyperalgesia. In contrast, hyperalgesia after inflammation of the skin overlying the masseter was attenuated by injection of AP-5 into the MDH but not Vi/Vc. Similar results were obtained by injecting glial inhibitors and IL-10, an anti-inflammatory cytokine, into the Vi/Vc or MDH (Shimizu *et al.* 2009b). These anatomical and behavioral observations support the view that there is differential involvement of trigeminal transition zone, and laminated subnucleus caudalis in orofacial deep and cutaneous hyperalgesia.

B. Visceral Input

The afferent projections to the ipsilateral dorsal Vi/Vc have been identified following HRP injection into the cervical vagus nerve (Gwyn *et al.*, 1985). Electrical stimulation of the vagus nerve induces expression of Fos-LI in the Vi/Vc transition zone (Gieroba and Blessing, 1994; Yousfi-Malki and Puizillout, 1994). The vagotomy produces a decrease in the masseteric inflammation-induced Fos-LI in the Vi/Vc transition zone (Imbe *et al.*, 1999). Taken together, a portion of the orofacial injury-induced Vi/Vc neuronal activation is likely a result of somatic-visceral integration that is mediated by vagal afferents to the brain.

C. Caudalis Input

The multiple lines of evidence indicate that neuronal activation in the transition zone, particularly the ventral pole, depends on input from the caudal Vc. Neurons in the caudal Vc project to rostral subnuclei of the spinal trigeminal nucleus (Ikeda *et al.*, 1982; Lovick and Wolstencroft, 1983; Jacquin *et al.*, 1990). The ascending pathway from caudal Vc modulates the activity of neurons in the more rostral subnuclei of the spinal trigeminal nucleus (Greenwood and Sessle, 1976; Scibetta and King 1969). Inhibition of caudal Vc affects Vi/Vc neuronal activity and evoked transmitter release (Bereiter *et al.*, 2002; Hirata *et al.*, 2003). Topical application of glutamate and morphine to the Vc/C1 region either facilitated or inhibited evoked activity of ~30% of corneal units tested in the Vi/Vc (Meng *et al.*, 1998). Following injection of the retrograde tracer Fluorogold into the Vi/Vc transition zone, retrogradely labeled cells were observed in the Vc/C1,2 region (Sato *et al.*, 2005). After lesions of the bilateral Vc, there is a selective reduction of inflammation-induced Fos-expressing neurons in the ventral Vi/Vc, but not in dorsal or intermediate Vi/Vc, or nucleus tractus solitarius (Sugiyo *et al.*, 2005). These findings support that trigeminal transition zone activity, particularly the ventral Vi/Vc, is modulated by the activation of the caudal laminated Vc zone.

D. Rostral Projections

Neurons in the spinal trigeminal complex project to a variety of rostral brain structures related to somatosensory, as well as somatoautonomic and somatovisceral processing. It has been shown that neurons in the ventral portion of the Vi/Vc transition zone have a major projection to the nucleus submedius of the thalamus (Sm) (Yoshida *et al.*, 1991). This Vi/Vc-Sm pathway is activated after orofacial injury. Through a combined Fluorogold retrograde tracing and Fos protein immunocytochemistry double labeling approach, rostrally projecting neurons that are activated after masseter inflammation can be identified (Ikeda *et al.*, 2003). In the ventral portion of the Vi/Vc transition zone, about 40 percent of neurons exhibiting inflammation-induced Fos-LI project to the Sm. However, very few Fos-labeled neurons in the dorsal Vi/Vc project to the Sm. Anesthesia alone also induces Fos expression in ventral Vi/Vc neurons but these neurons do not project to Sm (Ikeda *et al.*, 2003). About 20 percent of Fos-positive neurons in dorsal and ventral Vi/Vc project to the parabrachial nucleus and about 5 percent of Fos-positive neurons project to either the lateral hypothalamus or medial ventroposterior thalamic nucleus. The Sm plays a role in nociceptive processing, particularly related to aversive and emotional responses (Craig and Burton 1981). The parabrachial nucleus is involved in processing trigeminal nociceptive input

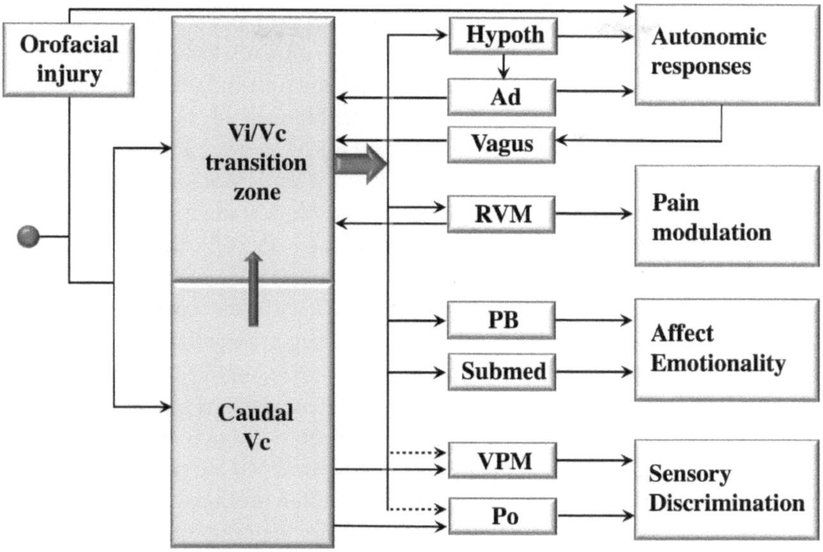

FIG. 3. Summary of the role of the trigeminal Vi/Vc transition zone in persistent orofacial pain. Orofacial injury-related inputs not only activate caudal Vc neurons, but also reach the Vi/Vc transition zone. The Vi/Vc output accesses hypothalamus (Hypoth), rostral ventromedial medulla (RVM), parabrachial nucleus (PB), and nucleus submedius of the thalamus (Submed) to play a role in autonomic responses to injury, descending pain modulation and pain-related emotionality. The Vi/Vc transition zone also receives input from RVM and Vi/Vc neuronal activation is regulated by caudal Vc through internuclear connections, the adrenal cortex (Ad) through circulating glucocorticoids and vagal afferents. Also shown is the Vc output that is relayed through the thalamic medial ventrolateral nucleus (VPM) and posterior thalamic nucleus (PO) for discriminative pain. The Vi/Vc transition zone may play a minor role in discriminative pain (dashed arrows).

and integrating emotional and autonomic responses (see Feil and Herbert 1995). The major projections from Vi/Vc are to the Sm and parabrachial nucleus, supporting the conclusion that this region plays a role in autonomic and hormonal functions and is emotionality related to persistent pain (Bereiter *et al.*, 1996; Ikeda *et al.*, 2003) (Fig. 3).

E. Reciprocal Interactions with the Brainstem Descending Circuitry

The rostral ventromedial medulla (RVM) is a key structure in descending pain modulation, which includes the midline nucleus raphe magnus and the adjacent reticular formation ventral to the gigantocellular reticular nucleus (Fields *et al.*, 2006). In addition to inhibitory descending input, RVM facilitates neuropathic pain, secondary hyperalgesia and persistent pain (Porreca *et al.*, 2002; Vanegas and Schaible, 2004; Ren and Dubner, 2008). The Vi/Vc transition zone has access to the RVM. Following the injection of Fluorogold into the RVM 7 days before injection of an inflammatory agent, Complete Freund's Adjuvant (CFA), into the masseter muscle and perfusion of the rat at 2-hour post-inflammation, a population of neurons in the ventral Vi/Vc exhibited Fluorogold/Fos double staining, suggesting the connection between Vi/Vc and RVM and the activation of the Vi/Vc-RVM pathway after inflammation. This Vi/Vc-RVM projection pathway appears selective for the ventral portion of the Vi/Vc since no double-labeled neurons were found in the dorsal Vi/Vc or laminae I–IV of Vc (Sugiyo *et al.*, 2005). Injection of an anterograde tracer, phaseolus vulgaris leucoagglutinin, into the RVM, resulted in labeling profiles overlapped with the region that showed Fluorogold/Fos double labeling in the Vi/Vc, suggesting that the connections between RVM and Vi/Vc are reciprocal. Excitotoxic lesions of the RVM or Vi/Vc with ibotenic acid led to the elimination or attenuation of masseter hyperalgesia/allodynia developed after masseter inflammation (Sugiyo *et al.*, 2005). Thus, there are reciprocal connections between the ventral Vi/Vc transition zone and RVM. The Vi/Vc-RVM pathway is activated after orofacial deep tissue injury and involved in descending facilitation of orofacial hyperalgesia.

III. Cellular and Chemical Mediators: Role of Neuron-Glia-Cytokine Interactions

Nerve signals arising from sites of tissue or nerve injury lead to long-term increases in excitability and plasticity in the central nervous system, often referred to as central sensitization. Central sensitization is brought about by a series of cellular events including neuronal depolarization, removal of the voltage-dependent magnesium block of the N-methyl-D-aspartate receptor (NMDAR); phosphorylation of NMDAR, alpha amino-3-hydroxy-5-methyl-4-isoxazolepropionate (AMPA), and neurokinin (NK) 1 receptors and an increase in synaptic strength (Dubner and Ren, 2004). Ample evidence indicates that central sensitization underlies mechanisms of persistent pain (Woolf and Salter, 2000; Dubner and Ren, 2004).

There has been an increasing awareness of neuroimmune interactions and their role in the etiology of diseases including chronic pain (Ren and Dubner, 2010). The neuroimmune interactions are reciprocal, or bi-directional, and involve central glial cells, cytokines, and neurotransmitters and their receptors. The emerging literature strongly implicates a role for glia and proinflammatory cytokines in the genesis and maintenance of persistent or chronic pain (Watkins and Maier, 2005).

The Vi/Vc transition zone contributes to central sensitization after orofacial injury. Sensitization of Vi/Vc neurons occurs after orofacial injury, which involves a cascade of cellular events including the activation of neurotransmitter receptors and neuron-glia-cytokine interactions. In response to orofacial tissue injury, glia in the Vi/Vc transition zone exhibit hyperactivity and inflammatory cytokines released, contributing to activity-dependent plasticity and hyperalgesia (Guo *et al.*, 2007).

A. Vi/Vc Glial Response to Injury

Following peripheral injury, microglia and astrocytes show increased levels of activity or a hyperactive state, and are often referred to as "activated". The specific expression of cellular markers is used to assess levels of glial activity. Among the most commonly used, glial fibrillary acidic protein (GFAP), an astrocytic intermediate cytoskeleton filament, is a marker of astrocytes and cluster of differentiation molecule 11b (CD11b), also known as Mac-1 or CR3, is the α-integrin marker of microglia. The monoclonal antibody OX-42 is commonly used to detect CD11b in brain microglia. Two calcium-binding peptides have been used as a functional marker of glia: S100B for astrocytes and Iba1 (ionized calcium-binding adapter molecule) for microglia.

Masseter inflammation induces glial hyperactivity in the Vi/Vc transition zone (Guo *et al.*, 2007). Following injection of the inflammatory agent CFA into the masseter muscle, reactive astrocytes were clearly seen in the Vi/Vc transition zone, indicated by GFAP immunostaining. The activated astrocytes typically exhibited hypertrophy with thicker processes and larger and densely stained cell bodies. The increase in GFAP levels is seen as early as at 0.5-hours and lasts for about one week after inflammation. The activation of astrocytes after inflammation is associated with upregulation of connexin 43 (Cx43), an astrocytic gap junction protein. Double immunohistochemistry shows that the Cx43-LI co-localizes with GFAP, but not with CD11b, a marker of microglia, NeuN, a neuronal marker, or Cx36, a neuronal gap junction protein. The levels of CD11b are also upregulated by masseter inflammation. The glial hyperactivity induced by masseter inflammation in the Vi/Vc transition zone correlates with the development of hyperalgesia (Sugiyo *et al.*, 2005; Watanabe *et al.*, 2005).

B. Role of Inflammatory Cytokine IL-1beta

The hyperactivity of glia induced by masseter inflammation is accompanied by an increase in the inflammatory cytokine levels. Compared to the naive rats, the immunostaining for interleukin-1beta (IL-1beta a prototypic proinflammatory cytokine, is increased significantly in the Vi/Vc transition zone (Guo *et al.*, 2007). Western blot shows the increase of IL-1beta in the Vi/Vc transition zone with a time course similar to that of astrocyte hypertrophy after masseter inflammation. Interestingly, IL-1beta is selectively induced in astrocytes, but not in microglia or neurons, in the ventral Vi/Vc transiton zone. The selective localization of IL-1beta in astrocytes has also been reported in other animal models, including bone cancer pain (Zhang *et al.*, 2005), tissue and nerve injury (Kawasaki *et al.*, 2008; Wei *et al.*, 2008; Weyerbacher *et al.*, 2010), and intracerebral hemorrhage (Wasserman *et al.*, 2007). These findings suggest that astrocytes provide an alternative source of IL-1beta, in addition to the known release of IL-1beta from microglia after injury (Clark *et al.*, 2006; Kawasaki *et al.*, 2008). The CFA-induced increases in IL-1beta levels are reduced after the treatment with propentofylline, a glial inhibitor (Guo *et al.*, 2007), suggesting that glial activation is upstream to cytokine induction in the Vi/Vc after inflammation.

The IL-1beta in the Vi/Vc plays a role in the development of orofacial hyperalgesia. The mechanical allodynia and hyperalgesia in the orofacial region can be assessed by applying a series of von Frey microfilaments to the skin. The response frequencies to a range of von Frey filament forces are determined. A stimulus-response frequency relationship is established and 50 perecnt effective force values are derived. The EF_{50} is defined as the force that induces 50 percent response frequency in rats. A significant reduction of EF_{50} vs. the baseline level indicates mechanical allodynia and hyperalgesia (Guo *et al.*, 2004). When an IL-1 receptor antagonist (IL-1ra) was administered intrathecally via osmotic pumps through a cannula implanted at the level of the obex prior to the induction of masseter inflammation, the behavioral allodynia and hyperalgesia were significantly attenuated (Guo *et al.*, 2007). Direct injection of IL-1beta into the ventral Vi/Vc transition zone produces mechanical allodynia and hyperalgesia (Shimizu *et al.*, 2009a).

C. Glia, Cytokine and NMDA Receptor Activation

The Vi/Vc glial hyperactivity and inflammatory cytokine release facilitates central sensitization through interactions with the NMDAR. NMDAR phosphorylation is widely accepted as an indication of synaptic plasticity and correlates with the time course of persistent pain (Guo *et al.*, 2002, 2004; Brenner *et al.*, 2004). IL-1beta facilitates NMDAR phosphorylation in an *ex vivo* medullary slice preparation (Guo *et al.*, 2007). Incubation of IL-1beta in the medullary slices induced a significant and dose-dependent increase in phospho-ser896-NR1 (P-NR1) levels in the Vi/Vc transition zone. In contrast, the application of TNF-alpha, the other prototypic inflammatory cytokine, does not affect P-NR1 levels at the dose tested (Guo *et al.*, 2007). Microinjection of IL-1beta into the ventral Vi/Vc transition zone *in vivo* also produced an increase in P-ser896-NR1 levels that is blocked by IL-1ra (Guo *et al.*, 2007).

The IL-1beta-induced NR1 phosphorylation is blocked by chelerythrine, a PKC inhibitor, confirming that PKC is involved in this effect. 2APB, a membrane permeable IP3 receptor antagonist also blocks IL-1beta-induced NR1 phosphorylation. The NMDAR channel blocker MK-801 does not affect the IL-1beta-induced increase in P-ser896-NR1 (Guo *et al.*, 2007). The involvement of the PKC inhibitor in IL-1beta-facilitated P-NR1 suggests that a key link between IL-1beta and subsequent activation of NMDAR involves phospholipases PLA2 or PLC, since PKC is a downstream effector of arachidonic acid and diacylglycerol. This hypothesis has been tested. The PLC inhibitor U73122 and PLA2 inhibitor AACOCF3 blocked the effect of IL-1beta on NMDAR phosphorylation in Vi/Vc. It is well known that IL-1R signaling leads to transcriptional regulation of cellular function (Martin and Wesche, 2002). These findings show that the effect of IL-1beta on NMDAR phosphorylation is attributable to the post-translational regulation through IL-1R signaling; and that the intermediate pathway involves PLC, PLA2 and subsequent PKC activation and intracellular Ca^{2+} release.

Direct administration of IL-1beta into the ventral trigeminal transition zone produced orofacial hyperalgesia that lasted for hours (Shimizu *et al.*, 2009a). Pretreatment with glial inhibitors does not block IL-1beta-induced hyperalgesia even with relatively high doses that have been shown to be effective in attenuating hyperalgesia after injury (Wei *et al.*, 2008; Shimizu *et al.*, 2009b). Although the glial inhibitor/modulator propentofylline do not block IL-1beta-induced hyperalgesia, propentofylline was able to attenuate hyperalgesia after masseter inflammation (Shimizu *et al.*, unpublished observations). Likewise, fluorocitrate is unable to block IL-1beta-induced NMDA receptor phosphorylation in the Vi/Vc transition zone *in vitro*, but attenuated masseter inflammatory hyperalgesia (Guo *et al.*, 2007). Thus, IL-1beta-induced hyperalgesia appears to be downstream to glial activity and involves activation of NMDAR. Direct application of IL-1beta bypasses glial cells, to produce neuronal hyperexcitability and hyperalgesia.

The NMDAR plays a major role in central sensitization and pain hypersensitivity, including orofacial hyperalgesia (Chiang *et al.*, 1997; Bereiter and Bereiter, 2000; Guo *et al.*, 2007; Wang *et al.*, 2009). Injection of the NMDAR antagonist into the Vi/Vc transition zone attenuates masseter inflammatory hyperalgesia (Wang *et al.*, 2006). The IL-1beta signaling facilitates NMDAR activity in neurons (Viviani *et al.*, 2003; Yang *et al.*, 2005; Guo *et al.*, 2007; Zhang *et al.*, 2008). IL-1beta exaggerates NMDA and glutamate-evoked hippocampal neuron death in the rat (Ma *et al.*, 2002-2003). Consistently, IL-1R colocalizes with the NMDAR NR1 subunit in Vi/Vc neurons (Guo *et al.*, 2007). Thus, IL-1R signaling may selectively regulate NMDAR function and increase synaptic strength via post-translational phosphorylation and contribute to inflammation-induced pain hypersensitivity. Collective evidence suggests that glial activation, inflammatory cytokine release and NMDAR activation are sequential events in the nervous system responses to injury, and that IL-1beta and its interaction with NMDA receptors plays a critical role in the central mechanisms of hyperalgesia.

IV. Functional Significance of Vi/Vc in Trigeminal Pain Processing

Noxious stimulation of the different dental and craniofacial regions induces bimodal neuronal activation in the spinal trigeminal complex. While the caudal peak of neuronal activity varies rostrocaudally and mediolaterally in the Vc according to somatotopy, the rostral peak is consistently located at the obex or the trigeminal transition zone level (Strassman and Vos, 1993). Further, anesthetic alone induces Fos protein expression and increased phosphorylation of the extracellular signal-regulated kinase in the Vi/Vc transition zone (Imbe *et al.*, 1999; Shoda *et al.*, 2009). These findings suggest that neuronal activation in the ventral Vi/Vc transition zone lacks somatotopy, although there are selective primary afferent inputs to the Vi/Vc transition zone (Klineberg, 1971; Shigenaga *et al.*, 1988; Pozo and Cervero 1993; Zhou *et al.*, 1999; Hirata *et al.*, 1999; Imbe *et al.*, 1999; Wang *et al.*, 2006). Evidence suggests that the Vi/Vc response, particularly the ventral Vi/Vc, to injury is related to the integration of somatosensory and visceral/autonomic functions, and the engagement of descending pain modulation, but less concerned with somatotopically organized pain behavior, that is mainly mediated by laminated Vc (Fig. 3).

A. Somatovisceral Somatoautonomic Integration

It is suggested that anesthetics-induced Fos expression in the brainstem nuclei could be explained at least in part by its cardiovascular effects, since they induce a decrease in the arterial blood pressure and heart rate (Rocha and Herbert, 1997). The administration of nitroglycerin, a vasodilator, also induces hypotension and bilateral Fos-LI in the ventral portion of Vi/Vc (Tassorelli and Joseph, 1995; Bereiter *et al.* 1994) show that mustard oil stimulation of the cornea induces Fos-LI in a group of neurons located in the ventral Vi/Vc and that local anesthesia of this area greatly attenuated the mustard oil-induced adrenal and autonomic responses. Vi/Vc neuronal activation is also related to injury-produced environmental stress and visceral input. Adrenalectomy and vagotomy selectively reduced Fos expression at the Vi/Vc transition zone with little effect on the caudal Fos peak (Imbe *et al.*, 1999), suggesting that Vi/Vc neuronal activation depends on the integrity of the adrenal cortex and vagus nerve. Thus, in addition to somatotopically organized nociceptive responses, orofacial injury is also coupled to somatovisceral and somatoautonomic activity that contributes to central neural activation mediated through the Vi/Vc.

B. Descending Modulation

Trigeminal neurons have connections with neurons in the nucleus raphe magnus, the major component of the RVM (Beitz *et al.*, 1983; Basbaum *et al.*, 1986). The spinal trigeminal nucleus receives serotonergic and enkephalinergic projections from the nucleus raphe magnus (Beitz, 1982; Beitz *et al.*, 1987). Pain modulating neurons in nucleus raphe magnus also have terminals in the spinal trigeminal nucleus (Mason and Fields, 1989), which may modulate trigeminal nociceptive transmission (Chiang *et al.*, 1994).

The Vi/Vc neurons also relay nociceptive input from the orofacial deep tissues to RVM neurons (Sugiyo *et al.*, 2005). Inflammation-activated neurons in the Vi/Vc transition zone project to the RVM and there is RVM neuronal activation after TMJ inflammation (Zhou *et al.*, 1999). An anterograde tracing study suggests that RVM neurons project to the area of the ventral trigeminal transition zone, where activated RVM projecting neurons are localized (Sugiyo *et al.*, 2005). This suggests reciprocal neural pathways between these two regions. These results further emphasize the importance of Vi/Vc neurons in engaging descending pain modulation.

Behavioral studies confirm the functional significance of the RVM-Vi/Vc connections (Sugiyo *et al.*, 2005; Shimizu *et al.*, 2009a). Unilateral CFA-induced inflammation of the masseter muscle produces mechanical allodynia and hyperalgesia in the orofacial region overlapping the masseter muscle. Excitotoxic lesions of the RVM or Vi/Vc transition zone lead to significant attenuation of behavioral hyperalgesia after masseter inflammation, indicating that modulatory inputs from the RVM enhance the hyperalgesia/allodynia, found after masseter inflammation. These results are consistent with the view that hyperalgesia in animal models of inflammatory and neuropathic pain are closely linked to the activation of descending pathways (Porreca *et al.*, 2002; Ren and Dubner, 2008; Vanegas and Schaible, 2004). Masseter inflammation-induced hyperalgesia is maintained by descending facilitatory drive that is recruited by the Vi/Vc-RVM circuitry, at least partially.

C. Deep vs. Cutaneous Injury

Deep orofacial tissue inflammation produces stronger central neuronal activation in the spinal trigeminal complex, including the Vi/Vc region than does cutaneous inflammation (Zhou *et al.*, 1999; Imbe *et al.*, 2001). Compared to cutaneous CFA injection, the injection of CFA into the TMJ produces a significantly stronger inflammation associated with greater Fos expression. It has been shown that mustard oil injections into the TMJ versus cutaneous tissues produces greater activation of masticatory muscles (Yu *et al.*, 1993) than the cutaneous mustard oil injections and that TMJ inflammation resulted in more widespread excitation of medullary dorsal horn neurons than perioral cutaneous inflammation (Iwata *et al.*, 1999).

There is also a differential involvement of the Vi/Vc transition zone in deep vs. cutaneous orofacial hyperalgesia. Injection of the NMDAR antagonist AP-5, anti-inflammatory cytokine IL-10 or glial inhibitors fluorocitrate and minocycline into the ventral Vi/Vc transition zone only attenuates hyperalgesia after masseter inflammation, without an effect on hyperalgesia associated with cutaneous injury (Wang *et al.*, 2006; Shimizu *et al.*, 2009b). In contrast, both masseter and cutaneous hyperalgesia are attenuated after the injection of these agents into the caudal Vc. Western blot analysis shows a selective enhancement of NMDAR phosphorylation and GFAP upregulation in the Vi/Vc transition zone after masseter, but not cutaneous inflammation (Shimizu *et al.*, 2009b). These observations indicate that, in addition to Vc, deep orofacial input engages Vi/Vc neurons in developing central sensitization and hyperalgesia. Noxious cutaneous or superficial input has access to the Vi/Vc (Strassman and Vos, 1993; Zhou *et al.*, 1999). The development of cutaneous hyperalgesia depends on caudal Vc and does not require coordination by Vi/Vc neurons (Shimizu *et al.*, 2009b; Chang *et al.*, 2010). Thus, while both deep and cutaneous orofacial nociceptive inputs are processed in the laminated Vc, the ventral pole of Vi/Vc is involved in the coordination of sensorimotor functions of the trigeminal system associated with the response to and recuperation from deep tissue injury. This response includes roles in nociceptive hyperexcitability involving glia and NMDAR, somatovisceral and somatoautomic integration, and descending pain modulation (also see Dubner and Ren, 2006).

Acknowledgments

The authors' work is supported by US National Institutes of Health grants DE11964, NS060735 and NS059028.

References

Arvidsson, J., Pfaller, K., and Gmeiner, S. (1992). The ganglionic origins and central projections of primary sensory neurons innervating the upper and lower lips in the rat Somatosens. *Mot. Res.* **9**, 199–209.

Arvidsson, J., and Raappana, P. (1989). An HRP study of the central projections from primary sensory neurons innervating the rat masseter muscle. *Brain Res.* **480**, 111–118.

Basbaum, A.I., Ralston, D.D., and Ralston, H.J.3rd. (1986). Bulbospinal projections in the primate: a light and electron microscopic study of a pain modulating system. *J. Comp. Neurol.* **250**, 311–323.

Beitz, A.J. (1982). The nuclei of origin of brainstem serotonergic projections to the rodent spinal trigeminal nucleus. *Neurosci. Lett.* **32**, 223–228.

Beitz, A.J., Clements, J.R., Ecklund, L.J., and Mullett, M.M. (1987). The nuclei of origin of brainstem enkephalin and cholecystokinin projections to the spinal trigeminal nucleus of the rat. *Neuroscience* **20**, 409–425.

Beitz, A.J., Wells, W.E., and Shepard, R.D. (1983). The location of brainstem neurons which project bilaterally to the spinal trigeminal nuclei as demonstrated by the double fluorescent retrograde tracer technique. *Brain Res.* **258**, 305–312.

Bereiter, D.A., and Bereiter, D.F. (2000). Morphine and NMDA receptor antagonism reduce c-Fos expression in spinal trigeminal nucleus produced by acute injury to the *TMJ region. Pain* **85**, 65–77.

Bereiter, D.A., Bereiter, D.F., and Hathaway, C.B. (1996). The NMDA receptor antagonist MK-801 reduces Fos-like immunoreactivity in central trigeminal neurons and blocks select endocrine and autonomic responses to corneal stimulation in the rat. *Pain* **64**, 179–189.

Bereiter, D.A., Hathaway, C.B., and Benetti, A.P. (1994). Caudal portions of the spinal trigeminal complex are necessary for autonomic responses and display Fos-like immunoreactivity after corneal stimulation in the cat. *Brain Res.* **657**, 73–82.

Bereiter, D.A., Hirata, H., and Hu, J.W. (2000). Trigeminal subnucleus caudalis: beyond homologies with the spinal dorsal horn. *Pain* **88**, 221–224.

Bereiter, D.A., Shen, S., and Benetti, A.P. (2002). Sex differences in amino acid release from rostral trigeminal subnucleus caudalis after acute injury to the TMJ region. *Pain* **98**, 89–99.

Brenner, G.J., Ji, R.R., Shaffer, S., and Woolf, C.J. (2004). Peripheral noxious stimulation induces phosphorylation of the NMDA receptor NR1 subunit at the PKC-dependent site, serine-896, in spinal cord dorsal horn neurons. *Eur. J. Neurosci.* **20**, 375–384.

Capra, N.F. (1987). Localization and central projections of primary afferent neurons that innervate the temporomandibular joint in cats. *Somatosens. Res.* **4**, 201–213.

Capra, N.F., and Dessem, D. (1992). Central connections of trigeminal primary afferent neurons: topographical and functional considerations. *Crit. Rev. Oral. Biol. Med.* **4**, 1–52.

Capra, N.F., and Wax, T.D. (1989). Distribution and central projections of primary afferent neurons that innervate the masseter muscle and mandibular periodontium: a double-label study. *J. Comp. Neurol.* **279**, 341–352.

Carstens, E., Saxe, I., and Ralph, R. (1995). Brainstem neurons expressing c-Fos immunoreactivity following irritant chemical stimulation of the rat's tongue. *Neuroscience* **69**, 939–953.

Chang, Z., Okamoto, K., Tashiro, A., and Bereiter, D.A. (2010). Ultraviolet irradiation of the eye and Fos-positive neurons induced in trigeminal brainstem after intravitreal or ocular surface transient receptor potential vanilloid 1 activation. *Neuroscience* **170**, 678–685.

Chattipakorn, S.C., Sigurdsson, A., Light, A.R., Narhi, M., and Maixner, W. (2002). Trigeminal c-Fos expression and behavioral responses to pulpal inflammation in ferrets. *Pain* **99**, 61–69.

Chattipakorn, S., Chattipakorn, N., Light, A.R., Narhi, M., and Maixner, W. (2005). Comparison of Fos expression within the ferret's spinal trigeminal nuclear complex evoked by electrical or noxious-thermal pulpal stimulation. *J. Pain* **6**, 569–580.

Chiang, C.Y., Hu, J.W., and Sessle, B.J. (1994). Parabrachial area and nucleus raphe magnus-induced modulation of nociceptive and non nociceptive trigeminal subnucleus caudalis neurons activated by cutaneous or deep inputs. *J. Neurophysiol.* **71**, 2430–2445.

Chiang, C.Y., Hu, J.W., and Sessle, B.J. (1997). NMDA receptor involvement in neuroplastic changes induced by neonatal capsaicin treatment in trigeminal nociceptive neurons. *J. Neurophysiol.* **78**, 2799–2803.

Clark, A.K., D'Aquisto, F., Gentry, C., Marchand, F., McMahon, S.B., and Malcangio, M. (2006). Rapid co-release of interleukin 1beta and caspase 1 in spinal cord inflammation. *J. Neurochem.* **99**, 868–880.

Coimbra, F., and Coimbra, A. (1994). Dental noxious input reaches the subnucleus caudalis of the trigeminal complex in the rat, as shown by c-Fos expression upon thermal or mechanical stimulation. *Neurosci. Lett.* **173**, 201–204.

Craig Jr., A.D., and Burton, H. (1981). Spinal and medullary lamina I projection to nucleus. submedius in medial thalamus: a possible pain center. *J. Neurophysiol.* **45**, 443–466.

Dubner, R., and Ren, K. (2004). Brainstem mechanisms of persistent pain following injury. *J. Orofacial. Pain* **18**, 299–305.

Dubner, R., and Ren, K. (2006). Pathophysiology of Persistent Orofacial Pain. In: Laskin, D.M., Greene, C.S., Hylander, W.L. (Eds.), *"Temporomandibular Disorders: An Evidence-Based Approach to Diagnosis and Treatment"*. Quintessence Publishing Co, Inc, Chicago, pp. 89–97.

Feil, K., and Herbert, H. (1995). Topographic organization of spinal and trigeminal somatosensory pathways to the rat parabrachial and Kölliker-Fuse nuclei. *J. Comp. Neurol.* **353**, 506–528.

Fields, H.L., Basbaum, A.I., and Heinricher, M.M. (2006). Central nervous system mechanisms of pain modulation. In: McMahon, S.B., Koltzenburg, M. (Eds.), *"Wall and Melzack's Textbook of Pain", 5th edit. Elsevier, Churchill Livingstone, pp. 125–142.*

Gieroba, Z.J., and Blessing, W.W. (1994). Fos-containing neurons in medulla and pons after unilateral stimulation of the afferent abdominal vagus in conscious rabbits. *Neuroscience* **59**, 851–858.

Gobel, S., Hockfield, S., and Ruda, M.A. (1981). Anatomical similarities between medullary and spinal dorsal horns. In: Kawamura, Y., Dubner, R. (Eds.), *"Oral-Facial Sensory and Motor Functions"*. Quintessence, Tokyo, pp. 211–223.

Greenwood, L.F., and Sessle, B.J. (1976). Inputs to trigeminal brain stem neurones from facial, oral, tooth pulp and pharyngolaryngeal tissues: II. *Role of trigeminal nucleus caudalis in modulating responses to innocuous and noxious stimuli. Brain Res.* **117**, 227–238.

Guo, W., Wang, H., Watanabe, M., Shimizu, K., Zou, S., LaGraize, S.C., Wei, F., Dubner, R., and Ren, K. (2007). Glial-cytokine-neuronal interactions underlying the mechanisms of persistent pain. *J. Neurosci.* **27**, 6006–6018.

Guo, W., Wei, F., Zou, S., Robbins, M.T., Sugiyo, S., Ikeda, T., Tu, J.C., Worley, P.F., Dubner, R., and Ren, K. (2004). Group I metabotropic glutamate receptor NMDA receptor coupling and signaling cascade mediate spinal dorsal horn NMDA receptor 2B tyrosine phosphorylation associated with inflammatory hyperalgesia. *J. Neurosci.* **24**, 9161–9173.

Guo, W., Zou, S., Guan, Y., Ikeda, T., Tal, M., Dubner, R., and Ren, K. (2002). Tyrosine phosphorylation of the NR2B subunit of the NMDA receptor in the spinal cord during the development and maintenance of inflammatory hyperalgesia. *J. Neurosci.* **22**, 6208–6217.

Gwyn, D.G., Leslie, R.A., and Hopkins, D.A. (1985). Observations on the afferent and efferent organization of the vagus nerve and the innervation of the stomach in the squirrel monkey. *J. Comp. Neurol.* **239**, 163–175.

Hathaway, C.B., Hu, J.W., and Bereiter, D.A. (1995). Distribution of Fos-like immunoreactivity in the caudal brainstem of the rat following noxious chemical stimulation of the temporomandibular joint. *J. Comp. Neurol.* **356**, 444–456.

Hirata, H., Hu, J.W., and Bereiter, D.A. (1999). Responses of medullary dorsal horn neurons to corneal stimulation by CO_2 pulses in the rat. *J. Neurophysiol.* **82**, 2092–2107.

Hirata, H., Okamoto, K., and Bereiter, D.A. (2003). GABA (A) receptor activation modulates corneal unit activity in rostral and caudal portions of trigeminal subnucleus caudalis. *J. Neurophysiol.* **90**, 2837–2849.

Ikeda, M., Matsushita, M., and Tanami, T. (1982). Termination and cells of origin of the ascending intranuclear fibers in the spinal trigeminal nucleus of the cat A study with the horseradish peroxidase technique. *Neurosci. Lett.* **31**, 215–220.

Ikeda, T., Terayama, R., Jue, S.S., Sugiyo, S., Dubner, R., and Ren, K. (2003). Differential rostral projection of caudal brainstem neurons receiving trigeminal input after masseter inflammation. *J. Comp. Neurol.* **465**, 220–233.

Imbe, H., Dubner, R., and Ren, K. (1999). Masseter inflammation-induced Fos protein expression in the trigeminal interpolaris/caudalis transition zone: contribution of somatosensory-vagal-adrenal integration. *Brain Res.* **845**, 165–175.

Imbe, H., Iwata, K., Zhou, Q.Q., Zou, S., Dubner, R., and Ren, K. (2001). Orofacial deep and cutaneous tissue inflammation and trigeminal neuronal activation: Implications for persistent temporomandibular pain. *Cells Tissues Organs* **169**, 238–247.

Iwata, K., Tsuboi, Y., Tashiro, A., Imai, T., Sumino, R., Dubner, R., and Ren, K. (1999). Enhancement and depression of medullary dorsal horn neuronal activity after noxious and non-noxious stimulation of the face in rats with persistent temporomandibular joint and cutaneous inflammation. *J. Neurophysiol.* **82**, 1244–1253.

Jacquin, M.F., Chiaia, N.L., Haring, J.H., and Rhoades, R.W. (1990). Intersubnuclear connections within the rat trigeminal brainstem complex. *Somatosens. Mot. Res.* **7**, 399–420.

Kawasaki, Y., Xu, Z.Z., Wang, X., Park, J.Y., Zhuang, Z.Y., Tan, P.H., Gao, Y.J., Roy, K., Corfas, G., Lo, E.H., and Ji, R.R. (2008). Distinct roles of matrix metalloproteases in the early- and late-phase development of neuropathic pain. *Nat. Med.* **14**, 331–336.

Klineberg, I. (1971). Structure and function of temporomandibular joint innervation. *Ann. R. Coll. Surg. Engl.* **49**, 268–288.

Lovick, T.A., and Wolstencroft, J.H. (1983). Projections from brain stem nuclei to the spinal trigeminal nucleus in the cat. *Neuroscience* **9**, 411–420.

Ma, X.C., Gottschall, P.E., Chen, L.T., Wiranowska, M., and Phelps, C.P. (2002). Role and mechanisms of interleukin-1 in the modulation of neurotoxicity. *Neuroimmunomodulation* **10**, 199–207.

Martin, M.U., and Wesche, H. (2002). Summary and comparison of the signaling mechanisms of the Toll/interleukin-1 receptor family. *Biochim. Biophys. Acta* **1592**, 265–280.

Mason, P., and Fields, H.L. (1989). Axonal trajectories and terminations of on- and off-cells in the cat lower brainstem. *J. Comp. Neurol.* **288**, 185–207.

Meng, I.D., Hu, J.W., and Bereiter, D.A. (1998). Differential effects of morphine on corneal-responsive neurons in rostral versus caudal regions of spinal trigeminal nucleus in the rat. *J. Neurophysiol.* **79**, 2593–2602.

Nishimori, T., Sera, M., Suemune, S., Yoshida, A., Tsuru, K., Tsuiki, Y., Akisaka, T., Okamoto, T., Dateoka, Y., and Shigenaga, Y. (1986). The distribution of muscle primary afferents from the masseter nerve to the trigeminal sensory nuclei. *Brain Res.* **372**, 375–381.

Oakden, E.L., and Boissonade, F.M. (1998). Fos expression in the ferret trigeminal nuclear complex following tooth pulp stimulation. *Neuroscience* **84**, 1197–1208.

Olszewski, J. (1950). On the anatomical and functional organization of the spinal trigeminal nucleus. *J. Comp. Neurol.* **92**, 401–413.

Porreca, F., Ossipov, M.H., and Gebhart, G.F. (2002). Chronic pain and medullary descending facilitation. *Trends Neurosci.* **25**, 319–325.

Pfaller, K., and Arvidsson, J. (1988). Central distribution of trigeminal and upper cervical primary afferents in the rat studied by anterograde transport of horseradish peroxidase conjugated to wheat germ agglutinin. *J. Comp. Neurol.* **268**, 91–108.

Pozo, M.A., and Cervero, F. (1993). Neurons in the rat spinal trigeminal complex driven by corneal nociceptors: receptive-field properties and effects of noxious stimulation of the cornea. *J. Neurophysiol.* **70**, 2370–2378.

Ren, K., and Dubner, R. (2008). Descending control mechanisms. In "The Senses: A Comprehensive Reference, Vol. 5, Pain" (A.I. Basbaum, A. Kaneko, G.M. Shepherd, and G. Westheimer, Eds.), Academic Press, San Diego. 723–762.

Ren, K., and Dubner, R. (2010). Interactions between the immune and nervous systems in pain. *Nat. Med.* in press.

Ro, J.Y., Harriott, A., Crouse, U., and Capra, N.F. (2003). Innocuous jaw movements increase c-Fos expression in trigeminal sensory nuclei produced by masseter muscle inflammation. *Pain* **104**, 539–548.

Rocha, M.J., and Herbert, H. (1997). Effects of anesthetics on Fos protein expression in autonomic brain nuclei related to cardiovascular regulation. *Neuropharmacology* **36**, 1779–1781.

Sato, T., Kitagawa, J., Ren, K., Tanaka, H., Tanabe, A., Watanabe, T., Mitsuhashi, Y., and Iwata, K. (2005). Activation of trigeminal intranuclear pathway in rats with temporomandibular joint inflammation. *J. Oral. Sci.* **47**, 65–69.

Scibetta, C.J., and King, R.B. (1969). Hyperpolarizing influence of trigeminal nucleus caudalis on primary afferent preterminals in trigeminal nucleus oralis. *J. Neurophysiol.* **32**, 229–238.

Sessle, B.J. (2000). Acute and chronic craniofacial pain: brainstem mechanisms of nociceptive transmission and neuroplasticity, and their clinical correlates. *Crit. Rev. Oral Biol. Med.* **11**, 57–91.

Shigenaga, Y., Chen, I.C., Suemune, S., Nishimori, T., Nasution, I.D., Yoshida, A., Sato, H., Okamoto, T., Sera, M., and Hosoi, M. (1986). Oral and facial representation within the medullary and upper cervical dorsal horns in the cat. *J. Comp. Neurol.* **243**, 388–408.

Shigenaga, Y., Sera, M., Nishimori, T., Suemune, S., Nishimura, M., Yoshida, A., and Tsuru, K. (1988). The central projection of masticatory afferent fibers to the trigeminal sensory nuclear complex and upper cervical spinal cord. *J. Comp. Neurol.* **268**, 489–507.

Shimizu, K., Chai, B., LaGraize, S.C., Wei, F., Dubner, R., and Ren, K. (2009a). Microinjection of IL-1beta into the trigeminal transition zone produces NMDA receptor-dependent orofacial hyperalgesia in rats. *The Open Pain Journal* **2**, 76–83.

Shimizu, K., Guo, W., Wang, H., Zou, S., LaGraize, S.C., Iwata, K., Wei, F., Dubner, R., and Ren, K. (2009b). Differential involvement of trigeminal transition zone and laminated subnucleus caudalis in orofacial deep and cutaneous hyperalgesia: the effects of interleukin-10 and glial inhibitors. *Mol. Pain* **5**, 75.

Shoda, E., Kitagawa, J., Suzuki, I., Nitta-Kubota, I., Miyamoto, M., Tsuboi, Y., Kondo, M., Masuda, Y., Oi, Y., Ren, K., and Iwata, K. (2009 b). Increased Phosphorylation of Extracellular Signal-Regulated Kinase in Trigeminal Nociceptive Neurons Following Propofol Administration in Rats. *J. Pain* **10**, 573–585.

Strassman, A.M., Mineta, Y., and Vos, B.P. (1994). Distribution of Fos-like immunoreactivity in the medullary and upper cervical dorsal horn produced by stimulation of dural blood vessels in the rat. *J. Neurosci.* **14**, 3725–3735.

Strassman, A.M., and Vos, B.P. (1993). Somatotopic and laminar organization of Fos-like immunoreactivity in the medullary and upper cervical dorsal horn induced by noxious facial stimulation in the rat. *J. Comp. Neurol.* **331**, 495–516.

Sugimoto, T., Hara, T., Shirai, H., Abe, T., Ichikawa, H., and Sato, T. (1994). c-Fos induction in the subnucleus cudalis following noxious mechanical stimulation of the oral mucous membrane. *Exp. Neurol.* **129**, 251–256.

Sugiyo, S., Takemura, M., Dubner, R., and Ren, K. (2005). Trigeminal transition zone/rostral ventromedial medulla connections and facilitation of orofacial hyperalgesia after masseter inflammation in rats. *J. Comp. Neurol.* **493**, 510–523.

Takemura, M., Sugimoto, T., and Sakai, A. (1987). Topographic organization of central terminal region of different sensory branches of the rat mandibular nerve. *Exp. Neurol.* **96**, 540–557.

Tashiro, A., Okamoto, K., Chang, Z., and Bereiter, D.A. (2010). Behavioral and neurophysiological correlates of nociception in an animal model of photokeratitis. *Neuroscience* **169**, 455–462.

Tassorelli, C., and Joseph, S.A. (1995). Systemic nitroglycerin induces Fos immunoreactivity in brainstem and forebrain structures of the rat. *Brain Res.* **682**, 167–181.

Vanegas, H., and Schaible, H.G. (2004). Descending control of persistent pain: inhibitory or facilitatory? *Brain Res. Rev.* **46**, 295–309.

Viviani, B., Bartesaghi, S., Gardoni, F., Vezzani, A., Behrens, M.M., Bartfai, T., Binaglia, M., Corsini, E., Di Luca, M., Galli, C.L., and Marinovich, M. (2003). Interleukin-1beta enhances NMDA receptor-mediated intracellular calcium increase through activation of the Src family of kinases. *J. Neurosci.* **23**, 8692–8700.

Wang, H., Wei, F., Dubner, R., and Ren, K. (2006). Selective distribution and function of primary afferent nociceptive inputs from deep muscle tissue to the brainstem trigeminal transition zone. *J. Comp. Neurol.* **498**, 390–402.

Wang, S., Lim, G., Mao, J., Sung, B., and Mao, J. (2009). Regulation of the trigeminal NR1 subunit expression induced by inflammation of the temporomandibular joint region in rats. *Pain* **141**, 97–103.

Wasserman, J.K., Zhu, X., and Schlichter, L.C. (2007). Evolution of the inflammatory response in the brain following intracerebral hemorrhage and effects of delayed minocycline treatment. *Brain Res.* **1180**, 140–154.

Watanabe, M., Guo, W., Zou, S., Sugiyo, S., Dubner, R., and Ren, K. (2005). Antibody array analysis of peripheral and blood cytokine levels in rats after masseter inflammation. *Neurosci. Lett.* **382**, 128–133.

Watkins, L.R., and Maier, S.F. (2005). Immune regulation of central nervous system functions: from sickness responses to pathological pain. *J. Intern. Med.* **257**, 139–155.

Wei, F., Guo, W., Zou, S., Ren, K., and Dubner, R. (2008). Supraspinal glial-neuronal interactions contribute to descending pain facilitation. *J. Neurosci.* **28**, 10482–10495.

Weyerbacher, A.R., Xu, Q., Tamasdan, C., Shin, S.J., and Inturrisi, C.E. (2010). N-Methyl-D-aspartate receptor (NMDAR) independent maintenance of inflammatory pain. *Pain* **148**, 237–246.

Woolf, C.J., and Salter, M.W. (2000). Neuronal plasticity: Increasing the gain in pain. *Science* **288**, 1765–1768.

Yang, S., Liu, Z.W., Wen, L., Qiao, H.F., Zhou, W.X., and Zhang, Y.X. (2005). Interleukin-1beta enhances NMDA receptor-mediated current but inhibits excitatory synaptic transmission. *Brain Res.* **1034**, 172–179.

Yoshida, A.K., Dostrovsky, J.O., Sessle, B.J., and Chiang, C.Y. (1991). Trigeminal projections to the nucleus submedius of the thalamus in the rat. *J. Comp. Neurol.* **307**, 609–625.

Yousfi-Malki, M., and Puizillout, J.J. (1994). Induction of Fos-like protein in neurons of the medulla oblongata after electrical stimulation of the vagus nerve in anesthetized rabbit. *Brain Res.* **635**, 317–322.

Yu, X.M., Sessle, B.J., and Hu, J.W. (1993). Differential effects of cutaneous and deep application of inflammatory irritant on mechanoreceptive field properties of trigeminal brain stem nociceptive neurons. *J. Neurophysiol.* **70**, 1704–1707.

Zhang, R., Yamada, J., Hayashi, Y., Wu, Z., Koyama, S., and Nakanishi, H. (2008). (200). Inhibition of NMDA-induced outward currents by interleukin-1beta in hippocampal neurons. *Biochem Biophys Res Commun* **372**, 816–820.

Zhang, R.X., Liu, B., Wang, L., Ren, K., Qiao, J.T., Berman, B.M., and Lao, L. (2005). Spinal glial activation in a new rat model of bone cancer pain produced by prostate cancer cell inoculation of the tibia. *Pain* **118**, 125–136.

Zhou, Q.Q., Imbe, H., Dubner, R., and Ren, K. (1999). Persistent trigeminal Fos protein expression after orofacial deep or cutaneous tissue inflammation in rats: implications for persistent orofacial pain. *J. Comp. Neurol.* **412**, 276–291.

PHYSIOLOGICAL MECHANISMS OF NEUROPATHIC PAIN: THE OROFACIAL REGION

Koichi Iwata[1], Yoshiki Imamura[2], Kuniya Honda[1,3] and Masamichi Shinoda[1]

[1]Department of Physiology,Nihon University School of Dentistry, 1-8-13 Kandasurugadai, Chiyoda-ku Tokyo, 101-8310, Japan
[2]Department of Oral Diagnosis, Nihon University School of Dentistry, 1-8-13 Kandasurugadai, Chiyoda-ku Tokyo, 101-8310, Japan
[3]Department of Physiology and Oral and Maxillofacial Surgery , Nihon University School of Dentistry, 1-8-13 Kandasurugadai, Chiyoda-ku Tokyo, 101-8310, Japan

I. Introduction

Peripheral nerve injury sometimes causes neuropathic pain, where there is a lowering of the pain threshold and increase in pain intensity (Fig. 1). Neuropathic pain is difficult to diagnose and treat because of the complexity of the neuronal mechanisms, underlying the neuropathic pain state (Sessle, 1999; Baron *et al.*,

INTERNATIONAL REVIEW OF
NEUROBIOLOGY, VOL. 97
DOI: 10.1016/B978-0-12-385198-7.00009-6

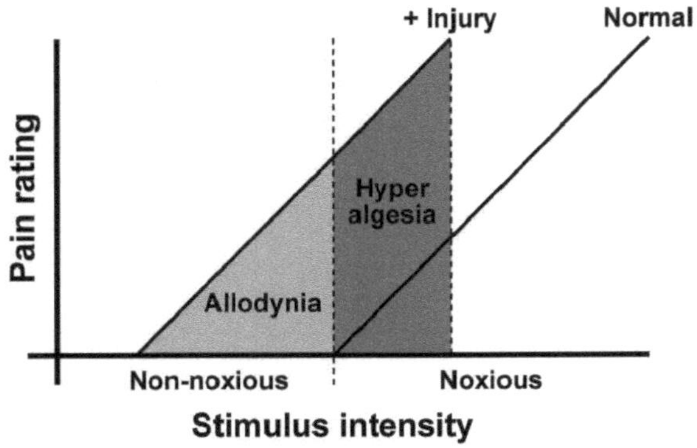

FIG. 1. The relationship between pain rating and stimulus intensity. After nerve injury non-noxious stimulation causes pain, and noxious stimulus causes stronger pain compared to the normal state.

2010; Maihofner *et al.*, 2010). Patients complain of severe pain under the neuropathic pain condition. In the orofacial region, tooth extraction, tooth pulp treatment or dental implantation sometimes causes trigeminal nerve injury, resulting in trigeminal neuropathic pain. Trigeminal neuropathic pain is known to cause pain abnormalities in the orofacial region such as allodynia or hyperalgesia. Allodynic neuropathic pain patients complain of severe pain normally following non-noxious mechanical or thermal stimulation of the extensive area innervated by the injured nerve. Hyperalgesic patients also complain of stronger pain compared with that of nociceptive pain. Neuroplastic changes both in the peripheral and central nervous systems are known to be important phenomena to generate and maintain pain abnormalities following peripheral nerve injury (Woolf and Salter, 2000). However, the detailed mechanisms underlying neuropathic pain in the orofacial region following trigeminal nerve injury is not fully understood. It is very important to know the neuronal mechanisms underlying trigeminal neuropathic pain following the trigeminal nerve injury to provide appropriate approaches to diagnose and treat neuropathic pain. Four animal models with trigeminal neuropathic pain were developed to examine the underlying mechanisms of trigeminal neuropathic pain and many studies have been conducted with many approaches using these animal models.

In this review, we introduce the inferior alveolar nerve injury (IANX) model, the infraorbital nerve ligation (ION-CCI) model, the inferior alveolar nerve regeneration (IANR) model and the cervical nerve transection (CNX) model, and discuss the recent findings of the peripheral and central mechanisms of trigeminal neuropathic pain. We also describe the clinical assessment of trigeminal neuropathic pain patients and the treatment of these patients in the last part of this chapter.

II. Peripheral Mechanisms

A. Trigeminal Neuropathic Pain Models

A number of experimental trigeminal neuropathic pain models have been developed, which are thought to be likely to induce the sensory disorders and to mimic trigeminal neuropathic pain that occurs in humans. First, the chronic sciatic nerve constriction injury as the animal model of neuropathic pain of legs had been developed (Bennett and Xie, 1988). In this model, the common sciatic nerve is exposed at the level of the middle of the thigh. About 7 mm of nerve is freed of adhering tissue and four ligatures by 4-0 chromic gut are tied loosely around it with 1 mm spacing. Heat and mechanical hyperalgesia occurs to the hind paw ipsilateral to ligated side and lasts for more than 2 months after nerve ligation. The degree of hyperalgesia declines gradually and the hind paws became hypoalgesic by 3–4 months. By applying this Bennett model, the experimental trigeminal neuropathic pain model on whisker pad skin was developed (Vos *et al.*, 1994). In this model, a midline scalp incision is made and the skull and nasal bone are exposed to give access to the infraorbital nerve (ION). The ION is dissected free at the infraorbital foramen. Two chromic gut (5-0) ligatures are loosely tied around the ION (2 mm apart) (Kayser *et al.*, 2002; Deseure *et al.*, 2003; Deseure *et al.*, 2004; Meunier *et al.*, 2005). The other researchers used two nylon (5-0) ligatures (2 mm apart) (Nakai *et al.*, 2010) or two silk (4-0) ligatures (2 mm apart) (Luiz *et al.*, 2010) around the ION instead of the chromic gut. Moreover, to induce the sensory disorders, the ION has been injured by irradiation with a tunable argon ion laser operating at 514 nm (Eriksson *et al.*, 2005; Dominguez *et al.*, 2009) and tight nerve ligation of one-third to one-half the diameter with silk (7-0) (Shinoda *et al.*, 2007; Xu *et al.*, 2008). The ligation criterion is that the ligature reduced the diameter of the nerve by a just noticeable amount and retarded, but did not interrupt, epineural circulation through the superficial vasculature (Bennett and Xie, 1988). Afterwards, to reduce an effect on orofacial tissue invasion to nocifensive behavior in the trigeminal neuropathic pain models, the ION was exposed by a small incision (approximately 1 cm in length) made intraorally along the gingivo-buccal margin proximal to the first molar, in order to keep the hair and skin on the snout and the vibrissae intact with the ION injury (Imamura *et al.*, 1997; Anderson *et al.*, 2003). Moreover, mechanical and thermal hypersensitivity of the whisker pad skin occurred with the inferior alveolar nerve (IAN) or mental nerve transection (Iwata *et al.*, 2001; Piao *et al.*, 2006; Okada-Ogawa *et al.*, 2009) (Fig. 2). A small incision was made on the surface of the facial skin over the masseter muscle. The alveolar bone surface was exposed and the bone surface covering the IAN was removed. The IAN was tightly ligated at two points of the nerve trunk at just

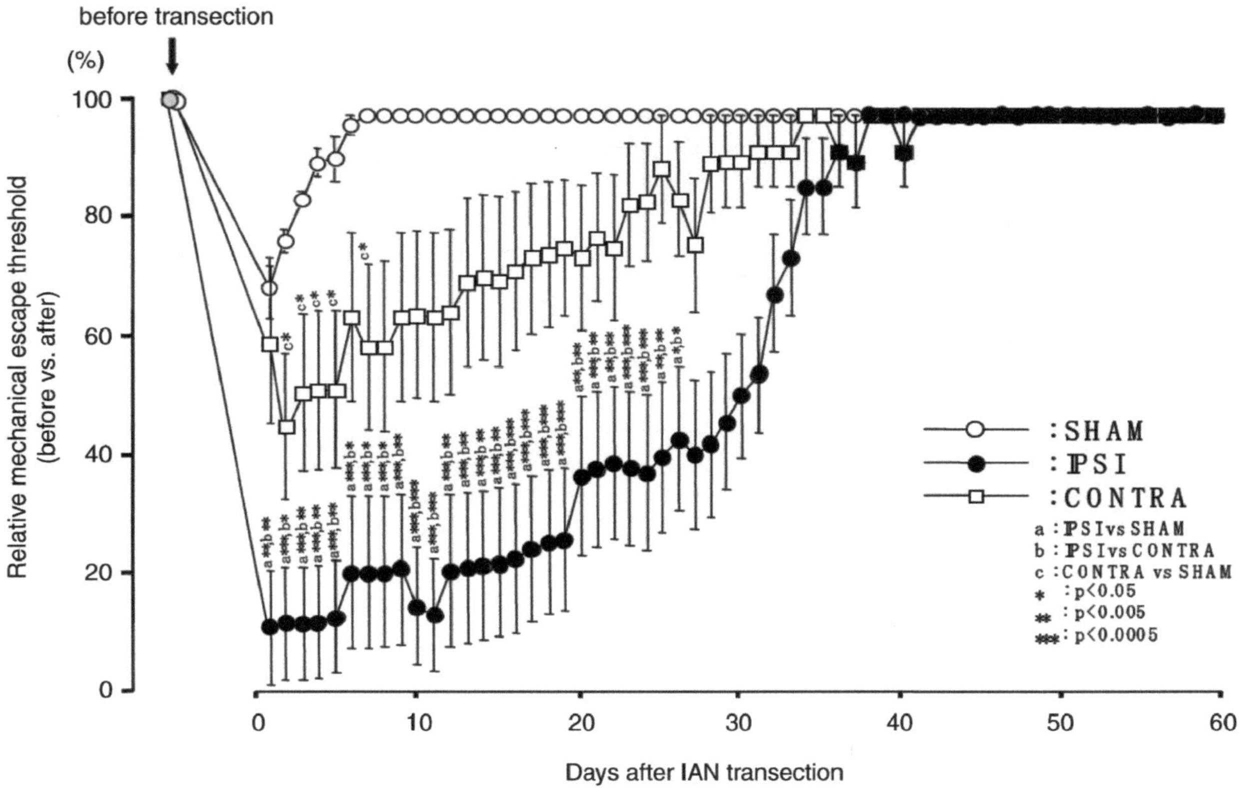

FIG. 2. Mechanical escape threshold in the IAN-transected rats. The change in threshold intensity was plotted as relative values where escape threshold values are compared before transection and at different periods after IAN transection. Sham: Sham-operated rats, contralateral: Changes of escape threshold from the mechanical stimulation applied to the contralateral side relative to the IAN transection, ipsilateral: changes of escape threshold from the mechanical stimulation applied to the ipsilateral side relative to the IAN transection. Modified from Iwata *et al.* (Iwata *et al.*, 2001).

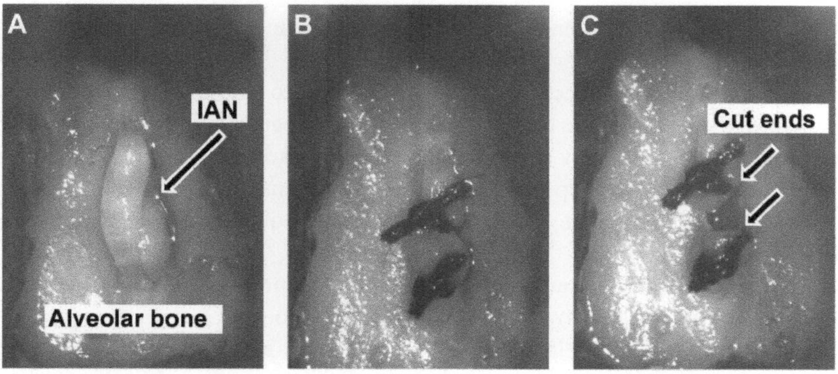

FIG. 3. Photographs of inferior alveolar nerve (IAN) transection and inferior orbital nerve (ION) ligation. A: intact IAN, B: tightly ligated IAN, C: transected IAN.

above the angle of the mandible, and 1 mm proximal to the angle of the mandibular bone (Fig. 3A, B and C).

The ION-injured model has not only been developed for trigeminal neuropathic pain on the whisker pad skin, but also trigeminal neuropathic pain on the mental skin. In the IAN-injured model, a small incision is made in the middle line under the chin, and the mental nerve is tightly ligated twice with silk sutures (Seino *et al.*, 2009).

Recently, C2-C4 spinal nerve transection models were also developed in our laboratory. An incision was made on the neck skin and the C2-C4 spinal nerves were exposed through the trapezius muscles. The C2-C4 spinal nerves were tightly ligated at two points of the nerve trunk and transected in the middle of the two ligations. Mechanical allodynia and thermal hyperalgesia occurred on the whisker pad skin, ipsilateral to the C2-C4 spinal nerve transection (Kobayashi *et al.*, 2011).

B. Primary Afferent Excitability

The modulation of spike discharges is obvious in the primary afferent neurons following peripheral nerve injury. In ION-injured animals established by IAN ligation of the chromic gut or transection, the ION fibers change their activity. High frequency burst or regular firings were observed in the injured sciatic nerve ligated by chromic gut (Kajander and Bennett, 1992; Bennett, 1993). The regular and burst firings in ION fibers ligated by chromic gut and with IAN fibers transection were also observed (Tsuboi *et al.*, 2004; Kitagawa *et al.*, 2006). The high frequency firings in primary afferents could be recorded for a long while in the rats with IAN transection and ION ligation by chromic gut. Because of the long-lasting abnormal spike generation in injured primary afferents for more than several weeks, primary afferent neurons were sensitized and the activation threshold in these neurons became lower compared to those of naive neurons (Kitagawa *et al.*, 2006). The high frequency burst or regular firing in the trigeminal nerve afferents also causes some substantial changes in the trigeminal ganglion (TG), such as the over-expression of channel proteins and intracellular protein kinase. These changes are thought to affect the frequency of trigeminal nerve firings.

The sodium channel accumulation in the TG neurons directly affects the spike generation of trigeminal primary afferent fibers. Over expression of a variety of sodium channels in the TG neurons are involved in an increase in the excitability of trigeminal nerve afferents (Eriksson *et al.*, 2005). The sodium currents have an important role in generating action potentials and are also involved in the modulation of primary afferent activity (Jackson, 1995). Therefore, the sodium currents are thought to be important for modulating the excitability of primary afferent neurons after nerve injury (Devor *et al.*, 1993; Rizzo *et al.*, 1996; Abdulla *et al.*, 2003).

The tetrodotoxin resistant (TTX-R) sodium channels and potassium channels are thought to be involved in an enhancement of TG neuronal activity following trigeminal nerve injury. Both TTX-R I_{Na} and -sensitive (TTX-S) I_{Na} densities of TG neurons were significantly larger, and there were significant differences in the background activity and mechanically evoked responses in Aδ-fibers between naive and IAN-transected rats. The after discharge was also significantly higher in the IAN-transected rats compared to naive rats (Nakagawa *et al.*, 2010) (Fig. 4). Our findings are consistent with the evidence that spike amplitudes of TG neurons were also significantly larger in the IAN-transected rats following current injection. The threshold current for spike generation was significantly smaller in IAN-transected rats than that of naive rats and current injection into TG neurons induced high-frequency spike discharges in rats with IAN transection. Because the increase in the magnitude of TTX-S I_{Na} was larger than that of TTX-R I_{Na} in the TG neurons after IAN transection, it is possible that the hyperexcitability of TG neurons innervated by the regenerated IAN is augmented by an increase in TTX-S sodium current densities, resulting in abnormal excitation of the CNS networks and nocifensive behavior.

The neuronal cross-talk between the injured IAN and intact ION has been also suggested as a possible mechanism for neuropathic pain of the whisker pad (Tsuboi *et al.*, 2004). The injured IAN underwent demyelination and the action potentials directly activate the adjacent intact fibers. It is also speculated that the demyelinated fibers sprout axon collaterals and make synapses in the presynaptic terminals of the intact fibers (Ueda, 2006). These peripheral neuroplastic changes are thought to be involved in the neuronal hyperexcitability of the intact ION neighboring the transected IAN.

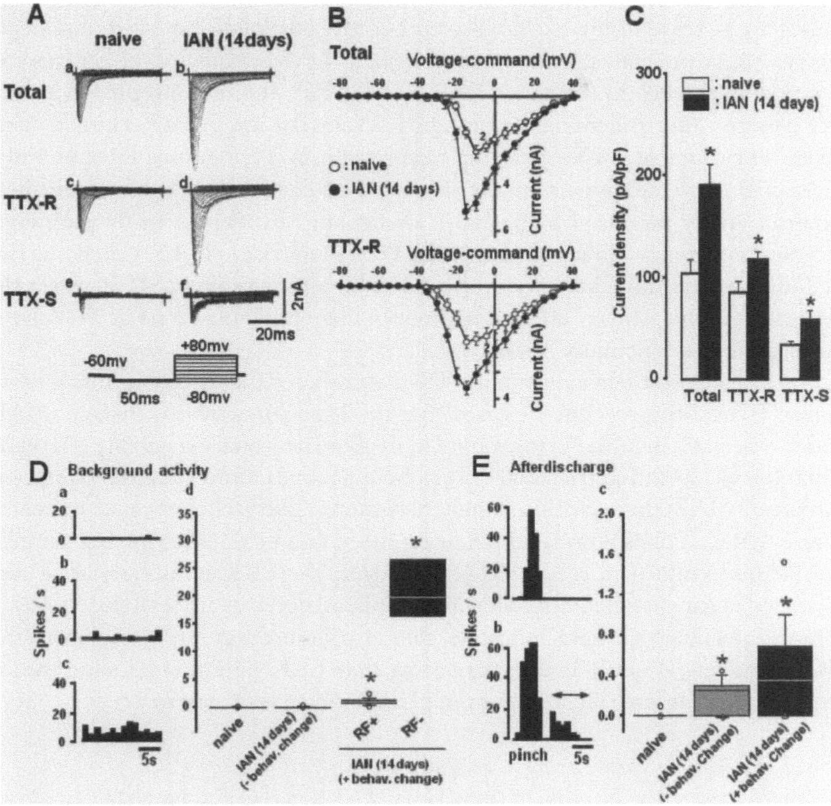

FIG. 4. Classification of TTX-S I_{Na} and TTX-R I_{Na}, Background activities and afterdischarges of Aδ-units to pressure, brushing or pinching of the receptive fields in IAN-transected rats. A: TTX-S I_{Na} was isolated by digitally subtracting TTX-R sodium current (I_{Na}) (in 1 μM TTX) from the total I_{Na} (without TTX). B: The current-voltage (I-V) relationship of total I_{Na} (without TTX) and TTX-R I_{Na} (in 1 μM TTX) in both naive and IAN-transected rats. Mean values (mean ± SEM) of total and TTX-R I_{Na} in TG neurons are illustrated in B. C: Peak current densities of total I_{Na}, TTX-R I_{Na}, and TTX sensitive (TTX-S) I_{Na} in naive and IAN-transected rats. Open column: naive rats. Solid column: rats with IAN transection. Da and Ea: IAN fibers in naive rats, Db and Eb: background activity (Db) and afterdischarge (Eb) of IAN fibers with receptive fields at 14 days after IAN transection, Dc: background activity of the IAN fiber without receptive field at 14 days after IAN transection, Dd and Ec: mean background activities and after discharges in naive, IAN-transected rats without behavioral changes and IAN-transected rats, respectively. Note that background activities and afterdischarges of A-units in IAN-transected rats showed significantly higher firing frequency than those of naive rats.* $p < 0.05$ (vs. naive) (Nakagawa *et al.*, 2010).

C. Molecular Changes in Trigeminal Ganglion (Tg) Neurons

The alteration of the molecules including neuropeptides, receptors, cytokines, and growth factors in TG neurons are thought to be a possible mechanism that causes an increase in the excitability of TG neurons following trigeminal nerve injury. Many previous reports have described the accumulation of a variety of neuropeptides, such as substance P(SP) and CGRP, and neurotrophic factors in TG neurons after trigeminal nerve injury (Wakisaka *et al.*, 1987; Harada *et al.*, 2003). For example, P2X3 receptor's expression in TG neurons increased in a trigeminal neuropathic pain model produced by partial ION ligation, and heat hypersensitivity produced by partial ION ligation was depressed by purinergic receptor antagonists (Shinoda *et al.*, 2007). Preprotachykinin mRNA encoding two well-known pain modulating neuropeptides, SP and neurokinin A, increases the expression in the primary afferent neurons in the mandibular zone in TG following trigeminal nerve injury (Tsuzuki *et al.*, 2003).

Intracellular protein kinase in the TG is also altered following trigeminal nerve injury. It has been recently reported that the Mitogen-activated Protein (MAP) kinase cascade is involved in the modulation of the neuronal excitability (Dai *et al.*, 2002; Ji *et al.*, 2002; Liu *et al.*, 2004). Peripheral noxious stimulus causes phosphorylation of MAP kinase within ganglion neurons. Extracellular-signal regulated kinase (ERK) is phosphorylated following the strong noxious peripheral stimulation within 5 min (Dai *et al.*, 2002). Moreover, the ERK phosphorylation also increased in ganglion neurons following peripheral nerve injury (Dai *et al.*, 2002). It is highly possible that ERK phosphorylation is induced in the TG neurons following trigeminal nerve injury, suggesting that ERK phosphorylation plays an important role in pain signaling in the peripheral nervous system.

D. Involvement of Non-Neuronal Glial Cells in TG Excitability

The TG is composed primary of neurons and satellite glial cells (SGCs). TG neurons are surrounded by a layer of SGCs. Similar to astrocytes in the central nervous system, glial fibrillary acidic protein (GFAP) is a signature maker for SGCs immunocytochemically. Dissimilar to astrocytes, GFAP cannot be detected in SGCs, in the resting state. Moreover, GFAP expression increases following nerve injury and becomes detectable by immunocytochemistry (Ohara *et al.*, 2009). Though it is not known whether the increase in GFAP in SGCs is associated with the same changes as those that increase of GFAP in astrocytes, an increase in extracellular glutamate causes the activation of astrocytes, as measured by a marked increase in GFAP *in vitro*. The increase in GFAP in SGCs after nerve injury may be triggered by increased glutamate released in the sensory ganglion, resulting from increased neuronal firing (Amir and Devor, 2003b, a).

The number of gap junctions between SGCs increases following nerve injury, suggesting that changes in SGC gap junctions with Cx43 is a factor in generating or maintaining neuropathic pain (Cherkas *et al.*, 2004; Ohara *et al.*, 2008). It is speculated that increase of neuromodulators transfer associated with pain signaling such as ATP through Cx43 between SGCs play a role in neuropathic pain (Dina *et al.*, 2005). Moreover, some molecules associated with pain modulating factors such as calcitonin gene-related peptide (CGRP), nerve growth factor, and vascular endothelial growth factors are released by neurons and SGCs following nerve injury (Chao *et al.*, 2008). Many of the factors released from SGCs will activate TG neurons following trigeminal nerve injury, resulting in pain abnormalities in the orofacial region.

III. Central Mechanisms of Trigeminal Neuropathic Pain

The strongly activated nociceptive neurons in the Vc affect the excitability of nociceptive neurons in the trigeminal ascending pain pathways (Ericson *et al.*, 1996; Park *et al.*, 2006; Zhang *et al.*, 2006). There are many projection neurons in the Vc projecting their axons to higher brain regions, and those relay noxious information to the higher CNS regions affecting the excitability of thalamic neurons, neurons in the limbic system and cortical neurons. In this chapter the modulation pattern nociceptive neurons in the ascending trigeminal pain pathways are reported, based on our animal studies (Iwata *et al.*, 1999; Iwata *et al.*, 2001).

A. Trigeminal Spinal Subnucleus Caudalis (Vc) and Upper Cervical Spinal Cord (C1-C2) Neurons

After the nerve injury, hyperexcitability of the primary afferent neurons sometimes lasts for more than several months. After the long-lasting hyperactivity of the primary afferent neurons, a barrage of action potentials is conveyed to the CNS neurons resulting in the sensitization of the CNS nociceptive neurons.

In the trigeminal system, hyperexcitability of nociceptive neurons occurs in the Vc followed by an extensive increase in the excitability of the trigeminal ganglion neurons (Iwata *et al.*, 2001). Nociceptive neurons receiving inputs from the orofacial region are organized within different laminae in the Vc and orofacial nociceptive neurons are functionally organized in each lamina of the Vc (Lam *et al.*, 2009b, a). Two types of nociceptive neurons are functionally identified in the Vc; i.e WDR and NS neurons (Iwata *et al.*, 1999). WDR neurons respond to both non-noxious and noxious stimulation of the receptive fields and increase in the firing frequency, following increase in the mechanical stimulus intensity. On the other hand, NS neurons extensively respond to noxious stimulation and only slightly increase in their firing following an increase in the stimulus intensity. Receptive field properties are also different between WDR and NS neurons the receptive field size being much larger in WDR neurons compared to NS neurons and also the center of the receptive fields in WDR neurons responds to non-noxious gentle mechanical stimulus (Iwata *et al.*, 1999; Iwata *et al.*, 2001). It is well documented that the excitability of WDR and NS neurons in the Vc is strongly modulated by the trigeminal nerve injury (Iwata *et al.*, 1999; Saito *et al.*, 2008). Following IAN transection, the background activity, mechanical and thermal evoked responses of WDR neurons in the Vc are strongly enhanced, and the receptive fields of WDR neurons are significantly expanded. This is not the case in NS neurons suggesting that the Vc WDR neurons are significantly involved in orofacial neuropathic pain (Iwata *et al.*, 1999). It has been also reported that Vc WDR and LTM neurons increase in their excitability after regeneration of the injured IAN (Saito *et al.*, 2008). These are very important observations because the low threshold non-noxious myelinated primary afferent neurons may be involved in orofacial neuropathic pain state following trigeminal nerve injury.

B. Synaptic Transmission in Vc Neurons

Glutamate is the major excitatory neurotransmitter in the Vc as well as spinal dorsal horn (51). N-methyl-D-aspartate (NMDA) receptor,α-amino-3-hydroxy-5-methyl-4-isoxazolepropionic acid (AMPA) receptor and kainate receptor as ligand-gated ionotrpic glutamate receptors, and G-protein coupled metabotropic glutamate receptors (mGluRs) are known to be differentially involved in neuronal transmission in the spinal dorsal horn and the Vc (Mitsikostas and Sanchez del Rio, 2001; Neugebauer, 2002; Garry *et al.*, 2004; Wang *et al.*, 2010). Once glutamate is released from the primary afferent terminals following a variety of peripheral stimuli, glutamate binds to these three glutamate receptors in the postsynaptic terminals. NMDA, AMPA and kainate receptors have four subtypes and for all these, synaptic transmission is excitatory (Fig. 5). The NMDA receptor is blocked by magnesium ions at the resting state, and when glutamate binds to the NMDA receptor slow excitatory depolarizing postsynaptic potentials (slow EPSPs) are produced. On the other hand, AMPA and kainate receptors open when glutamate binds to these receptors the fast excitatory postsynaptic potentials (fast EPSPs) are produced in the postsynaptic terminals. Slow EPSPs are also evoked by G-protein coupled receptor activation. Following sustained strong stimulation of the peripheral tissues, neuropeptides such as substance P or CGRP are released with glutamate, and bind to the receptors in the postsynaptic terminals (Chesselet, 1984). Furthermore, long-lasting activation of primary afferent neurons causes phosphorylation of the NMDA receptor and it's excitability in the postsynaptic nociceptive neurons. Eight mGluRs have been identified and these are segregated into three

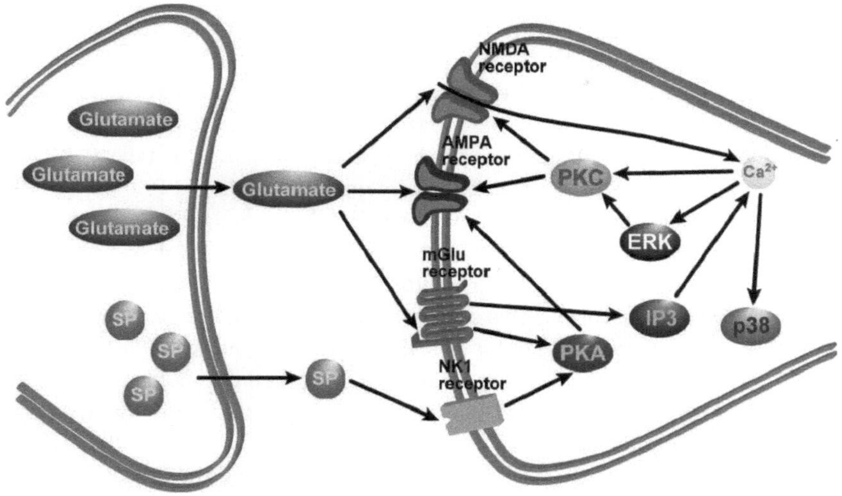

FIG. 5. Synaptic transmission and intracellular molecular cascades in Vc neurons. (For interpretation of the references to color in this figure legend, the reader is referred to the Web version of the chapter.).

groups. Group I mGluR (GluR1 and GluR5) is located in the presynaptic terminal and post synaptic membrane affecting the excitability of nociceptive neurons in the Vc. These three glutamate receptors have important functions to modulate Vc neuronal excitability. Following the trigeminal nerve injury, AMPAR, NMDAR, and group 1mGlu R are strongly activated in Vc nociceptive neurons. Prolonged strong activation of these receptors enhances the generation of action potentials in Vc nociceptive neurons, resulting in the sensitization of Vc nociceptive neurons. The central sensitization of Vc nociceptive neurons is thought to be involved in neuroplastic changes in Vc neurons, resulting in the trigeminal neuropathic pain.

C. Map Kinase and Fos in Vc Neurons

The MAPKs have three cascades in neurons, ERK, p38 and JNK. These three cascades are thought to be involved in the modulation of neuronal excitability (Cano and Mahadevan, 1995; Seger and Krebs, 1995). ERK and p38 in dorsal horn neurons or glial cells are phosphorylated following a variety of strong stimuli applied to peripheral structures (Zhuang *et al.*, 2005; Zhang and Dellon, 2008). The ERK in the spinal dorsal horn and Vc neurons is phosphorylated within 10 min following peripheral noxious stimuli (Dai *et al.*, 2002; Liu *et al.*, 2004). The number of phosphorylated ERK (pERK)-immunoreactive (LI) cells increases in the DRG and spinal DH with increase in the noxious stimulus intensity (Dai *et al.*, 2002; Liu *et al.*, 2004). Recently, it has been reported that ERK is phosphorylated in many neurons distributed in the superficial laminae of Vc and C1-C2 within

5 min following the noxious stimulation (Noma *et al.*, 2008). It has also been reported that the number of pERK-LI cells in the Vc is increased following increase in the mechanical and thermal noxious stimulus intensity applied to the facial skin (Honda *et al.*, 2008). These results strongly suggest that the activation of neurons following noxious stimuli of the trigeminal structures is reflected by the phosphorylation of ERK in Vc and C1-C2 neurons (Fig. 6).

The ERK phosphorylation is also observed in Vc and C1-C2 neurons following non-noxious mechanical or thermal stimulation of the facial skin in cervical nerve transection rats (Kobayashi *et al.* submitted). The number of pERK-LI cells following non-noxious mechanical and thermal stimuli was significantly greater in CNX rats as compared to sham rats. Furthermore, the number of pERK-LI cells in C1-C2 was graded following increases in the facial stimulus intensity, suggesting that ERK phosphorylation in C1-C2 neurons is involved in the sensory discrimination of trigeminal neuropathic pain.

The FOS protein is also well known to be expressed in the dorsal horn after noxious stimulation of the hind paw (Hunt *et al.*, 1987). The strong expression of FOS protein-LI cells are also reported in the superficial and deep laminae of the Vc and C1-C2 region 1–2 hours after following non-noxious and noxious mechanical stimulation of the facial skin in rats with IAN transection (Noma *et al.*, 2008). The number of FOS-LI cells increased both in the superficial and deep laminae of Vc and C1-C2 following increases in the stimulus intensity. The pERK and FOS

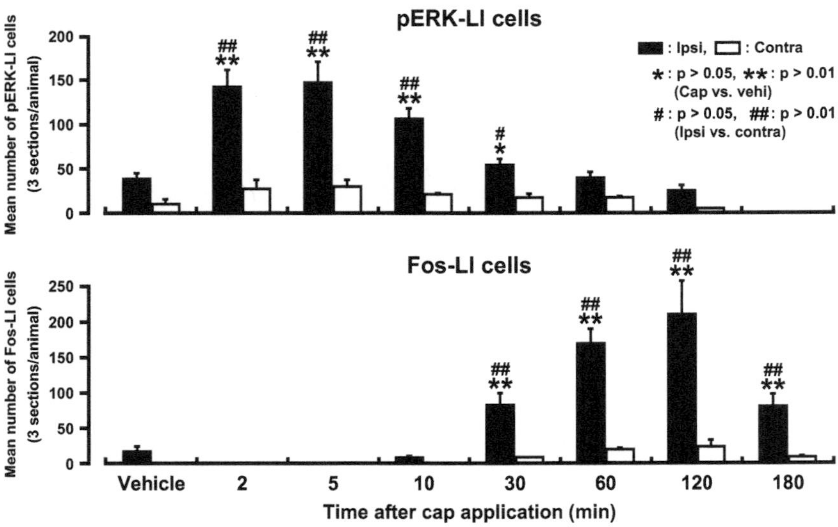

FIG. 6. Time-course differences in expression of pERK-LI cells and FOS protein-LI cells following capsaicin stimulation of the face. Note that ERK phosphorylation occurs within 5 min whereas FOS protein expression takes more than 30 min. Modified from Noma *et al.* (Noma *et al.* 2008).

protein expression is obviously different in expression pattern and time course (Fig. 6). The ERK phosphorylation occurred in Vc neurons both with and without FOS expression following noxious stimulation of the face. This suggests that several intracellular cascades, including MAP kinase, are involved in FOS expression in Vc neurons.

D. Ectopic Pain Abnormalities In The Orofacial Region

It has been reported that IAN transection causes an extensive increase in the neuronal excitability of Vc nociceptive neurons as well as in TG neurons (Iwata *et al.*, 2002; Nomura *et al.*, 2002; Tsuboi *et al.*, 2004; Okada-Ogawa *et al.*, 2009). The excitability of TG neurons innervated by the 2nd branch of the trigeminal nerve significantly increases following IAN (3rd branch) transection as described previously (Tsuboi *et al.*, 2004). A barrage of action potentials is conveyed to Vc neurons resulting in the strong activation of Vc neurons (Iwata *et al.*, 2002). Okada-Ogawa *et al.* reported that the hyperactive astroglial cells in Vc were significantly involved in the modulation of Vc nociceptive neurons (Okada-Ogawa *et al.*, 2009). The hyperactive astroglial cells were in the Vc following IAN transection, and Vc neuronal activity was enhanced. This suggests that hyperactive astroglial cells release glutamine which is taken at the primary afferent terminals via glutamate transporters, resulting in an increase in the glutamate release at the synaptic cleft. This mechanism is known as the glutamine-glutamate shuttle (Chiang *et al.*, 2007; Chiang *et al.*, 2008; Okada-Ogawa *et al.*, 2009) (Fig. 7). The microglial cell activation is also observed in the Vc following IAN transection (Piao *et al.*, 2006). The

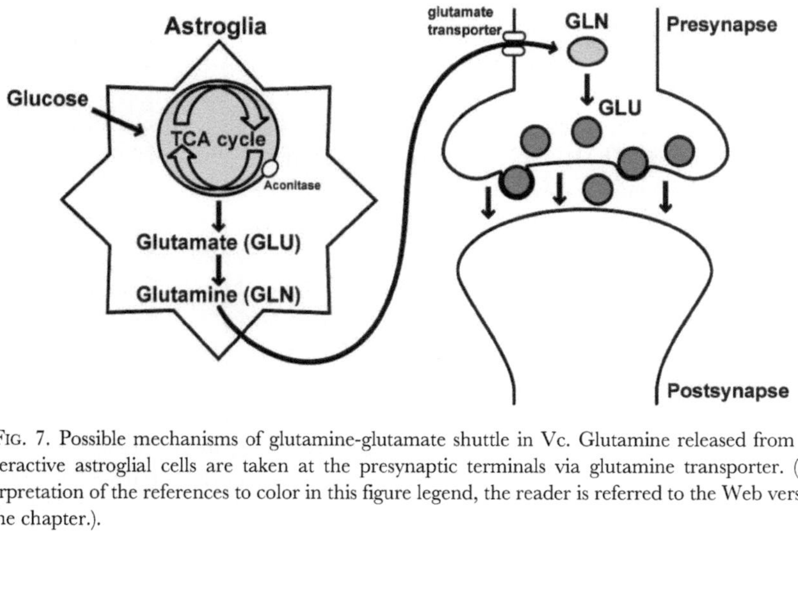

Fig. 7. Possible mechanisms of glutamine-glutamate shuttle in Vc. Glutamine released from the hyperactive astroglial cells are taken at the presynaptic terminals via glutamine transporter. (For interpretation of the references to color in this figure legend, the reader is referred to the Web version of the chapter.).

activation is much faster in microglial cells in the Vc compared with that of the astroglial cells. The microglial cells are activated 1–3 days after IAN transection, whereas the activation of astroglial cells takes 7–14 days after that. It has recently been reported that astroglial and microglial cells have specific interactions and communicate with each other. The astroglial and microglial cell interactions may be involved in the hyper-activation of Vc nociceptive neurons following trigeminal nerve injury. It is also important that microglial and astroglial cell activation are observed in a wide area in the Vc after trigeminal nerve injury. This suggests that activation of glial cells in a wide area in the Vc is involved in the activation of nociceptive neurons distributed in the wide area in the Vc. The glia-glia interaction and neuron-glial cell interaction are thought to have an important function involved in ectopic pain abnormalities in the orofacial region, following trigeminal nerve injury.

E. CNS Pain Pathways

Orofacial noxious inputs are conveyed to Vc nociceptive neurons through three branches of the trigeminal nerve. Trigeminal nerve injury produces an extensive increase in primary afferent activity. The barrage of action potentials generated in the injured nerve fibers is conveyed to the Vc. Action potentials reaching the Vc affect the neuronal excitability of Vc nociceptive neurons, and cause an increase in the background activity, and evoked responses to mechanical and/or thermal stimuli. The hyperexcitability of Vc nociceptive neurons are further conveyed to the higher CNS regions through two ascending CNS pathways; i.e., medial and lateral thalamic pathways. The medial pathway consists of medial thalamic nuclei, central medial thalamic nuclei, intralaminar nucleus and nucleus sub-medius in the thalamus (Fig. 8). The nociceptive neurons in these thalamic subnuclei are also classified as WDR and NS neurons as observed in the Vc.

The orofacial noxious inputs are conveyed to the ventro-posterior medial thalamic nucleus (VPM) and intralaminar thalamic nucleus via the Vc. Many WDR and NS neurons are encountered in the VPM receive inputs from the orofacial region (Sessle *et al.*, 1986; Sessle, 1999; Zhang *et al.*, 2006; Chiang *et al.*, 2008). Guilbaud *et al.* has reported that WDR and NS neurons in the ventro-posterior lateral thalamic nucleus (VPL) increase their excitability and receptive fields in rats following CCI of the sciatic nerve (Guilbaud *et al.*, 1990). This suggests that nociceptive neurons in the VPM also become hyperexcitable following trigeminal nerve injury as observed in VPL neurons. Nociceptive neurons in the primary somatosensory cortex or limbic system may also increase their excitability following trigeminal nerve injury, resulting in the orofacial neuropathic pain. However, we have no data how the nociceptive neurons in cortices are modulated following the trigeminal nerve injury.

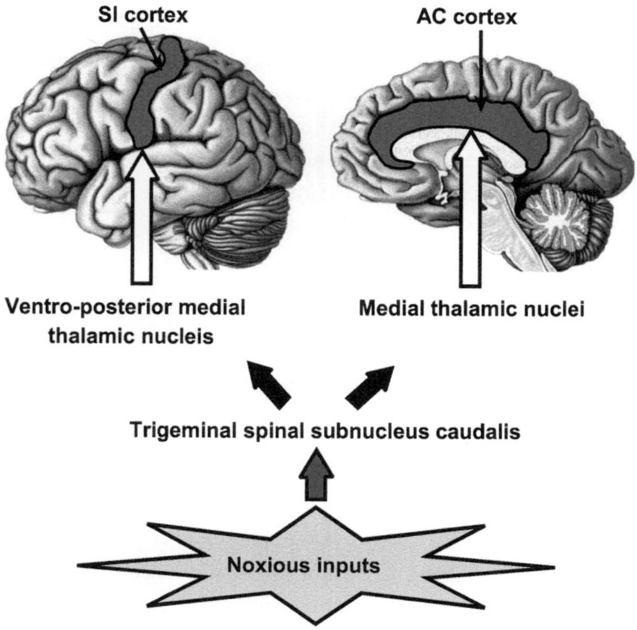

FIG. 8. Schematic illustration of medial and lateral pain ascending pathways in the trigeminal system.

IV. Clinical Management of Orofacial Neuropathic Pain

A. Clinical Manifestations

When we talk about orofacial neuropathic pain, we should consider two distinct groups of neuropathic pain conditions. The first one is paroxysmal (idiopathic) cranial neuralgias and the other is continuous neuropathic pain disorders. Although these two types of orofacial neuropathic pain disorders are classified into the same category, they have typically different clinical manifestations and pathologies.

B. Paroxysmal Cranial Neuralgias

Paroxysmal cranial neuralgias include trigeminal neuralgia, glossopharyngeal neuralgia, intermediate neuralgia, and they have unique common modalities. Pain can be precipitated by sensory inputs and motion. Stimuli that elicit precipitation are usually gentle inputs from exteroceptive and proprioceptive receptors, such as light touch to the facial skin and oropharyngeal mucosa and/or movement of face, jaw, tongue, and pharynx. Common activity in daily living such as eating, drinking, brushing teeth, washing face, combing, shaving, making up, and conversation can induce pain paroxysm. The pain is characterized as having a sudden onset and being short lasting (seconds to minutes), and described as being like lightening or electric shock. The most distinct difference from continuous neuropathic pain is the lack of both sensory changes and continuous burning pain. Patients do not complain about symptoms between pain paroxysms.

C. Continuous Neuropathic Pain Disorders

In general, continuous neuropathic pain is characterized by continuous burning sensation with or without pain precipitation and altered pain sensitivity (allodynia and hyperalgesia). Continuous neuropathic pain disorders can be induced by some systemic diseases (e.g., diabetic painful neuropathy, Sjögren syndrome and Bechet disease), viral infections (e.g., herpes zoster, postherpetic neuralgia and AIDS), traumatic events and some unknown causes (e.g., burning mouth syndrome and atypical odontalgia). Continuous pain is represented as burning, tingling or throbbing in nature. Other manifestations such as local sensory changes (hypoesthesia, paresthesia, and dysesthesia) and changes in skin color, temperature and/or sweating may be observed. In the trigeminal territory, clinical manifestations of continuous neuropathic pain disorders are considered rather different from that of the extremities. Sensory changes and burning pain are frequently observed, whereas sympathetic symptoms and jaw mobility impairment are rarely present (Garza, 2008). Although some dental practices require nerve avulsion (e.g., pulpectomy and tooth extraction) more frequently than other medical treatment in the extremities and the trunk, patients seldom complain of deafferentation pain after the procedures. Some researchers suppose that there should be certain mechanisms that prevent neuropathic conditions in dental pulp and periodontal tissue injury (Bennett, 2004). Indeed, there are few case reports of complex regional pain syndrome (CRPS) in the trigeminal territory that fulfill its diagnostic criteria, whereas it is one of the most apparent conditions of neuropathic pain (Sakamoto *et al.*). However, some patients surely complain of inveterate pain after dental practice, and it is believed that orofacial neuropathic pain conditions can be caused by some dental procedures and pathologies (Benoliel and Eliav, 2008).

Clinical researches have proposed a possibility of neuropathic etiology in some non-odontogenic pain conditions. Eliav *et al.* (Eliav *et al.*, 2007) showed injury of the chorda tympani nerve in burning mouth syndrome, and List *et al.* (List *et al.*, 2008) suggested trigeminal nerve dysfunction in atypical odontalgia. Most of the studies have assessed the neuropathic profile of orofacial pain disorders by observing sensory changes (Forssell *et al.*, 2002; Jaaskelainen, 2004; Granot and Nagler, 2005), although some recent works have reported morphological or immunohistochemical changes in biopsied tongue specimens (Lauria *et al.*, 2005; Yilmaz *et al.*, 2007; Beneng *et al.*, 2010). The failure in distinguishing neuropathic pain conditions from dental or other orofacial organic diseases may require further invasive procedures that probably aggravate patient's signs and symptoms, and therefore should be prevented.

D. Clinical Assessment and Diagnosis of Continuous Orofacial Neuropathic Pain

It is extremely important to observe and record precise signs and symptoms to share and understand the pathology of orofacial neuropathic pain conditions, especially in rare conditions like CRPS associated with trigeminal innervations (Sakamoto *et al.* 2010). The orofacial neuropathic pain in general is not such a rare condition as believed, and should not be overlooked (Truelove, 2004). The most common finding in neuropathic pain conditions both in the extremities and the orofacial region is sensory changes (Jaaskelainen, 2004). Although there is an exception for the classic microneuroma formation of dental pulp or periapical nerves in the alveolar bone, that explains neuropathic pain after endodontic therapy (Bradlaw, 1936), most neuropathic pain conditions are considered to present sensory changes in the oral mucosa or the facial skin.

The German Research Network on Neuropathic Pain has recently developed a comprehensive quantitative sensory testing (QST) protocol for neuropathic pain (Rolke *et al.*, 2006). There were a couple of attempts to adapt this protocol into the orofacial region (Maier *et al.*, 2010; Pigg *et al.*, 2010), and the Orofacial Pain Special Interested Group of the International Association for the Study of Pain is preparing guidelines and recommendations for orofacial neuropathic pain assessment using this protocol. The protocol includes the following measurements: thermal detection thresholds (warm and cold: WDT and CDT), thermal sensory limen (TSL), paradoxical heat sensations (PHS) during the limen procedure, thermal pain thresholds (heat and cold: HPT and CPT), mechanical detection threshold (MDT), mechanical pain threshold (MPT), mechanical pain sensitivity (MPS) for pinprick stimuli, dynamic mechanical allodynia (DMA), wind-up ratio (WUR) for pin-prick stimuli (hyperpathia), vibration detection threshold (VDT), and pressure pain threshold (PPT). TDT and TPT are measured using a stimulator. The thermal stimulation is applied with an intraoral probe equipped a 0.9×0.9 mm Peltier element with a thermode and the increasing and decreasing ramp is set for 1C/sec. Baseline temperature is 37C for the intraoral examination and 32C for the extraoral one. WDT/CDT and HPT/CPT are determined by heat or cold thermal stimuli that are applied starting from the baseline temperature. The cut-off temperature for heat stimulation is set at 51C and cold 10C. Each threshold is calculated by averaging data of three temperature measurements. In the thermal limen procedure, bidirectional heating or cooling stimulation is alternately applied between the thresholds that patients feel changes in temperature and PHS during this procedure is recorded. MDT is measured using von Frey filaments with the "method of limits" technique. A series of filaments is applied in an ascending fashion from the thinnest to thicker ones until the patient detects (upper limit), then in a descending fashion to thinner ones until he or she fails to detect (lower limit). This ascending and descending measurement is repeated five times, and a mean value is obtained from five upper and five lower limits. In determining MPT a series of pinprick stimulators that are made to deliver 8, 16, 32, 64, 128, 256, and 512 mN are applied in the same manner to which used in obtaining MDT. MPS is determined by rating the intensity of pain sensation when a series of seven pinprick stimulators are applied. The patients are asked to rate it with the numerical rating scale (NRS). DMA can be observed by applying three kinds of materials as mechanical stimulation: cotton wisp, cotton wool tip, and tooth brush; which are designed to exert a force of ~3, ~100, and ~200 mN upon light stroking, respectively. WUR represents temporal summation of mechanical stimulation. Using a specific pinprick stimulator that exerts "light pricking" sensation to each testing site (the specific stimulator differs from site to site: It is already determined in MPS measurement procedure), a train of ten consecutive pinprick stimuli with a rate of 1 Hertz are applied following preceding single pin prick. Patients rate pain intensity for single pinprick first, and then rate after completion of the train of pin prick stimuli using NRS. This procedure is repeated five times and an average of NRS ratio (pain intensity for a train of ten pinpricks/single pinprick) for five series of trains is calculated for the wind-up ratio. VDT is determined using a 64 Hz, 8-scale graded fork. The vibrating fork is placed on a testing site and the patient is asked to tell when the vibration is no longer sensed. The intensity of vibration is rated in a 0–8 scale. A digital pressure algometer is used for measuring PPT. A 0.18 cm^2 sized probe is used for intraoral examination and 1 cm^2 sized probe for extraoral examination.

In thermal QSTs, CDT, and HPT are considered to be mediated by Aδ fibers and WDT by C fibers. CPT and PPT may represent both Aδ- and C-fiber function. Aβ-fiber function is represented by MDT and VDT.

E. Treatment of Orofacial Neuropathic Pain

1. *Paroxysmal Cranial Neuralgias*

Treatment of paroxysmal cranial neuralgias comprises of a two-step strategy: The first is conservative medication therapy and the second includes invasive treatment procedures. The first line medication includes carbamazepine and oxycabazepine. When these drugs have failed in medical management, baclofen, lamotrigine, and valproic acid are used as second line drugs. A combination of carbamazepine and baclofen or lamotrigine improves success rate of pain management (Sindrup and Jensen, 2002). When satisfactory pain control cannot be obtained with the first step conservative medical treatment, or an unacceptable side effect is observed, patients undergo ablative procedures. This second step treatment includes micro-vascular decompression, gamma knife surgery, radiofrequency thermo-coagulation and trigeminal ganglion balloon compression.

2. *Continuous Orofacial Neuropathic Pain Disorders*

Local treatment of continuous orofacial neuropathic pain includes topical application of agents and local injection of anesthetics. Agents frequently used for this purpose are capsaicin, lidocaine, and clonazepam. A lidocaine patch has been approved in some countries to treat postherpetic neuralgia in the spinal nerve territories. There is another commercial lidocaine patch originally designed for local anesthesia in the oral cavity during dental practice, although its safety in continuous usage for chronic orofacial pain treatment has not been established. An acrylic resin stent is employed to apply ointments topically to the oral mucosa on the bone. An ointment made of 0.025% capsaicin with 5% lidocaine is frequently used with a stent, whereas a systematic review has revealed that there is a lack of evidence in the effectiveness of topical capsaicin for neuropathic pain. 5% plain lidocaine ointment can be used instead of this mixture. Effectiveness of topical clonazepam has been reported in the treatment of burning mouth syndrome (Gremeau-Richard *et al.*, 2004). In this treatment, a clonazepam tablet is sucked and soaked in the saliva and kept in the mouth near painful site for three minutes, then spit out.

Systemic medication for continuous orofacial neuropathic pain is the same as in neuropathic pain in the extremities and the trunk. Systematic reviews (Dworkin *et al.*, 2007; Moulin *et al.*, 2007) recommend tryciclic antidepressants (amitryptiline and nortriptyline) and calcium channel alpha-delta ligand anticonvulsants (gabapentin and pregabaline) as first line medicines, followed by serotonin noradrenaline reuptake inhibitors, tramadol, and sustained releasing opioids. Mexiletine, cannabinoids, methadone, lamotrigine, topiramate, valproic acid, NMDA receptor blockers are next options.

Acknowledgments

This study was supported in part by Research Grants from Sato and Uemura Funds from Nihon University School of Dentistry, and a grant from the Dental Research Center, Nihon University School of Dentistry; Nihon

University multidisciplinary research grant for KI; grants from the Ministry of Education, Culture, Sports, Science, and Technology to promote multidisciplinary research project "Translational Research Network on Orofacial Neurological Disorders", at Nihon University School of Dentistry; the Japan-Canada Joint Health Research Program 167458, NIH grant (DE04786), and CHIR grants (MOP-43095), (MOP-82831).

References

Abdulla, F.A., Moran, T.D., Balasubramanyan, S., and Smith, P.A. (2003). Effects and consequences of nerve injury on the electrical properties of sensory neurons. *Can. J. Physiol. Pharmacol.* **81**, 663–682.

Amir, R., and Devor, M. (2003a). Extra spike formation in sensory neurons and the disruption of afferent spike patterning. *Biophys. J.* **84**, 2700–2708.

Amir, R., and Devor, M. (2003b). Electrical excitability of the soma of sensory neurons is required for spike invasion of the soma, but not for through-conduction. *Biophys. J.* **84**, 2181–2191.

Anderson, L.C., Vakoula, A., and Veinote, R. (2003). Inflammatory hypersensitivity in a rat model of trigeminal neuropathic pain. *Arch. Oral Biol.* **48**, 161–169.

Baron, R., Binder, A., and Wasner, G. (2010). Neuropathic pain: diagnosis, pathophysiological mechanisms, and treatment. *Lancet. Neurol.* **9**, 807–819.

Beneng, K., Yilmaz, Z., Yiangou, Y., McParland, H., Anand, P., and Renton, T. (2010). Sensory purinergic receptor P2X3 is elevated in burning mouth syndrome. *Int. J. Oral Maxillofac. Surg.* **39**, 815–819.

Bennett, G.J. (1993). An animal model of neuropathic pain: a review. *Muscle Nerve* **16**, 1040–1048.

Bennett, G.J. (2004). Neuropathic pain in the orofacial region: clinical and research challenges. *J. Orofac. Pain.* **18**, 281–286.

Bennett, G.J., and Xie, Y.K. (1988). A peripheral mononeuropathy in rat that produces disorders of pain sensation like those seen in man. *Pain* **33**, 87–107.

Benoliel, R., and Eliav, E. (2008). Neuropathic orofacial pain. *Oral Maxillofac. Surg. Clin. North Am.* **20**, 237–254 vii.

Bradlaw, R. (1936). The Innervation of Teeth: (Section of Odontology). *Proc. R. Soc. Med.* **29**, 507–518.

Cano, E., and Mahadevan, L.C. (1995). Parallel signal processing among mammalian MAPKs. *Trends Biochem. Sci.* **20**, 117–122.

Chao, T., Pham, K., Steward, O., and Gupta, R. (2008). Chronic nerve compression injury induces a phenotypic switch of neurons within the dorsal root ganglia. *J. Comp. Neurol.* **506**, 180–193.

Cherkas, P.S., Huang, T.Y., Pannicke, T., Tal, M., Reichenbach, A., and Hanani, M. (2004). The effects of axotomy on neurons and satellite glial cells in mouse trigeminal ganglion. *Pain* **110**, 290–298.

Chesselet, M.F. (1984). Presynaptic regulation of neurotransmitter release in the brain: facts and hypothesis. *Neuroscience* **12**, 347–375.

Chiang, C.Y., Li, Z., Dostrovsky, J.O., Hu, J.W., and Sessle, B.J. (2008). Glutamine uptake contributes to central sensitization in the medullary dorsal horn. *Neuroreport* **19**, 1151–1154.

Chiang, C.Y., Wang, J., Xie, Y.F., Zhang, S., Hu, J.W., Dostrovsky, J.O., and Sessle, B.J. (2007). Astroglial glutamate-glutamine shuttle is involved in central sensitization of nociceptive neurons in rat medullary dorsal horn. *J. Neurosci.* **27**, 9068–9076.

Dai, Y., Iwata, K., Fukuoka, T., Kondo, E., Tokunaga, A., Yamanaka, H., Tachibana, T., Liu, Y., and Noguchi, K. (2002). Phosphorylation of extracellular signal-regulated kinase in primary afferent neurons by noxious stimuli and its involvement in peripheral sensitization. *J. Neurosci.* **22**, 7737–7745.

Deseure, K., Koek, W., Adriaensen, H., and Colpaert, F.C. (2003). Continuous administration of the 5-hydroxytryptamine1A agonist (3-Chloro-4-fluoro-phenyl)-[4-fluoro-4-[[(5-methyl-pyridin-2-ylmethyl) -amino]-methyl]piperidin-1-yl]-methadone (F 13640) attenuates allodynia-like behavior in a rat model of trigeminal neuropathic pain. *J. Pharmacol. Exp. Ther.* **306**, 505–514.

Deseure, K.R., Adriaensen, H.F., and Colpaert, F.C. (2004). Effects of the combined continuous administration of morphine and the high-efficacy 5-HT1A agonist F 13640 in a rat model of trigeminal neuropathic pain. *Eur. J. Pain.* **8**, 547–554.

Devor, M., Govrin-Lippmann, R., and Angelides, K. (1993). Na + channel immunolocalization in peripheral mammalian axons and changes following nerve injury and neuroma formation. *J. Neurosci.* **13**, 1976–1992.

Dina, O.A., Hucho, T., Yeh, J., Malik-Hall, M., Reichling, D.B., and Levine, J.D. (2005). Primary afferent second messenger cascades interact with specific integrin subunits in producing inflammatory hyperalgesia. *Pain* **115**, 191–203.

Dominguez, C.A., Kouya, P.F., Wu, W.P., Hao, J.X., Xu, X.J., and Wiesenfeld-Hallin, Z. (2009). Sex differences in the development of localized and spread mechanical hypersensitivity in rats after injury to the infraorbital or sciatic nerves to create a model for neuropathic pain. *Gend. Med.* **2**(6 Suppl); 225–234.

Dworkin, R.H., O'Connor, A.B., Backonja, M., Farrar, J.T., Finnerup, N.B., Jensen, T.S., Kalso, E.A., Loeser, J.D., Miaskowski, C., Nurmikko, T.J., Portenoy, R.K., Rice, A.S., Stacey, B.R., Treede, R. D., Turk, D.C., and Wallace, M.S. (2007). Pharmacologic management of neuropathic pain: evidence-based recommendations. *Pain* **132**, 237–251.

Eliav, E., Kamran, B., Schaham, R., Czerninski, R., Gracely, R.H., and Benoliel, R. (2007). Evidence of chorda tympani dysfunction in patients with burning mouth syndrome. *J. Am. Dent. Assoc.* **138**, 628–633.

Ericson, A.C., Blomqvist, A., Krout, K., and Craig, A.D. (1996). Fine structural organization of spinothalamic and trigeminothalamic lamina I terminations in the nucleus submedius of the cat. *J. Comp. Neurol.* **371**, 497–512.

Eriksson, J., Jablonski, A., Persson, A.K., Hao, J.X., Kouya, P.F., Wiesenfeld-Hallin, Z., Xu, X.J., and Fried, K. (2005). Behavioral changes and trigeminal ganglion sodium channel regulation in an orofacial neuropathic pain model. *Pain* **119**, 82–94.

Forssell, H., Jaaskelainen, S., Tenovuo, O., and Hinkka, S. (2002). Sensory dysfunction in burning mouth syndrome. *Pain* **99**, 41–47.

Garry, E.M., Jones, E., and Fleetwood-Walker, S.M. (2004). Nociception in vertebrates: key receptors participating in spinal mechanisms of chronic pain in animals. *Brain Res. Brain Res. Rev.* **46**, 216–224.

Garza, I. (2008). The trigeminal trophic syndrome: an unusual cause of face pain, dysaesthesias, anaesthesia and skin/soft tissue lesions. *Cephalalgia* **28**, 980–985.

Granot, M., and Nagler, R.M. (2005). Association between regional idiopathic neuropathy and salivary involvement as the possible mechanism for oral sensory complaints. *J. Pain* **6**, 581–587.

Gremeau-Richard, C., Woda, A., Navez, M.L., Attal, N., Bouhassira, D., Gagnieu, M.C., Laluque, J. F., Picard, P., Pionchon, P., and Tubert, S. (2004). Topical clonazepam in stomatodynia: a randomised placebo-controlled study. *Pain* **108**, 51–57.

Guilbaud, G., Benoist, J.M., Jazat, F., and Gautron, M. (1990). Neuronal responsiveness in the ventrobasal thalamic complex of rats with an experimental peripheral mononeuropathy. *J. Neurophysiol.* **64**, 1537–1554.

Harada, F., Hoshino, N., Hanada, K., Kawano, Y., Atsumi, Y., Wakisaka, S., and Maeda, T. (2003). The involvement of brain-derived neurotrophic factor (BDNF) in the regeneration of periodontal Ruffini endings following transection of the inferior alveolar nerve. *Arch. Histol. Cytol.* **66**, 183–194.

Honda, K., Kitagawa, J., Sessle, B.J., Kondo, M., Tsuboi, Y., Yonehara, Y., and Iwata, K. (2008). Mechanisms involved in an increment of multimodal excitability of medullary and upper cervical dorsal horn neurons following cutaneous capsaicin treatment. *Mol. Pain* **4**, 59.

Hunt, S.P., Pini, A., and Evan, G. (1987). Induction of c-fos-like protein in spinal cord neurons following sensory stimulation. *Nature* **328**, 632–634.

Imamura, Y., Kawamoto, H., and Nakanishi, O. (1997). Characterization of heat-hyperalgesia in an experimental trigeminal neuropathy in rats. *Exp. Brain Res.* **116**, 97–103.

Iwata, K., Tashiro, A., Tsuboi, Y., Imai, T., Sumino, R., Morimoto, T., Dubner, R., and Ren, K. (1999). Medullary dorsal horn neuronal activity in rats with persistent temporomandibular joint and perioral inflammation. *J. Neurophysiol.* **82**, 1244–1253.

Iwata, K., Imai, T., Tsuboi, Y., Tashiro, A., Ogawa, A., Morimoto, T., Masuda, Y., Tachibana, Y., and Hu J,,Hu J. (2001). Alteration of medullary dorsal horn neuronal activity following inferior alveolar nerve transection in rats. *J. Neurophysiol.* **86**, 2868–2877.

Iwata, K., Fukuoka, T., Kondo, E., Tsuboi, Y., Tashiro, A., Noguchi, K., Masuda, Y., Morimoto, T., and Kanda, K. (2002). Plastic changes in nociceptive transmission of the rat spinal cord with advancing age. *J. Neurophysiol.* **87**, 1086–1093.

Jaaskelainen, S.K. (2004). Clinical neurophysiology and quantitative sensory testing in the investigation of orofacial pain and sensory function. *J. Orofac. Pain* **18**, 85–107.

Jackson, M.B. (1995). Presynaptic excitability. *Int. Rev. Neurobiol.* **38**, 201–251.

Ji, R.R., Befort, K., Brenner, G.J., and Woolf, C.J. (2002). ERK MAP kinase activation in superficial spinal cord neurons induces prodynorphin and NK-1 upregulation and contributes to persistent inflammatory pain hypersensitivity. *J. Neurosci.* **22**, 478–485.

Kajander, K.C., and Bennett, G.J. (1992). Onset of a painful peripheral neuropathy in rat: a partial and differential deafferentation and spontaneous discharge in A beta and A delta primary afferent neurons. *J. Neurophysiol.* **68**, 734–744.

Kayser, V., Aubel, B., Hamon, M., and Bourgoin, S. (2002). The antimigraine 5-HT 1B/1D receptor agonists, sumatriptan, zolmitriptan and dihydroergotamine, attenuate pain-related behaviour in a rat model of trigeminal neuropathic pain. *Br. J. Pharmacol.* **137**, 1287–1297.

Kitagawa, J., Takeda, M., Suzuki, I., Kadoi, J., Tsuboi, Y., Honda, K., Matsumoto, S., Nakagawa, H., Tanabe, A., and Iwata, K. (2006). Mechanisms involved in modulation of trigeminal primary afferent activity in rats with peripheral mononeuropathy. *Eur. J. Neurosci.* **24**, 1976–1986.

Kobayashi, A., Shinoda, M., Sessle, B.J., Honda, K., Imamura, Y., Hitomi, S., Tsuboi, Y., Okada-Ogawa, A., and Iwata, K. (2011). Mechanisms involved in extraterritorial facial pain following cervical spinal nerve injury in rats. *Mol Pain* **10**, 12.

Lam, D.K., Sessle, B.J., and Hu, J.W. (2009a). Glutamate and capsaicin effects on trigeminal nociception II: activation and central sensitization in brainstem neurons with deep craniofacial afferent input. *Brain Res.* **1253**, 48–59.

Lam, D.K., Sessle, B.J., and Hu, J.W. (2009b). Glutamate and capsaicin effects on trigeminal nociception I: Activation and peripheral sensitization of deep craniofacial nociceptive afferents. *Brain Res.* **1251**, 130–139.

Lauria, G., Majorana, A., Borgna, M., Lombardi, R., Penza, P., Padovani, A., and Sapelli, P. (2005). Trigeminal small-fiber sensory neuropathy causes burning mouth syndrome. *Pain* **115**, 332–337.

List, T., Leijon, G., and Svensson, P. (2008). Somatosensory abnormalities in atypical odontalgia: A case-control study. *Pain* **139**, 333–341.

Liu, Y., Obata, K., Yamanaka, H., Dai, Y., Fukuoka, T., Tokunaga, A., and Noguchi, K. (2004). Activation of extracellular signal-regulated protein kinase in dorsal horn neurons in the rat neuropathic intermittent claudication model. *Pain* **109**, 64–72.

Luiz, A.P., Schroeder, S.D., Chichorro, J.G., Calixto, J.B., Zampronio, A.R., and Rae, G.A. (2010). Kinin B(1) and B(2) receptors contribute to orofacial heat hyperalgesia induced by infraorbital nerve constriction injury in mice and rats. *Neuropeptides* **44**, 87–92.

Maier, C et al., (2010). Quantitative sensory testing in the German Research Network on Neuropathic Pain (DFNS): somatosensory abnormalities in 1236 patients with different neuropathic pain syndromes. *Pain* **150**, 439–450.

Maihofner, C., Nickel, F.T., and Seifert, F. (2010). [Neuropathic pain and neuroplasticity in functional imaging studies]. *Schmerz* **24**, 137–145.

Meunier, A., Latremoliere, A., Mauborgne, A., Bourgoin, S., Kayser, V., Cesselin, F., Hamon, M., and Pohl, M. (2005). Attenuation of pain-related behavior in a rat model of trigeminal neuropathic pain by viral-driven enkephalin overproduction in trigeminal ganglion neurons. *Mol. Ther.* **11**, 608–616.

Mitsikostas, D.D., and Sanchez del Rio, M. (2001). Receptor systems mediating c-fos expression within trigeminal nucleus caudalis in animal models of migraine. *Brain Res. Brain Res. Rev.* **35**, 20–35.

Moulin, D.E et al., (2007). Pharmacological management of chronic neuropathic pain - consensus statement and guidelines from the Canadian Pain Society. *Pain Res. Manag.* **12**, 13–21.

Nakagawa, K., Takeda, M., Tsuboi, Y., Kondo, M., Kitagawa, J., Matsumoto, S., Kobayashi, A., Sessle, B.J., Shinoda, M., and Iwata, K. (2010). Alteration of primary afferent activity following inferior alveolar nerve transection in rats. *Mol. Pain* **6**, 9.

Nakai K, Nakae A, Oba S, Mashimo T, Ueda K, (2010) 5-HT2C receptor agonists attenuate pain-related behaviour in a rat model of trigeminal neuropathic pain. *Eur. J. Pain* in press.

Neugebauer, V. (2002). Metabotropic glutamate receptors–important modulators of nociception and pain behavior. *Pain* **98**, 1–8.

Noma, N., Tsuboi, Y., Kondo, M., Matsumoto, M., Sessle, B.J., Kitagawa, J., Saito, K., and Iwata, K. (2008). Organization of pERK-immunoreactive cells in trigeminal spinal nucleus caudalis and upper cervical cord following capsaicin injection into oral and craniofacial regions in rats. *J. Comp. Neurol.* **507**, 1428–1440.

Nomura, H., Ogawa, A., Tashiro, A., Morimoto, T., Hu, J.W., and Iwata, K. (2002). Induction of Fos protein-like immunoreactivity in the trigeminal spinal nucleus caudalis and upper cervical cord following noxious and non-noxious mechanical stimulation of the whisker pad of the rat with an inferior alveolar nerve transection. *Pain* **95**, 225–238.

Ohara, P.T., Vit, J.P., Bhargava, A., and Jasmin, L. (2008). Evidence for a role of connexin 43 in trigeminal pain using RNA interference in vivo. *J. Neurophysiol.* **100**, 3064–3073.

Ohara, P.T., Vit, J.P., Bhargava, A., Romero, M., Sundberg, C., Charles, A.C., and Jasmin, L. (2009). Gliopathic pain: when satellite glial cells go bad. *Neuroscientist* **15**, 450–463.

Okada-Ogawa, A., Suzuki, I., Sessle, B.J., Chiang, C.Y., Salter, M.W., Dostrovsky, J.O., Tsuboi, Y., Kondo, M., Kitagawa, J., Kobayashi, A., Noma, N., Imamura, Y., and Iwata, K. (2009). Astroglia in medullary dorsal horn (trigeminal spinal subnucleus caudalis) are involved in trigeminal neuropathic pain mechanisms. *J. Neurosci.* **29**, 11161–11171.

Park, S.J., Zhang, S., Chiang, C.Y., Hu, J.W., Dostrovsky, J.O., and Sessle, B.J. (2006). Central sensitization induced in thalamic nociceptive neurons by tooth pulp stimulation is dependent on the functional integrity of trigeminal brainstem subnucleus caudalis but not subnucleus oralis. *Brain Res.* **1112**, 134–145.

Piao, Z.G., Cho, I.H., Park, C.K., Hong, J.P., Choi, S.Y., Lee, S.J., Lee, S., Park, K., Kim, J.S., and Oh, S.B. (2006). Activation of glia and microglial p38 MAPK in medullary dorsal horn contributes to tactile hypersensitivity following trigeminal sensory nerve injury. *Pain* **121**, 219–231.

Pigg, M., Baad-Hansen, L., Svensson, P., Drangsholt, M., and List, T. (2010). Reliability of intraoral quantitative sensory testing (QST). *Pain* **148**, 220–226.

Rizzo, M.A., Kocsis, J.D., and Waxman, S.G. (1996). Mechanisms of paresthesiae, dysesthesiae, and hyperesthesiae: role of Na + channel heterogeneity. *Eur. Neurol.* **36**, 3–12.

Rolke, R., Magerl, W., Campbell, K.A., Schalber, C., Caspari, S., Birklein, F., and Treede, R.D. (2006). Quantitative sensory testing: a comprehensive protocol for clinical trials. *Eur. J. Pain* **10**, 77–88.

Saito, K., Hitomi, S., Suzuki, I., Masuda, Y., Kitagawa, J., Tsuboi, Y., Kondo, M., Sessle, B.J., and Iwata, K. (2008). Modulation of trigeminal spinal subnucleus caudalis neuronal activity following regeneration of transected inferior alveolar nerve in rats. *J. Neurophysiol.* **99**, 2251–2263.

Sakamoto E, Shiiba S, Noma N, Okada-Ogawa A, Shinozaki T, Kobayashi A, Kamo H, Koike K, Imamura Y A possible case of complex regional pain syndrome in the orofacial region. *Pain Med* **11** 274–280.

Seger, R., and Krebs, E.G. (1995). The MAPK signaling cascade. *FASEB J.* **9**, 726–735.

Seino, H., Seo, K., Maeda, T., and Someya, G. (2009). Behavioural and histological observations of sensory impairment caused by tight ligation of the trigeminal nerve in mice. *J. Neurosci. Methods* **181**, 67–72.

Sessle, B.J. (1999). Neural mechanisms and pathways in craniofacial pain. *Can. J. Neurol. Sci.* **3**(26 Suppl); S7–11.

Sessle, B.J., Hu, J.W., Amano, N., and Zhong, G. (1986). Convergence of cutaneous, tooth pulp, visceral, neck and muscle afferents onto nociceptive and non-nociceptive neurones in trigeminal subnucleus caudalis (medullary dorsal horn) and its implications for referred pain. *Pain* **27**, 219–235.

Shinoda, M., Kawashima, K., Ozaki, N., Asai, H., Nagamine, K., and Sugiura, Y. (2007). P2X3 receptor mediates heat hyperalgesia in a rat model of trigeminal neuropathic pain. *J. Pain* **8**, 588–597.

Sindrup, S.H., and Jensen, T.S. (2002). Pharmacotherapy of trigeminal neuralgia. *Clin. J. Pain* **18**, 22–27.

Truelove, E. (2004). Management issues of neuropathic trigeminal pain from a dental perspective. *J. Orofac. Pain* **18**, 374–380.

Tsuboi, Y., Takeda, M., Tanimoto, T., Ikeda, M., Matsumoto, S., Kitagawa, J., Teramoto, K., Simizu, K., Yamazaki, Y., Shima, A., Ren, K., and Iwata, K. (2004). Alteration of the second branch of the trigeminal nerve activity following inferior alveolar nerve transection in rats. *Pain* **111**, 323–334.

Tsuzuki, K., Fukuoka, T., Sakagami, M., and Noguchi, K. (2003). Increase of preprotachykinin mRNA in the uninjured mandibular neurons after rat infraorbital nerve transection. *Neurosci. Lett.* **345**, 57–60.

Ueda, H. (2006). Molecular mechanisms of neuropathic pain-phenotypic switch and initiation mechanisms. *Pharmacol. Ther.* **109**, 57–77.

Vos, B.P., Strassman, A.M., and Maciewicz, R.J. (1994). Behavioral evidence of trigeminal neuropathic pain following chronic constriction injury to the rat's infraorbital nerve. *J. Neurosci.* **14**, 2708–2723.

Wakisaka, S., Ichikawa, H., Nishikawa, S., Matsuo, S., Takano, Y., and Akai, M. (1987). The distribution and origin of calcitonin gene-related peptide-containing nerve fibres in feline dental pulp Relationship with substance P-containing nerve fibres. *Histochemistry* **86**, 585–589.

Wang, Y., Wu, J., Wu, Z., Lin, Q., Yue, Y., and Fang, L. (2010). Regulation of AMPA receptors in spinal nociception. *Mol. Pain* **6**, 5.

Woolf, C.J., and Salter, M.W. (2000). Neuronal plasticity: increasing the gain in pain. *Science* **288**, 1765–1769.

Xu, M., Aita, M., and Chavkin, C. (2008). Partial infraorbital nerve ligation as a model of trigeminal nerve injury in the mouse: behavioral, neural, and glial reactions. *J. Pain* **9**, 1036–1048.

Yilmaz, Z., Renton, T., Yiangou, Y., Zakrzewska, J., Chessell, I.P., Bountra, C., and Anand, P. (2007). Burning mouth syndrome as a trigeminal small fibre neuropathy: Increased heat and capsaicin receptor TRPV1 in nerve fibres correlates with pain score. *J. Clin. Neurosci.* **14**, 864–871.

Zhang, S., Chiang, C.Y., Xie, Y.F., Park, S.J., Lu, Y., Hu, J.W., Dostrovsky, J.O., and Sessle, B.J. (2006). Central sensitization in thalamic nociceptive neurons induced by mustard oil application to rat molar tooth pulp. *Neuroscience* **142**, 833–842.

Zhang, Z., and Dellon, A.L. (2008). Facial pain and headache associated with brachial plexus compression in the thoracic inlet. *Microsurgery* **28**, 347–350.

Zhuang, Z.Y., Gerner, P., Woolf, C.J., and Ji, R.R. (2005). ERK is sequentially activated in neurons, microglia, and astrocytes by spinal nerve ligation and contributes to mechanical allodynia in this neuropathic pain model. *Pain* **114**, 149–159.

NEUROBIOLOGY OF ESTROGEN STATUS IN DEEP CRANIOFACIAL PAIN

David A Bereiter and Keiichiro Okamoto

Department of Diagnostic and Biological Sciences, University of Minnesota School of Dentistry, Minneapolis, MN 55455 USA

I. Introduction

The impact of craniofacial pain on society is considerable both in terms of reduced quality of life and financial burden (Macfarlane *et al.*, 2002; Riley *et al.*, 2003). Despite a high incidence and evidence that multiple factors are involved, one likely risk factor for developing chronic craniofacial pain is female gender and/or sex hormone status (Lipton *et al.*, 1993; LeResche, 1997). Diverse conditions such as migraine headache (Bingefors and Isacson, 2004), burning mouth (Forssell *et al.*, 2002), atypical odontalgia (List *et al.*, 2007), trigeminal neuralgia (Katusic *et al.*, 1991) and temporomandibular joint disorders (TMJD, LeResche, 1997) share the common feature of being significantly more prevalent in females than males.

II. Painful Temporomandibular Joint Disorders (TMJD)

This review focuses on the role of estrogen status and sex-related differences in TMJD pain. TMJD represents a family of conditions that present with pain in the temporomandibular joint (TMJ) region and muscles of mastication and is the most common non-dental chronic craniofacial pain syndrome (Maixner, 2009). Development of the Research Diagnostic Criteria for TMJD (RDC/TMD) has

INTERNATIONAL REVIEW OF NEUROBIOLOGY, VOL. 97
DOI: 10.1016/B978-0-12-385198-7.00010-2

greatly aided the classification and diagnosis of this complex, often idiopathic, pain condition (Dworkin and LeResche, 1992). The RDC/TMD relies on measurements along two axes: Axis I assesses the physical/biological status, while Axis II assesses the psychological status. TMJD patients fall into three broad subclasses based on Axis I criteria: Pain involving masticatory muscles (Group I), disk displacement (Group II) and arthralgia, or arthritic conditions (Group III). Recent validation of the RDC/TMD indicates that the vast majority of patients (>80%) present with some form of Group I (myofascial pain) disability (Schiffman *et al.*, 2010). Thus, animal models that involve masticatory muscles as well as the TMJ proper are valid components of experimental models for TMJD pain. Feedback from jaw motor function may also influence TMJD pain; however, current evidence suggests that the origin of TMJD pain cannot be explained by muscle hyperactivity alone (Svensson, 2007; Svensson and Graven-Nielsen, 2001) and is not considered further in this review.

Chronic non-rheumatoid TMJD patients often describe their pain as spontaneous, fluctuating and non-progressive (Ohrbach and Dworkin, 1998; Rammelsberg *et al.*, 2003). Pain sensation can be either aching or sharp, often poorly localized to the jaw region with spreading outside the trigeminal dermatomes to the neck and shoulders (Turp *et al.*, 1998). Several risk factors to develop chronic TMJD pain have been identified: Psychological stress, co-occurrence of a second chronic pain condition such as headache or irritable bowl and genetic susceptibility (Huang *et al.*, 2002; Slade *et al.*, 2007; Diatchenko *et al.*, 2006). However, the most consistent and likely risk factor for chronic idiopathic TMJD pain is female gender or sex hormone status. Table I indicates

Table I
FEMALE: MALE PREVALENCE RATIOS FOR PAINFUL TMD IN ADULTS REPORTED FROM POPULATION AND CLINIC STUDIES.

Study	Study type	N	Female:male
Gesch *et al.*, (2004)	P	4289	2.4
Goncalves *et al.*, (2010)	P	1230	2.1
Isong *et al.*, (2008)	P	30978	2.3
Lipton *et al.*, (1993)	P	42370	2.1
Rauhala *et al.*, (2000)	P	1371	1.3
Rutkiewicz *et al.*, (2006)	P	6335	2.1
Bush *et al.*, (1993)	C	165	5.2
Davis *et al.*, (2010)	C	251	8.7
Manfredini *et al.*, (2006)	C	144	4.3
List and Dworkin (1996)	C	343	3.8
Rammelsberg *et al.*, (2003)	C	235	3.7

C = clinic data; P = population or community-derived data.

that the female: male prevalence ratio for TMJD is nearly 2:1 in the general population, whereas in clinical populations it can exceed 8:1. The neurobiological basis for this high female prevalence is not known and likely involves peripheral as well as central mechanisms. Four lines of evidence support the notion that estrogen status plays a significant role in TMJD pain. First, the expression of TMJD pain follows a pattern consistent with the development and regression of the ovarian production of estrogens. That is, the prevalence and severity of TMJD pain in females is similar to males prior to puberty, when estrogen production is low, rises during the reproductive years and diminishes after menopause (List and Dworkin, 1996; Gesch *et al.*, 2004; LeResche *et al.*, 2005a; Goncalves *et al.*, 2010). Second, natural variations in estrogen production over the menstrual cycle (Isselee *et al.*, 2002; LeResche *et al.*, 2003; Landi *et al.*, 2005) and during pregnancy (LeResche *et al.*, 2005b) influence TMJD pain. Third, the estrogen replacement therapy after menopause increases TMJD pain (LeResche *et al.*, 1997). Fourth, genetic polymorphisms of the estrogen receptor alter the susceptibility to develop TMJD pain in women (Kang *et al.*, 2007; Ribeiro-DaSilva *et al.*, 2009). This review examines peripheral and central neural mechanisms involving the activational, as opposed to organizational, effects of estrogens that may contribute to TMJD-related pain in humans and nociception in animals. We also discuss selected pathways for estrogen actions in the brain and draw attention to some pathways that have received little attention in TMJ research.

III. Estrogens and Estrogen Receptors (ER) and TMJD

Estrogens bind at multiple receptors and act on diverse physiological systems within and outside the nervous system that could impact the expression of chronic TMJD pain (Gruber *et al.*, 2002; Ciana *et al.*, 2003). Effects on basic physiological systems such as energy homeostasis (Shi *et al.*, 2009; Foryst-Ludwig and Kintscher, 2010), cardiovascular regulation (Miller and Duckles, 2008), bone and cartilage metabolism (Galal *et al.*, 2008; Tanko *et al.*, 2008; Frenkel *et al.*, 2010) and inflammation (Straub, 2007) indicate that maintenance of proper estrogen status is critical to the overall health of females. Ovarian production of estradiol (E2), the principal biologically active form of estrogen, is secreted in a species-specific rhythmic and pulsatile pattern. Considerable evidence suggests that the pattern of E2 secretion is a key factor in the neural response to E2, and that failure to account for this pattern could confound the interpretation of experimental results in unpredictable ways (Grundt *et al.*, 2010; Kramer and Bellinger, 2009). For example, in the hippocampus long-term potentiation (LTP) and pyramidal cell excitability varies over the estrous cycle in intact female rats (Woolley, 1999; Scharfman *et al.,* 2003) and is replicated in ovariectomized (OvX) rats by administering physiological levels of E2 in a sequential pattern (Scharfman *et al.,* 2007). However, animals treated chronically for 2 weeks by daily injections of E2 display minimal changes in hippocampus neuronal excitability (Barraclough *et al.,* 1999). Similarly, the efficacy of E2 to lessen cognitive deficits in aging female rats is significantly greater after intermittent, than chronic administration (Markowska and Savonenko, 2002). In spinal dorsal root ganglion (DRG) neurons long-term E2 replacement in OvX rats *reduces* the expression of trkA, the specific receptor for nerve growth factor (NGF, Liuzzi *et al.,* 1999a), whereas short-term administration for 2 days increases trkA expression (Liuzzi *et al.,* 1999b). These examples suggest that long-term exposure to E2 can have unexpected consequences that confound the interpretation of results from animal models designed to link estrogen status and TMJD pain. Accordingly, the design of experimental investigations of estrogen actions in whole animals should consider both the normal timing, as well as the magnitude of exposure to estrogens.

Estrogens act through rapid membrane-initiated and genomic nuclear-initiated signaling pathways to alter neuronal excitability, gene expression, and behavior (McEwen, 2001; Scharfman and MacLusky, 2006; Woolley, 2007; Micevych and Mermelstein, 2008). Intracellular nuclear ERs consist of two major subtypes, ER alpha (ERa) and ER beta (ERb) that, upon binding estrogens, form dimers that activate nuclear response elements and alter gene transcription. By contrast, the basis for membrane-initiated signaling is less certain and may involve nuclear ERs as well as G protein-coupled receptors such as GPR30 (Levin, 2009). Importantly, it is now understood that membrane- and nuclear-initiated pathways are not independent, but rather interact to modify neural function (Vasudevan and Pfaff, 2007; Roepke *et al.,* 2009). Thus, changes in behavior after acute administration of E2 in steroid-depleted OvX animals should be viewed with some limitations since normal cycling females are exposed to E2 in a continuous, but variable pattern.

The role of estrogens on neural function generally has been pursued along three converging lines of inquiry (McEwen, 2001). First, the anatomical approaches have identified the distribution of receptors and sites for specific binding in peripheral tissues and the CNS. Second, pharmacological agonists and antagonists have probed the functional significance of estrogens and ERs in modifying behavior. Third, the cell and molecular approaches have assessed signaling pathways for effects on neuronal excitability, synapse formation, and plasticity. Although these lines of inquiry are far from complete, each has made a significant contribution to understanding of the role of estrogens in TMJD pain.

IV. Estrogen Status and Peripheral Mechanisms in TMJD

Estrogen status affects the composition of TMJ-related tissues in normal cycling animals (Abubaker *et al.,* 1996; Mariotti *et al.,* 2000) and following E2 treatment in OvX animals (Hashem *et al.,* 2006). Estrogens alter the expression patterns of bone morphogenetic proteins (Min *et al.,* 2007) consistent with the pattern of specific binding in articular tissues (Aufdemorte *et al.,* 1986; Milam *et al.,* 1987). Although ERa and ERb are expressed in fibrocartilage cells of TMJ tissues (Nozawa-Inoue *et al.,* 2003; Yamada *et al.,* 2003; Puri *et al.,* 2009; Wang *et al.,* 2009; Yu *et al.,* 2009), evidence for specific staining of neural elements in the TMJ is weak. Similarly, ERa has been reported in male and female TMJ tissues in some human studies (Abubaker *et al.,* 1993), whereas others found no nuclear staining for E2 (Campbell *et al.,* 1993) or E2 binding (Henry *et al.,* 2008). Based on the analyzes of E2 binding and expression of ER subtypes, evidence that E2-induced effects on TMJ afferents are due to direct actions through classical ER subtypes expressed in neurons, is not consistent.

The sensory innervation of the TMJ region is more complex than other body areas and consists of three distinct sources of primary afferent neurons: trigeminal root ganglion (TRG) neurons from the mandibular and maxillary trigeminal nerve branches,DRG neurons from upper cervical spinal rootlets and nodose ganglion (NG) neurons that give rise to the auricular branch of the vagus nerve (Denny-Brown and Yanagisawa, 1973; Widenfalk and Wiberg, 1990; Kido *et al.,* 1991; Uddman *et al.,* 1998; Casatti *et al.,* 1999). Although ERa and ERb (Papka *et al.,* 1997; Bereiter *et al.,* 2005; Puri *et al.,* 2005a) and GPR30 (Dun *et al.,* 2009; Liverman *et al.,* 2009) are expressed in significant numbers of TRG, cervical DRG and NG neurons, it is not known what percentage of ER-positive cells also supply the TMJ region.

The relationship between estrogen status and peripheral neural mechanisms in TMJD pain is confounded further by the fact that a significant percentage of joint and muscle C-fiber afferents are so-called silent nociceptors that become active only after injury (Schaible and Grubb, 1993; Mense, 1993; Schaible *et al.,* 2009). This is problematic for developing animal models since chronic non-rheumatoid TMJD pain patients generally do not display overt signs of injury (Ohrbach and Dworkin, 1998) or consistent elevation of neuropeptide levels in synovial fluid (2005; 2007). If estrogens act peripherally to maintain TMJD pain, then E2 treatment should modify the activity of TMJ and muscle afferents consistent with known features of peripheral sensitization such as increased spontaneous activity, lower thresholds and increased responses to applied stimuli. Indeed, recordings from TMJ (Cairns *et al.,* 2001b) and masseter muscle afferents (Cairns *et al.,* 2001a; Cairns *et al.,* 2002; Dong *et al.,* 2007) revealed greater responses to local injections of glutamate receptor agonists in females than males, although the responses to other excitants such as 5HT and NGF were similar (Sung *et al.*, 2008; Svensson *et al.*, 2010). Importantly, mechanical sensitivity and thresholds to detect chemical excitants by TMJ and muscle afferents were not altered by estrogen status in any of these studies. This suggests that if estrogens act peripherally to modify TMJ pain, they do so through mechanisms somewhat different from those attributed to more classical views of peripheral sensitization. This conclusion is tempered, however, by the fact that C-fibers were not recorded in these studies, and the knowledge that C-fibers represent the largest fraction of sensory afferents that supply the TMJ (Kido *et al.*, 1995). Indeed, *in vitro* recording from TMJ-labeled TRGs in female rats found <25% were myelinated and although chronic E2 increased neuronal excitability, the majority of cells were not responsive to capsaicin (Flake *et al.*, 2005). It also is possible that E2 acts indirectly to alter TRG excitability since E2 increases the expression of prolactin in TRPV1-positive neurons, increases phosphorylation of TRPV1 receptors and capsaicin-evoked current (Diogenes *et al.*, 2006), increases phospho-extracellular signal-regulated kinase (pERK)–positive TRG neurons (Puri *et al.*, 2005b) and the expression of NMDA receptors (Dong *et al.*, 2007) in female rats. An anti-hyperalgesic effect is suggested by the co-injection of E2 into the TMJ reduced formalin-evoked nociceptive behavior, (Favaro-Moreira *et al.*, 2009), this may be explained by the anti-inflammatory actions of E2 (Straub, 2007). Recent reviews indicate no consensus that chronic TMJD pain patients benefit significantly from the anti-inflammatory drug treatment (List and Axelsson, 2010). This would appear to limit the usefulness of severe TMJ inflammation in animals as a model for chronic TMJD pain in humans. In summary, anatomical, physiological, and behavioral studies in animals suggest that estrogen status may, under some conditions, modulate sensory neuron activity relevant to TMJD. However, future studies need to better define the phenotype of TMJ sensory neurons and determine if E2 delivered at physiological levels in a pulsatile pattern similar to cycling females, is sufficient to alter neuronal activity.

Quantitative sensory testing (QST) provides critical information on sensory function and supplements results from the clinical examination. However, the influence of estrogen status on QST results in TMJD patients has been limited since this factor is not documented routinely at the time of testing. Sex difference comparisons in chronic TMJD also have been limited since few men are included in most of the clinic populations. The pain-free female subjects generally had lower tactile detection thresholds at facial skin sites than males (Komiyama and De Laat 2005; Chen *et al.*, 1995). Other studies found no sex differences in mechanical or electrical stimulation detection thresholds from skin overlying the TMJ, while repetitive electrical stimulation of the TMJ increased thresholds in both groups (Ayesh et al., 2007a). Hypertonic saline infusion into masseter muscle also reduced cutaneous sensitivity in males and females, although pain rating during saline infusion was greater in females (Stohler *et al.*, 2001). Glutamate injection into masseter muscle evoked greater overall muscle pain in females than males; however, the threshold concentrations of glutamate required to evoke pain sensation were quite high and not different between sexes (Cairns *et al.,* 2001a).

The most consistent finding from QST studies in TMJD patients is a reduction in pain thresholds or tolerance, especially for pressure, but not in sensory detection thresholds (see Sarlani and Greenspan, 2003). Pressure pain thresholds (PPT) over the TMJ region was lower in female TMJD patients than control subjects (Reid *et al.,* 1994; Svensson *et al.,* 1995). Although hypertonic saline infusion into masseter muscle evoked greater pain ratings and lower PPTs over the TMJ in patients than controls, heat pain thresholds were similar and no sex differences were reported (Svensson *et al.,* 2001). In mainly female subjects, PPTs over the TMJ were lower in TMJD patients than controls, while tactile detection thresholds were similar (Michelotti *et al.,* 2008; Pfau *et al.,* 2009) and TMJD patients were able to detect and discriminate small increments in temperature as well as control subjects (Maixner *et al.,* 1998). In female TMJD patients PPTs at the TMJ region (Isselee *et al.,* 2002) and ischemic pain rating varied as a function of stage of the menstrual cycle (Sherman *et al.,* 2005). The TMJD patients had lower pain, but not sensory, detection thresholds in response to intra-TMJ electrical stimulation, and no sex-related differences were noted (Ayesh *et al.,* 2007b). Laser evoked potentials (LEPs) allows discrete assessment of small fiber function in sensory systems in clinical settings (Treede, 2003). Although LEP amplitude after facial skin stimulation was reduced in TMJD patients compared to controls, at low intensity stimulation it was sufficient to assess perception thresholds no group differences were seen (Romaniello *et al.,* 2003). These data suggest that PPTs overlying the TMJ are lower in TMJD patients, and are modulated by estrogen status. By contrast, there is less evidence that sensory detection thresholds, a measure of peripheral sensitization, are altered in chronic TMJD.

A second line of evidence regarding estrogen status, peripheral neural mechanisms, and TMJD pain concerns the effectiveness of local intra-articular (IA) administration of analgesic and anesthetic drugs. In studies that comprised mainly of females, IA morphine alone had little effect on TMJD pain (List *et al.,* 2001) or pain following arthroscopy (Bryant *et al.,* 1999). The IA lidocaine reduced ongoing pain in female TMJD patients either briefly (Danzig *et al.,* 1992) or not all (Ayesh *et al.,* 2007a), although in the latter study application to the auriculotemporal nerve provided pain relief for at least 30 min. Similarly, local anesthetic injection into trigger points in the female myofascial pain patients had only minor effects on pressure pain thresholds, while controls displayed significant increases (McMillan and Blasberg, 1994). Although injection of pharmacological doses of glutamate into masseter muscle evoked greater pain scores in women than men (Cairns *et al.,* 2001a), local blockade of NMDA receptors in masseter muscle (Castrillon *et al.,* 2008) or TMJ (Ayesh *et al.,* 2008) did not improve pain scores in female patients.

In summary, while there is clear evidence that E2 binds and acts peripherally to alter some properties of neurons that transmit sensory signals from the TMJ region, the functional significance of these contributions to ongoing chronic pain remains uncertain. The results from QST studies and local anesthetic/analgesic treatments in patients suggest that peripheral sensitization and estrogen-modulation of peripheral sensory neurons alone cannot explain the signs and symptoms of chronic TMJD pain or the higher prevalence in women.

V. Estrogen Status and Central Mechanisms in TMJD

There is considerable evidence from clinical and experimental studies that support the notion of a central neural dysfunction, often presenting as central sensitization.(Diatchenko *et al.*, 2006; Yunus, 2007). This is supported by evidence of widespread pain beyond the TMJ region (Reid *et al.*, 1994; Turp *et al.*, 1998; John *et al.*, 2003; Fernandez-de-las-Penas *et al.*, 2009) and enhanced spatial and temporal summation to painful stimuli (Maixner *et al.*, 1998; Svensson *et al.*, 2001; Sarlani and Greenspan, 2005). Enhanced sensitivity in TMJD patients appears specific to noxious stimuli, since sensitivity to vibrotactile stimulation is reduced (Hollins *et al.*, 1996; Hollins *et al.*, 2001), while responses to visual (Maixner *et al.*, 1998) and auditory stimuli (Hollins *et al.*, 2009) are not affected. Neuroimaging studies indicate significant structural changes in trigeminal and limbic brain areas of female patients consistent with a CNS dysfunction (Younger *et al.*, 2010). The vast majority of subjects in these studies were women; however, since estrogen status per se was not assessed, a specific role for sex steroids in CNS mechanisms related to chronic TMJD pain remains uncertain. In a recent study, repetitive mechanical stimuli presented at short intervals, produced progressive increases in pain perception in female but not male TMJD patients, suggesting a sex-related difference in temporal summation and central nociceptive processing (Sarlani *et al.*, 2007).

The literature on sex-related factors and the neurobiological basis of pain processing is extensive and expanding rapidly (Fillingim *et al.*, 2009). Anatomical, physiological, and behavioral studies in animals and humans provide strong evidence that estrogens act on multiple targets in the CNS to modify pain pathways. Three levels of action within the CNS are discussed below for the estrogens to influence TMJ nociceptive processing: 1) Effects on cellular and synaptic function at the initial stage of integration in the trigeminal brainstem nuclear complex (TBNC), 2) Effects on descending supraspinal networks that modulate TBNC activity and 3) Effects on autonomic nervous system function or outflow. To frame this discussion we propose the existence of a TMJ pain matrix

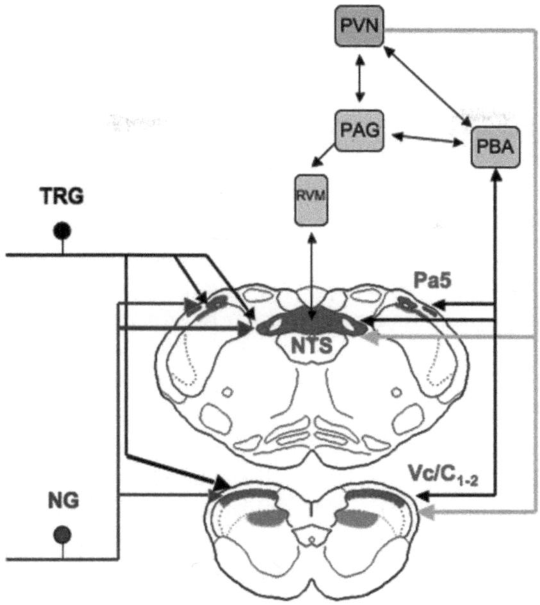

FIG. 1. Proposed model for a "TMJ pain matrix". The proposed matrix centers around three highly interconnected regions of the lower brainstem: Vc/C_{1-2} junction, Pa5 and caudal NTS. These regions share several structural and functional features that may impact TMJD pain signaling and its modulation by estrogen status: 1) Significant direct input from trigeminal (black) and vagal afferent fibers (blue), 2) High density of estrogen receptors, 3) Strong synaptic modulation by GABA, and 4) Significant direct input from higher centers (green) that underlie endogenous pain and central autonomic control circuits. Abbreviations: NG, nodose ganglion; NTS, nucleus tractus solitarii; Pa5, dorsal paratrigeminal nucleus; PAG, periaqueductal gray; PBA, parabrachial area; PVN, paraventricular hypothalamus; RVM, rostroventromedial medulla; Vc/C_{1-2}, trigeminal subnucleus caudalis/upper cervical spinal cord junction region. (For interpretation of the references to color in this figure legend, the reader is referred to the Web version of the chapter.).

(Fig. 1), along the lines of previous proposals for pain integration (see Melzack, 2005; Tracey and Mantyh, 2007). The TMJ pain matrix integrates sensory signals from the TMJ proper and associated masticatory muscles, as well as inputs from CNS regions that underlie endogenous pain modulation and control of autonomic outflow. Although input from higher brain centers certainly influences the activity of TMJ-responsive neurons, for simplicity, the discussion of the TMJ pain matrix centers on three interconnected nuclear regions in the lower brainstem, the paratrigeminal nucleus (Pa5), Vc/C_{1-2} junction and caudal nucleus tractus solitarii (NTS). The Pa5, Vc/C_{1-2} junction and caudal NTS each receives direct input from the mandibular branch of the trigeminal nerve (Jacquin *et al.*, 1983; Nomura *et al.*, 1984; Takemura *et al.*, 1987; Shigenaga *et al.*, 1988; Marfurt and Rajchert, 1991; Morch *et al.*, 2007), in contrast to spinal afferents that first terminate in the spinal cord before ascending to the NTS. Thus, trigeminal connections with NTS are likely to be stronger than spinal inputs since they derive both from primary afferents in TRG and second-order neurons in Pa5 and Vc. Direct trigeminal afferent input to NTS may underlie the marked effects of nerve stimulation on parasympathetic nervous system (PaNS) outflow, described as the trigeminal depressor reflex (Kumada *et al.,* 1977) and clinically as the trigemino-cardiac reflex (Schaller *et al.,* 2009). Second, vagal afferents also project directly to Pa5, Vc/C1-2 and NTS (Nomura *et al.,* 1984; Gwyn *et al.,* 1985; McNeill *et al.,* 1991; Berthoud and Neuhuber, 2000; Ma *et al.,* 2007). Convergence of trigeminal and visceral sensory afferents onto common second-order neurons in Pa5, Vc/C1-2 and NTS may contribute to the high rate of comorbidity for TMJD and visceral pain (Diatchenko, *et al.,* 2006; Maixner, 2009). A third feature is a significant direct descending input to the Pa5, Vc/C1-2 junction and caudal NTS from monoaminergic neurons in the periaqueductal gray-rostroventromedial medulla (PAG-RVM, (Beitz, 1982; Thor and Helke, 1987) and oxytocinergic neurons in the paraventricular hypothalamus (PVN, Sofroniew, 1983; Schorscher–Petcu *et al.,* 2009; Geerling *et al.,* 2010). Two distinguishing cellular features of the TMJ pain matrix are significant expression levels of the classical ER subtypes and evidence of associated local GABAergic control of synaptic function. We propose that an estrogen-GABA interaction at synapses within the TMJ pain matrix is a key feature of the neural network that integrates TMJD pain signals.

Nuclear ERa and ERb subtypes display a wide, generally non-overlapping, neuronal distribution in the CNS with moderate to high density expression in regions that process sensory and autonomic information (Shughrue *et al.,* 1997; Merchenthaler *et al.,* 2004; Vanderhorst *et al.,* 2005; Vanderhorst *et al.,* 2009). Within the TBNC dense ERa staining is restricted to Vc (see Fig. 2b) mainly localized to superficial laminae (Amandusson *et al.,* 1996; Bereiter *et al.,* 2005), while ERb is more evenly distributed across all laminae, as in spinal dorsal horn (Papka *et al.,* 2001). With the exception of the trigeminal motor nucleus, few ER-positive neurons are found in the regions of TBNC rostral to the Pa5 and Vc (Bereiter *et al.,* 2005; Vanderhorst *et al.,* 2005). In general, the expression of ERa matches well with the zones of termination of trigeminal afferents that supply the TMJ region based on transganglionic transport and c-Fos immunohistochemistry studies (Jacquin *et al.,* 1983; Takemura *et al.,* 1987; Shigenaga *et al.,* 1988; Hathaway *et al.,* 1995; Bereiter, 2001; Dessem *et al.,* 2007; Okamoto *et al.,* 2008). Figure 2 demonstrates the overlapping pattern of expression for c-Fos protein after TMJ stimulation (Fig. 2A), ERa-positive neurons (Fig. 2B) and GABA (Fig. 2C) in the Vc/C_{1-2} junction region of the female rat.

Nuclear regions outside the TBNC likely to influence the TMJ pain matrix also express a significant level of ER staining: PVN, PAG-RVM, parabrachial area (PBA) and NTS (Shughrue *et al.,* 1997; Shughrue and Merchenthaler, 2001; Merchenthaler *et al.,* 2004). Although the phenotype of ER-positive neurons has

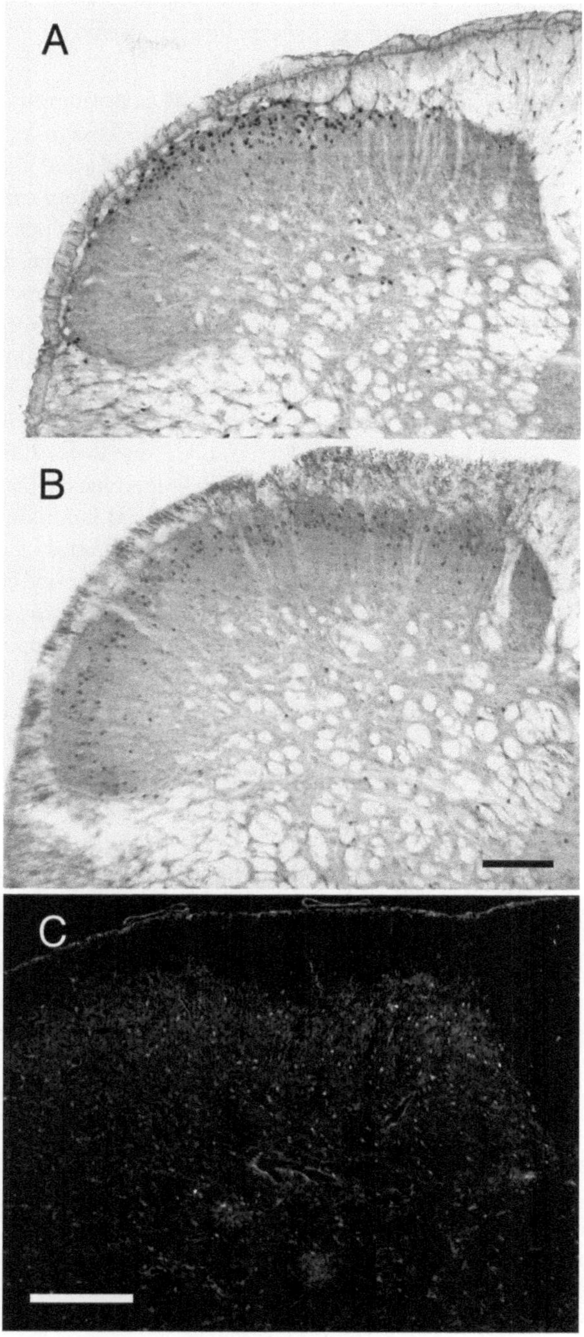

FIG. 2. Examples of staining in the Vc/C_{1-2} junction region of the female rat for A) c-Fos protein after intra-TMJ injection of bradykinin, B) Estrogen receptor alpha, and C) GABA (red). Calibration = 100 μm (A and B), 150 μm (C). (For interpretation of the references to color in this figure legend, the reader is referred to the Web version of the chapter.).

not been confirmed in all cases, co-expression of ER in presumptive GABAergic neurons occurs throughout the brain (Blurton-Jones and Tuszynski, 2002) including the Pa5, Vc/C_{1-2} region and NTS (Vanderhorst *et al.,* 2005; Bereiter *et al.,* 2007; Spary *et al.,* 2010). The estrogen status modifies GABAergic function in the female brain and alters diverse systems such as psychomotor behavior (Lovick, 2006), reproduction (Wagner *et al.,* 2001) and synaptic plasticity in limbic and forebrain areas (Murphy *et al.,* 1998; Nakamura *et al.,* 2004; Kurunczi *et al.,* 2009). A second feature of ER-positive neurons is the high percentage of co-localization in monoamine containing neurons in midbrain and lower brainstem such as noradrenergic neurons of the NTS, rostral ventrolateral medulla and locus ceruleus (LC) and 5HT-containing neurons in raphe nuclei (Herbison *et al.,* 2000; Vanderhorst *et al.,* 2005; Wang *et al.,* 2006; Vanderhorst *et al.,* 2009). The CNS distribution of the G protein-coupled ER, GPR30, is less well described; however, a network of fibers and cell somata is seen in superficial laminae of spinal and medullary dorsal horns as well as the PVN, LC and NTS (Brailoiu *et al.,* 2007; Dun *et al.,* 2009). These studies indicate a moderate to high density of ER-positive neurons in CNS regions associated with endogenous pain pathways and autonomic control circuits. The adaptive functions of endogenous pain modulatory and cardiovascular regulatory pathways indicate a shared central neural substrate, while it has been proposed that an uncoupling of these pathways contributes to chronic pain (Bruehl and Chung, 2004). This uncoupling may be critical for pain conditions that are more prevalent in females such as complex region pain syndrome (Bruehl, 2010), Raynaud's syndrome (Heidrich, 2010) and TMJD (Mohn *et al.,* 2008; Light *et al.,* 2009).

The cellular and molecular basis for E2-induced modulation of synaptic plasticity at the level of the dorsal horn is not well defined. By contrast, estrogen status has been studied extensively in relation to learning and memory, and was found to have marked effects on neuronal structure and excitability (Dalla and Shor, 2009). C-fiber evoked central sensitization in spinal neurons and long-term potentiation (LTP) in hippocampus share many features and pharmacology (Ji *et al.,* 2003; Sandkuhler, 2009). N-methyl-D-aspartate (NMDA) receptors are critical for the sensitization of spinal dorsal horn neurons in arthritic pain models (Schaible *et al.,* 2002) and LTP in spinal neurons (Drdla and Sandkuhler, 2008). In the hippocampal CA1 subfield, 24 hour after exposure to E2 increases were seen in dendritic spine density, glutamate binding, and magnitude of LTP that occur in an NMDA receptor-dependent manner, effects that were mimicked by natural changes in E2 levels over the estrous cycle (Woolley *et al.,* 1997; Smith *et al.,* 2009). High E2 conditions enhanced the NMDA contribution to TMJ sensory processing, as seen by TMJ-evoked c-Fos expression at the Pa5 and Vc/C1-2 junction regions (Okamoto *et al.,* 2008). In neural recording studies, high E2 conditions in normal cycling females or 48 hour after E2 in OvX rats markedly enhanced the activity of TMJ-responsive units in superficial laminae at the Vc/C1-2 region (Okamoto *et al.*, 2003; Tashiro *et al.*, 2007). The enhancement of TMJ-evoked activity under high E2, but not low E2, conditions was reduced significantly by the topical application of a selective NMDA antagonist to the dorsal Vc/C1-2 surface (Tashiro *et al.*, 2009a), whereas estrogen status did not affect the inhibition of TMJ-evoked responses by non-NMDA receptor antagonists. Estrogen status may also affect the availability of glutamate at the Vc/C1-2 region as well as the postsynaptic activity after TMJ stimulation. Microdialysis samples collected from sites in the Vc/C1-2 region of male and female rats revealed similar glutamate levels after TMJ stimulation; however, perfusion of a glutamate-aspartate reuptake inhibitor through the dialysis probe caused a prompt elevation in glutamate in females under high E2 conditions but not in males (Bereiter and Benetti, 2006). TMJ stimulation also increases glutamate concentration in dialysis samples collected at the trigeminal interpolaris/caudal transition region (Vi/Vc); however, this response was blocked completely by inhibition of the $Vc/C_{1\text{-}2}$ region by local perfusion of the GABAa receptor agonist muscimol (Bereiter *et al.*, 2002b). These studies suggest that the Vc/C1-2 region is critical for TMJ nociceptive processing, estrogen status alters glutamate action and/or availability at Vc/C1-2 region and NMDA receptors play a key role in this system.

NMDA receptor activation results in central sensitization of second-order neurons and activation of transcription pathways. Downstream effects of NMDA receptor activation include increased mitogen-activated protein kinase/extracellular regulated kinase (MAPK/ERK) activity in spinal dorsal horn relevant for nociceptive processing (Ji *et al.*, 2003; Kawasaki *et al.*, 2004). Estrogen status significantly influences MAPK/ERK activation in limbic regions (Bi *et al.*, 2001; Manella and Brinton, 2006; Szego *et al.*, 2006) and mediates long-term changes in synaptic function relevant in learning and memory (Fernandez *et al.*, 2008). The roles of MAPK/ERK activation, estrogen status, and inflammation were assessed on TMJ-responsive neurons at the Vc/C1-2 region and showed that naïve rats under high E2, but not low E2, conditions displayed a marked sensitivity to the local inhibition of MAPK/ERK, whereas under inflamed conditions sensitivity to MAPK inhibition was independent of estrogen status (Tashiro *et al.*, 2009b). This suggests that estrogen status and inflammation share a common MAPK/ERK-dependent signaling pathway to influence TMJ nociceptive processing at the $Vc/C_{1\text{-}2}$ junction region. There is also evidence of sex differences in jaw-related nociception, since jaw movement-evoked increases in c-Fos expression at the Vc/C1-2 region requires RDG integrins in female, but not male rats (Bereiter *et al.*, 2006). Limited range of jaw movement and movement-induced pain are common clinical features in chronic TMJD (List and Dworkin, 1996; Svensson and Graven-Nielsen, 2001; Gesch *et al.*, 2004). The amplification of excitatory amino acid transmission likely plays a significant role in TMJD pain; however, other promising pathways have received little attention. For example, C fiber-evoked LTP in spinal dorsal horn involves both the NMDA receptors and

T-type calcium channels (Drdla and Sandkuhler, 2008). Estrogen up-regulates low threshold T-type channels in hypothalamus (Qiu *et al.*, 2006); however, this pathway has not been assessed in medullary or spinal dorsal horn.

Loss of GABAergic function in spinal dorsal horn also contributes to synaptic plasticity in nociceptive processing through NMDA-dependent mechanisms (Baba *et al.*, 2003; Torsney and MacDermott, 2006). GABAergic function is closely associated with estrogen status in several brain regions. In hippocampus, high E2 conditions leads to depression of GABA function, and loss of terminals on inhibitory synapses resulting in enhanced magnitude of LTP (Rudick and Woolley, 2001; Ledoux and Woolley, 2005). In the TBNC a high density of GABAergic neurons are seen in Pa5 and caudal Vc (Fig. 2C) with lesser numbers in more rostral subnuclei (Ginestal and Matute, 1993; Avendano *et al.*, 2005). At the Vc/C1-2 region ~50% of ERa-positive neurons in superficial laminae in female rats co-express either preproenkephalin-A mRNA (Amandusson *et al.*, 1996) or GABA (Bereiter *et al.*, 2007). In male rats, trigeminothalamic (DiFiglia and Aronin, 1990) and trigemino-parabrachial (Wang *et al.*, 2001) projection neurons receive strong connections from the intrinsic GABAergic neurons suggesting a high level of local circuit modulation for craniofacial nociceptors. Systemic administration of GABAa receptor antagonists block TMJ-evoked EMG activity (Seo *et al.*, 2001) and GABA receptor agonists reduce muscle hyperalgesia in male rats (Yokoyama *et al.*, 2007). The role of estrogen status on local GABAergic neurons within the TBNC on TMJ or muscle nociception is not yet known. Cutaneous allodynia is not a common symptom in chronic TMJD (Michelotti *et al.*, 2008; Pfau *et al.*, 2009) suggesting that if estrogen status modulates TMJ input by altering local GABAergic function at the Vc/C_{1-2} region, then it likely involves mechanisms different from the classic view of GABA dis-inhibition in which low threshold fiber input to superficial dorsal horn neurons is facilitated (Woolf and Salter, 2000, Baba *et al.*, 2003). This is supported by recording studies in which high E2 conditions do not enhance the responses of TMJ units at the Vc/C_{1-2} region to brushing the skin, whereas responses to TMJ stimulation are increased (Okamoto *et al.*, 2003; Tashiro *et al.*, 2007).

VI. Estrogen Status and Endogenous Pain Control Systems

Although chronic TMJD pain may be accompanied by changes in peripheral afferent drive and/or central processing by local dorsal horn inter-neurons, considerable evidence supports the hypothesis that recruitment or efficacy of descending endogenous pain modulatory controls are also compromised (Yunus, 2007; Maixner, 2009). The diffuse noxious inhibitory controls (DNIC), defined as a decrease in pain rating evoked by a second noxious stimulus at a remote site, was less effective or even increases the pain in chronic (mainly female) TMJD patients compared to control subjects (Maixner *et al.,* 1995a; King *et al.,* 2009). After sensations, but not peak pain onset, also were enhanced in TMJD patients following repetitive noxious mechanical stimulation (Sarlani *et al.,* 2004) or hypertonic saline infusion into masseter muscle compared to sex matched controls (Svensson *et al.,* 2001). The basis for reduced endogenous pain controls in chronic TMJD is not certain and may depend on the body region of the test site and the modality of the provocative stimulus. For example, in pain-free subject's neck or leg muscle PPTs were elevated in men but not women, after noxious stimulation of remote sites (Ge *et al.,* 2004; Arendt-Nielsen *et al.,* 2008). However, no sex differences were seen for masseter muscle PPT after noxious stimulation of the forehead (Wang *et al.,* 2010) or intraoral pain threshold after noxious stimulation of the hand (Baad-Hansen *et al.,* 2005).

Two mechanisms to explain group differences in pain sensitivity in chronic TMJD patients are altered opioidergic transmission and cardiovascular/autonomic regulation, both of which are well established as factors that influence pain sensation. Mental stress-evoked increases in beta-endorphin were positively correlated with ischemic pain tolerance in pain-free women, but negatively correlated in female TMJD patients, while pain free men displayed no correlation (Bragdon *et al.,* 2002). Pain-free men also had a strong negative correlation between systolic blood pressure and ischemic pain thresholds and tolerance, while pain-free women displayed no correlation and female TMJD patients displayed a positive correlation. These data suggested that in pain-free subjects, men rely more on autonomic mechanisms to modulate pain while women rely more on endogenous opioidergic transmission; however, the ability to recruit autonomic controls via opioid pathways may be deficient in female TMJD patients. This notion was suggested by an earlier study in which ischemic pain tolerance in TMJD patients was not affected by naloxone, whereas pain-free controls displayed a significant decrease (Maixner *et al.,* 1995b).

There is an extensive literature supporting a significant relationship between estrogen status and opioidergic mechanisms in pain processing at the cellular as well as systems level (see Craft *et al.,* 2004; Fillingim *et al.,* 2009). At the cellular level, high E2 conditions and noxious stimulation share the common feature of increasing enkephalin gene expression in dorsal horn (Holtzman *et al.,* 1997; Amandusson *et al.,* 1999). This may have significant consequences for E2 and pain processing since a localized increase in endogenous opioids causes internalization of opioid receptors (Eckersell *et al.,* 1998; Trafton *et al.,* 2000) that, in turn, may limit the recruitment of endogenous pain controls or efficacy of exogenous opioids. Indeed, estrogen status significantly affects the availability of endogenous opioid receptors during acute masseter muscle stimulation (Zubieta *et al.,* 2002; Smith *et al.,* 2006). Opioid receptor subtypes display high levels of expression in the nuclear regions of the TMJ pain matrix: Pa5, superficial laminae of the Vc/C1-2 region and caudal NTS (Ding *et al.*, 1996; Mansour *et al.*, 1996). In recording studies in female rats high E2 conditions greatly reduces the inhibitory effects of systemic morphine on TMJ-evoked single units in superficial laminae at the Vc/C1-2 junction in a naloxone-reversible manner compared to units recorded during low E2 conditions. Importantly, the direct application of morphine to the dorsal surface of Vc/C1-2 region inhibits TMJ-evoked unit activity independent of estrogen status suggesting the site for critical interaction between estrogen status and exogenous opioids TMJ nociceptive processing in superficial laminae at the Vc/C1-2 region is outside the medullary dorsal horn (Tashiro *et al.*, 2008). A possible site for an estrogen-opioid receptor interaction in pain modulation is the PAG-RVM, a dominant pain modulatory system that expresses a high level of ERs (Vanderhorst *et al.*, 2005) and opioid receptors (Ding *et al.*, 1996). PAG-RVM outflow is under tonic GABAergic control and differs in males and females (Bobeck *et al.*, 2009). GABA receptor function in the PAG varies over the estrous cycle (Lovick, 2008), a factor that may contribute to the sexually dimorphic aspects of pain modulation in some animal species (Loyd and Murphy, 2009). It is not known that if estrogen-GABA interactions play a role in the conversion of descending pain inhibitory to facilitatory effects that may influence nociceptive processing in chronic pain states such as TMJD (Heinricher *et al.*, 2009).

A second descending pain modulatory pathway, that has received little attention regarding chronic joint or muscle pain is the hypothalamic oxytocin system. The neurons in paraventricular hypothalamus (PVN) are the sole source of oxytocin in the lower brainstem and spinal cord and are markedly influenced by estrogen status (Shughrue *et al.*, 2002). Oxytocinergic neurons project directly to the dorsal horn and high levels of oxytocin binding are seen in superficial laminae of caudal Vc (Schorscher-Petcu *et al.*, 2009). Blockade of the PVN enhanced nociceptive spinal reflexes in arthritic rats (Pinto-Ribeiro *et al.*, 2008), while chronic arthritis elevated oxytocin levels in lower brainstem samples (Millan *et al.*, 1985) suggesting a role for oxytocin in modulation of joint pain. Interestingly, oxytocin-induced antinociception at the spinal levels is reported to act through a GABAergic mechanism in superficial laminae (Breton *et al.*, 2009; Condes-Lara *et al.*, 2009) consistent with the common theme among nuclear regions in the TMJ pain matrix. Elevated levels of oxytocin would be consistent with a reduction in pain severity in chronic TMJD near the end of pregnancy (LeResche *et al.*, 2005b).

The brain regions that control endogenous pain autonomic and endocrine regulatory systems are closely linked and share many features (Millan, 2002; Saper, 2002; Bruehl and Chung, 2004) including a high level of expression of ER subtypes. Psychological stress (Slade *et al.*, 2007) and altered regulation of stress hormones (Korszun *et al.*, 2002; Quartana *et al.*, 2010) and autonomic nervous system function (Maixner *et al.*, 1997; Mohn *et al.*, 2008; Light *et al.*, 2009) are common signs in chronic TMJD. Importantly, other functional vascular-pain disorders, such as complex regional pain syndrome and Raynaud's syndrome also are more prevalent in women than men (Schwartzman *et al.*, 2009; Heidrich, 2010). Several lines of evidence indicate a strong association between the control of cardiovascular function and estrogen status (Miller and Duckles, 2008). Mental stress-induced increases in sympathetic nervous system (SNS) activity varies over the menstrual cycle in pain-free subjects (Carter and Lawrence, 2007), while beta adrenergic receptor blockade causes a prompt decrease in total clinical pain rating in chronic TMJD patients (Light *et al.*, 2009). A genetic basis for adrenergic receptor involvement in chronic pain is suggested by results indicating that variations in haplotypes for catechol-*O*-methyl transferase (COMT), a major catabolic enzyme for catecholamines in peripheral tissues and CNS, predict the likelihood to develop TMJD in women (Diatchenko *et al.*, 2005). Sex differences have been reported for COMT expression in cortical and limbic brain regions of mice (Segall *et al.*, 2010) and acute blockade of COMT alters spinal C-fiber evoked LTP in female rats (Jacobsen *et al.*, 2010). Estrogen treatment reduces the inhibitory effect of parabrachial nucleus (PBA) stimulation on trigeminal-evoked nociception, an effect that is mediated by adrenergic receptor mechanisms (Nag and Mokha, 2004). Estrogens also have long-term trophic effects on central monoaminergic pathways that could influence pain sensation and autonomic outflow. For example, pulsatile, but not constant, administration of E2 increases tyrosine hydroxylase gene expression in NTS and LC in female rats (Sabban *et al.*, 2010). The TMJ and masticatory muscles receive a rich supply from autonomic nerves that often terminate on or near blood vessels (Uddman *et al.*, 1998; Casatti *et al.*, 1999; Kido *et al.*, 2001). Furthermore, E2 treatment increases the density of sensory CGRP-containing nerve fibers that appose small arterioles (Blacklock *et al.*, 2004) and increases the cutaneous receptive field areas of TRG neurons in female rats (Bereiter and Barker, 1980), an effect that was mimicked by chemical or surgical sympathectomy (Bereiter *et al.*, 1980). A close association of sensory nerves with blood vessels in cutaneous (Bowsher *et al.*, 2009) and deep tissue (Brunsden *et al.*, 2007) has been proposed as a pathway capable of causing conscious perceptions. Convergence of autonomic and sensory fibers onto common regions of peripheral blood vessels may allow local changes in blood flow or release of endothelium-derived neuroactive agents to modify sensory nerve activity. The administration of E2 elevates plasma epinephrine and causes hyperalgesia (Khasar *et al.*, 2005) and increases masseter muscle blood flow by a beta adrenergic mechanism (Ishii *et al.*, 2009a). This suggests that modulation of sensory neuron-vascular relations via adrenergic receptors may be a novel mechanism by which estrogen status and stress interact to enhance jaw pain. It is not known if these putative mechanisms impact chronic TMJD pain.

Equally important to craniofacial functions are contributions from the parasympathetic nervous system (PaNS) that is complex, displays unique anatomical and functional features, and may be different in males and females. The trigemino-cardiac reflex is characterized by sudden bradycardia, hypotension, and hypermobility of the gastrointestinal tract (Schaller *et al.,* 2009) and can occur during surgery of the TMJ (Chuong and Piper, 1991; Morey and Bjoraker, 1996). Stimulation of the lingual nerve in rats increases masseter (Ishii *et al.,* 2005) and diagastric muscle blood flow and depends on a relay in superior salivatory nucleus, activation of postganglionic neurons in the otic ganglion and causes a presumptive increase in PaNS outflow (Sudo *et al.,* 2009). The PaNS-dependent reflexes may be organized differently in males and in females, since lingual nerve-evoked increases in masseter muscle and carotid arterial blood flow are reduced by cholinergic antagonists in females, but not males (Ishii *et al.,* 2009b). This suggests a higher level of cholinergic tone to masseter muscles in females, a notion that is supported by studies indicating vagal control of the heart also is under greater cholinergic control in females than males (Du *et al.,* 1994). Since some properties and classes of vagal afferents are unique to females (Li *et al.,* 2008) and vagal afferents influence masticatory muscle blood flow (Ishii *et al.,* 2010), it will be important to determine if this afferent system contributes to sex differences in TMJD pain. The vagus nerve has long been implicated in pain modulation (Randich and Gebhart, 1992). Vagal sensory neurons originating from the nodose ganglion (NG) innervate the TMJ region (Denny-Brown and Yanagisawa, 1973; Uddman *et al.,* 1998; Casatti *et al.,* 1999) and terminate centrally in the Vc/C_{1-2} region and Pa5 (Nomura and Mizuno, 1984; Gwyn *et al.,* 1985; McNeill *et al.,* 1991). The Pa5 is thought to be a critical integrative center for somato-autonomic relations (Saxon and Hopkins, 1998). Vagus nerve stimulation (VNS) modifies trigeminal-evoked Pa5 neural activity after TMJ injury (Yamazaki *et al.,* 2008) and excites Vc/C1-2 neurons with receptive fields overlying the jaw (Chandler *et al.,* 1996; Qin *et al.,* 2001). VNS is commonly used to manage intractable seizure activity and neuropsychiatric disorders (Groves and Brown, 2005; Nemeroff *et al.,* 2006). Clinical studies further support the notion of vagal afferent contributions to TMJD pain since one side effect of VNS is pain referred to the lower jaw (Myers, 2008). Vagal afferents also have been implicated in the pain referred to the lower jaw in lung cancer (Sarlani *et al.,* 2003) and cardiac ischemia (Kreiner *et al.,* 2007), the latter condition being more prevalent in women than men. It is well established that vagal afferents contribute to the cardiovascular and analgesic effects of exogenous opioid drugs (Randich and Gebhart, 1992). A reduction in TMJ-evoked c-Fos staining in TBNC by morphine is blunted by prior vagotomy in males and diestrous, but not proestrous female rats suggesting a significant role for estrogen status in vagus nerve-opioid interactions relevant for experimental jaw pain (Bereiter *et al.,* 2002a). Estrogens may act peripherally as well as centrally to influence vagal contributions to TMJ nociception since nuclear ER (Papka *et al.,* 1997) and opioid receptors (Buzas and Cox, 1997) are expressed in NG neurons as well as in brainstem regions (i.e., Pa5, Vc/C1-2 and NTS) that receive direct vagal afferent input (Amandusson et el. 1996; Ding *et al.,* 1996; Bereiter *et al.,* 2005; Vanderhorst *et al.,* 2005).

Convergence of trigeminal and vagal afferents at multiple sites within the TMJ pain matrix may contribute to the high comorbidity of chronic TMJD patients with gastrointestinal dysfunctions (Maixner, 2009).

VII. Summary and Conclusions

Considerable evidence supports the hypothesis of estrogen status as a significant factor in the development and expression of chronic TMJD pain. Since estrogens act at multiple targets in the periphery and brain and do so through pathways that couple rapid membrane-initiated events to long-term nuclear receptor-initiated genomic effects lasting hours or days, it seems unlikely that a unique mechanism will explain the role of estrogen status in chronic TMJD pain.

To address the issue of central organization and estrogen-dependent modulation of TMJ nociceptive processing, we propose a structural model, the TMJ pain matrix (Fig. 1), comprised of three lower brainstem regions (i.e., Pa5, Vc/C1-2, and NTS) that display strong anatomical connections and share key cellular features. The TMJ pain matrix receives strong input from supra-spinal brain regions (PAG-RVM, PBA, PVN) known to mediate endogenous pain modulation and control of autonomic outflow, expresses moderate to high levels of nuclear ER subtypes and displays evidence of local GABAergic control of synaptic function (Hirata *et al.*, 2003; Boscan *et al.*, 2002; Potts, 2006). Convergence of nociceptor and baroreceptor input onto common neurons in the TMJ pain matrix and its modulation by local GABAergic interneurons may be necessary to reset cardiovascular reflex gain and preserve normal function in the face of ongoing pain. The relationship between estrogens and GABAergic function in the TMJ pain matrix is likely complex. Although there are no reliable pharmacological therapies to adequately treat pain in chronic TMJD (List and Axelsson, 2010), the proposed model identifies key targets in the CNS relevant for TMJ nociceptive processing that could be tested for responsiveness to drugs developed as putative selective estrogen receptor modulators (SERM) in brain (Zhao *et al.*, 2005) or as having sex-specific actions (Gillies and McArthur, 2010). Experimental models for TMJD in animals have been limited by relying on severe joint injury and behaviors that do not assess jaw function. It is time now to move beyond "first generation" injury models, and include features in animal studies that better translate to pain conditions in TMJD patients. The TMJ pain matrix provides a structural foundation to begin testing the effects of factors that may influence chronic TMJD pain.

Acknowledgments

The authors were supported by a grant from the National Institutes of Health (DE12758) and the Office of Research on Womens Health. The authors thank Dr. Z. Chang for assistance in preparation of the manuscript.

References

Abubaker, A.O., Hebda, P.C., and Gunsolley, J.N. (1996). Effects of sex hormones on protein and collagen content of the temporomandibular joint disc of the rat. *J. Oral Maxillofac. Surg.* **54**, 721–727.

Abubaker, A.O., Raslan, W.F., and Sotereanos, G.C. (1993). Estrogen and progesterone receptors in temporomandibular joint discs of symptomatic and asymptomatic persons: a preliminary study. *J. Oral Maxillofac. Surg.* **51**, 1096–1100.

Amandusson, A., Hallbeck, M., Hallbeck, A.L., Hermanson, O., and Blomqvist, A. (1999). Estrogen-induced alterations of spinal cord enkephalin gene expression. *Pain* **83**, 243–248.

Amandusson, A., Hermanson, O., and Blomqvist, A. (1996). Colocalization of oestrogen receptor immunoreactivity and preproenkephalin mRNA expression to neurons in the superficial laminae of the spinal and medullary dorsal horn of rats. *Eur. J. Neurosci.* **8**, 2440–2445.

Arendt-Nielsen, L., Sluka, K.A., and Nie, H.L. (2008). Experimental muscle pain impairs descending inhibition. *Pain* **140**, 465–471.

Aufdemorte, T.B., Sickels, J.E.V., Dolwick, M.F., Sheridan, P.J., Holt, G.R., Aragon, S.B., and Gates, G.A. (1986). Estrogen receptors in the temporomandibular joint of the baboon (Papio cynocephalus): an autoradiographic study. *Oral Surg. Oral Med. Oral Pathol. Oral Radiol. Endod.* **61**, 307–314.

Avendano, C., Machin, R., Bermejo, P.E., and Lagares, A. (2005). Neuron numbers in the sensory trigeminal nuclei of the rat: A GABA- and glycine-immunocytochemical and stereological analysis. *J. Comp. Neurol.* **493**, 538–553.

Ayesh, E.E., Ernberg, M., and Svensson, P. (2007a). Effects of local anesthetics on somatosensory function in the temporomandibular joint area. *Exp. Brain Res.* **180**, 715–725.

Ayesh, E.E., Jensen, T.S., and Svensson, P. (2007b). Somatosensory function following painful repetitive electrical stimulation of the human temporomandibular joint and skin. *Exp. Brain Res.* **179**, 415–425.

Ayesh, E.E., Jensen, T.S., and Svensson, P. (2008). Effects of intra-articular ketamine on pain and somatosensory function in temporomandibular joint arthralgia patients. *Pain* **137**, 286–294.

Baad-Hansen, L., Poulsen, H.F., Jensen, H.M., and Svensson, P. (2005). Lack of sex differences in modulation of experimental intraoral pain by diffuse noxious inhibitory controls (DNIC). *Pain* **116**, 359–365.

Baba, H., Ji, R.R., Kohno, T., Moore, K.A., Ataka, T., Wakai, A., Okamoto, M., and Woolf, C.J. (2003). Removal of GABAergic inhibition facilitates polysynaptic A fiber-mediated excitatory transmission to the superficial spinal dorsal horn. *Mol. Cell. Neurosci.* **24**, 818–830.

Barraclough, D.J., Ingram, C.D., and Brown, M.W. (1999). Chronic treatment with oestradiol does not alter in vitro LTP in subfield CA1 of the female rat hippocampus. *Neuropharmacology* **38**, 65–71.

Beitz, A.J. (1982). The nuclei of origin of brainstem serotonergic projections to the rodent spinal trigeminal nucleus. *Neurosci. Lett.* **32**, 223–228.

Bereiter, D.A. (2001). Sex differences in brainstem neural activation after injury to the TMJ region. *Cells Tissues Organs* **169**, 226–237.

Bereiter, D.A., and Barker, D.J. (1980). Hormone-induced enlargement of receptive fields in trigeminal mechanoreceptive neurons. I. Time course, hormone, sex and modality specificity. *Brain Res.* **184**, 395–410.

Bereiter, D.A., and Benetti, A.P. (2006). Amino acid release at the spinomedullary junction after inflammation of the TMJ region in male and female rats. *Pain* **126**, 175–183.

Bereiter, D.A., Bereiter, D.F., and Ramos, M. (2002a). Vagotomy prevents morphine-induced reduction in Fos-like immunoreactivity in spinal trigeminal nucleus produced after TMJ injury in a sex-dependent manner. *Pain* **96**, 205–213.

Bereiter, D.A., Cioffi, J.L., and Bereiter, D.F. (2005). Oestrogen receptor-immunoreactive neurons in the trigeminal sensory system of male and cycling female rats. *Arch. Oral Biol.* **50**, 971–979.

Bereiter, D.A., Cioffi, J.L., Bereiter, D.F., Zardeneta, G., and Milam S.B.,,Milam S.B.. (2006). Local blockade of integrins in the temporomandibular joint region reduces Fos-positive neurons in trigeminal subnucleus caudalis of female rats produced by jaw movement. *Pain* **125**, 65–73.

Bereiter, D.A., Shen, S., and Benetti A.P.,,Benetti A.P.. (2002b). Sex differences in amino acid release from rostral trigeminal subnucleus caudalis after acute injury to the TMJ region. *Pain* **98**, 89–99.

Bereiter, D.A., Simone, P., and Thompson, R. (2007). Estrogen receptor alpha and GABA coexpression in trigeminal subnucleus caudalis neurons in the rat. *Soc. Neurosci. Abstr.* No. 824.13

Bereiter, D.A., Stanford, L.R., and Barker, D.J. (1980). Hormone-induced enlargement of receptive fields in trigeminal mechanoreceptive neurons. II. Possible mechanisms. *Brain Res.* **184**, 411–423.

Berthoud, H.R., and Neuhuber, W.L. (2000). Functional and chemical anatomy of the afferent vagal system. *Autonom. Neurosci. Basic Clin.* **85**, 1–17.

Bi, R., Foy, M.R., Voimba, R.M., Thompson, R.F., and Baudry, M. (2001). Cyclic changes in estradiol regulate synaptic plasticity through the MAP kinase pathway. *Proc. Nat. Acad. Sci.* **98**, 13391–13395.

Bingefors, K., and Isacson, D. (2004). Epidemiology, co-morbidity, and impact on health-related quality of life of self-reported headache and muscolskeletal pain – a gender perspective. *Eur. J. Pain* **8**, 435–450.

Blacklock, A.D., Cauveren, J.A., and Smith, P.G. (2004). Estrogen selectively increases sensory nociceptor innervation of arterioles in the female rat. *Brain Res.* **1018**, 55–65.

Blurton-Jones, M., and Tuszynski, M.H. (2002). Estrogen receptor-beta colocalizes extensively with parvalbumin-labeled inhibitory neurons in the cortex, amygdala, basal forebrain, and hippocampal formation of intact and ovariectomized adult rats. *J. Comp. Neurol.* **452**, 276–287.

Bobeck, E.N., McNeal, A.L., and Morgan, M.M. (2009). Drug dependent sex-differences in periaqueducatal gray mediated antinociception in the rat. *Pain* **147**, 210–216.

Boscan, P., Pickering, A.E., and Paton J.F.,,Paton J.F.. (2002). The nucleus of the solitary tract: an integrating station for nociceptive and cardiorespiratory afferents. *Exp. Physiol.* **87**, 259–266.

Bowsher, D., Geoffrey Woods, C., Nicholas, A.K., Carvalho, O.M., Haggett, C.E., Tedman, B., Mackenzie, J.M., Crooks, D., Mahmood, N., Twomey, J.A., Hann, S., Jones, D., Wymer, J.P., Albrecht, P.J., Argoff, C.E., and Rice, F.L. (2009). Absence of pain with hyperhidrosis: a new syndrome where vascular afferents may mediate cutaneous sensation. *Pain* **147**, 287–298.

Bragdon, E.E., Light, K.C., Costello, N.L., Sigurdsson, A., Bunting, S., Bhalang, K., and Maixner, W. (2002). Group differences in pain modulation: pain-free women compared to pain-free men and to women with TMD. *Pain* **96**, 227–237.

Brailoiu, E., Dun, S.L., Brailoiu, G.C., Mizuo, K., Sklar, L.A., Oprea, T.I., Prossnitz, E.R., and Dun, N.J. (2007). Distribution and characterization of estrogen receptor G protein-coupled receptor 30 in the rat central nervous system. *J. Endocrinol.* **193**, 311–321.

Breton, J.D., Poisbeau, P., and Darbon, P. (2009). Antinociceptive action of oxytocin involves inhibition of potassium channel currents in lamina II neurons of the rat spinal cord. *Mol. Pain* **5**, 63.

Bruehl, S. (2010). An update on the pathophysiology of complex regional pain syndrome. *Anesthesiology* **113**, 713–725.

Bruehl, S., and Chung, O.Y. (2004). Interactions between the cardiovascular and pain regulatory systems: an updated review of mechanisms and possible alterations in chronic pain. *Neurosci. Biobehav. Rev.* **28**, 395–414.

Brunsden, A.M., Brookes, S.J., Bardhan, K.D., and Grundy, D. (2007). Mechanisms underlying mechanosensitivity of mesenteric afferent fibers to vascular flow. *Am J. Physiol. Gastrointest. Liver Physiol.* **293**, G422–428.

Bryant, C.J., Harrison, S.D., Hopper, C., and Harris, M. (1999). Use of intra-articular morphine for postoperative analgesia following TMJ arthroscopy. *Br. J. Oral. Maxillofac. Surg.* **37**, 391–396.

Bush, F.M., Harkins, S.W., Harrington, W.G., and Price, D.D. (1993). Analysis of gender effects on pain perception and symptom presentation in temporomandibular pain. *Pain* **53**, 73–80.

Buzas, B., and Cox, B.M. (1997). Quantitative analysis of mu and delta opioid receptor gene expression in rat brain and peripheral ganglia using competitive polymerase chain reaction. *Neuroscience* **76**, 479–489.

Cairns, B.E., Gambarota, G., Svensson, P., Arendt-Nielsen, L., and Berde, C.B. (2002). Glutamate-induced sensitization of rat masseter muscle fibers. *Neuroscience* **109**, 389–399.

Cairns, B.E., Hu, J.W., Arendt-Nielsen, L., Sessle, B.J., and Svensson, P. (2001a). Sex-related differences in human pain and rat afferent discharge evoked by injection of glutamate into the masseter muscle. *J. Neurophysiol.* **86**, 782–791.

Cairns, B.E., Sessle, B.J., and Hu, J.W. (2001b). Characteristics of glutamate-evoked temporomandibular joint afferent activity in the rat. *J. Neurophysiol.* **85**, 2446–2454.

Campbell, J.H., Courey, M.S., Bourne, P., and Odziemiec, C. (1993). Estrogen receptor analysis of human temporomandibular disc. *J. Oral Maxillofac. Surg.* **51**, 1101–1105.

Carter, J.R., and Lawrence, J.E. (2007). Effects of the menstrual cycle on sympathetic neural responses to mental stress in humans. *J. Physiol.* **585**, 635–641.

Casatti, C.A., Frigo, L., and Bauer, J.A. (1999). Origin of sensory and autonomic innervation of the rat temporomandibular joint: a retrograde axonal tracing study with the fluorescent dye Fast Blue. *J. Dent. Res.* **78**, 776–783.

Castrillon, E.E., Cairns, B.E., Ernberg, M., Wang, K., Sessle, B.J., Arendt-Nielsen, L., and Svensson, P. (2008). Effect of peripheral NMDA receptor blockade with ketamine on chronic myofascial pain in temporomandibular disorder patients: a randomized, double-blinded, placebo-controlled trial. *J. Orofac. Pain* **22**, 122–130.

Chandler, M.J., Zhang, J., and Foreman, R.D. (1996). Vagal, sympathetic and somatic sensory inputs to upper cervical (C1-C3) spinothalamic tract neurons in monkeys. *J. Neurophysiol.* **76**, 2555–2567.

Chen, C.C., Essick, G.K., Kelly, D.G., Young, M.G., Nestor, J.M., and Masse, B. (1995). Gender-, side- and site-dependent variations in human perioral spatial resolution. *Arch. Oral Biol.* **40**, 539–548

Chuong, R., and Piper, M.A. (1991). Sinus bradycardia related to temporomandibular joint surgery. *Oral Surg. Oral Med. Oral. Pathol.* **71**, 423–425.

Ciana, P., Raviscioni, M., Mussi, P., Vegeto, E., Que, I., Parker, M.G., Lowik, C., and Maggi, A. (2003). In vivo imaging of transcriptionally active estrogen receptors. *Nature Med.* **9**, 82–86.

Condes-Lara, M., Rojas-Piloni, G., Martinez-Lorenzana, G., Lopez-Hidalgo, M., and Rodriguez-Jimenez, J. (2009). Hypothalamospinal oxytocinergic antinociception is mediated by GABAergic and opiate neurons that reduce A-delta and C fiber primary afferent excitation of spinal cord cells. *Brain Res.* **1247**, 38–49.

Craft, R.M., Mogil, J.S., and Aloisi, A.M. (2004). Sex differences in pain and analgesia: the role of gonadal hormones. *Eur. J. Pain* **8**, 397–411.

Dalla, C., and Shors, T.J. (2009). Sex differences in learning processes of classical and operant conditioning. *Physiol. Behav.* **97**, 229–238.

Danzig, W., May, S., McNeill, C., and Miller, A. (1992). Effect of an anesthetic injected into the temporomandibular joint space in patients with TMD. *J. Craniomandib. Disord.* **6**, 288–295.

Davis, C.E., Carlson, C.R., Studts, J.L., Curran, S.L., Hoyle, R.H., Sherman, J.J., and Okeson, J.P. (2010). Use of a structural equation model for prediction of pain symptoms in patients with orofacial pain and temporomandibular disorders. *J. Orofac. Pain* **24**, 89–100.

Denny-Brown, D., and Yanagisawa, N. (1973). The function of the descending root of the fifth nerve. *Brain* **96**, 783–814.

Dessem, D., Moritani, M., and Ambalavanar, R. (2007). Nociceptive craniofacial muscle primary afferent neurons synapse in both the rostral and caudal brain stem. *J. Neurophysiol.* **98**, 214–223.

Diatchenko, L., Nackley, A.G., Slade, G.D., Fillingim, R.B., and Maixner, W. (2006). Idiopathic pain disorders–pathways of vulnerability. *Pain* **123**, 226–230.

Diatchenko, L., Slade, G.D., Nackley, A.G., Bhalang, K., Sigurdsson, A., Belfer, I., Goldman, D., Shabalina, S.A., Shagin, D., Max, M.B., Makarov, S.S., and Maixner, W. (2005). Genetetic basis for individual variations in pain perception and the development of a chronic pain condition. *Human Mol. Genet.* **14**, 135–143.

DiFiglia, M., and Aronin, N. (1990). Synaptic interactions between GABAergic neurons and trigeminothalamic cells in the rat trigeminal nucleus caudalis. *Synapse* **6**, 358–363.

Ding, Y.-Q., Kaneko, T., Nomura, S., and Mizuno, N. (1996). Immunohistochemical localization of μ-opioid receptors in the central nervous system of the rat. *J. Comp. Neurol.* **367**, 375–402.

Diogenes, A., Patwardhan, A.M., Jeske, N.A., Ruparel, N.B., Goffin, V., Akopian, A.N., and Hargreaves, K.M. (2006). Prolactin modulates TRPV1 in female rat trigeminal sensory neurons. *J. Neurosci.* **26**, 8126–8136.

Dong, X.D., Mann, M.K., Kumar, U., Svensson, P., Arendt-Nielsen, L., Hu, J.W., Sessle, B.J., and Cairns, B.E. (2007). Sex-related differences in NMDA-evoked rat masseter muscle afferent discharge result from estrogen-mediated modulation of peripheral NMDA receptor activity. *Neuroscience* **146**, 822–832.

Drdla, R., and Sandkuhler, J. (2008). Long-term potentiation at C-fibre synapses by low-level presynaptic activity in vivo. *Mol. Pain* **4**, 18.

Du, X.J., Dart, A.M., and Riemersma, R.A. (1994). Sex differences in the parasympathetic nerve control of rat heart. *Clin. Exp. Pharmacol. Physiol.* **21**, 485–493.

Dun, S.L., Brailoiu, G.C., Gao, X., Brailoiu, E., Arterburn, J.B., Prossnitz, E.R., Oprea, T.I., and Dun, N.J. (2009). Expression of estrogen receptor GPR30 in the rat spinal cord and in autonomic and sensory ganglia. *J. Neurosci. Res.* **87**, 1610–1619.

Dworkin, S.F., and LeResche, L. (1992). Research diagnostic criteria for temporomandibular disorders: review, criteria, examinations and specifications. *J. Craniomandib. Disord.* **6**, 301–355.

Eckersell, C.B., Popper, P., and Micevych, P.E. (1998). Estrogen-induced alteration of m-opioid receptor immunoreactivity in the medial preoptic nucleus and medial amygdala. *J. Neurosci.* **18**, 3967–3976.

Favaro-Moreira, N.C., Torres-Chavez, K.E., Fischer, L., and Tambeli, C.H. (2009). Peripheral estradiol induces temporomandibular joint antinociception in rats by activating the nitric oxide/cyclic guanosine monophosphate signaling pathway. *Neuroscience* **164**, 724–732.

Fernandez, S.M., Lewis, M.C., Pechenino, A.S., Harburger, L.L., Orr, P.T., Gresack, J.E., Schafe, G. E., and Frick, K.M. (2008). Estradiol-induced enhancement of object memory consolidation involves hippocampal extracellular signal-regulated kinase activation and membrane-bound estrogen receptors. *J. Neurosci.* **28**, 8660–8667.

Fernandez-de-las-Penas, C., Galan-del-Rio, F., Fernandez-Carnero, J., Pesquera, J., Arendt-Nielsen, L., and Svensson, P. (2009). Bilateral widespread mechanical pain sensitivity in women with myofascial temporomandibular disorder: evidence of impairment in central nociceptive processing. *J. Pain* **10**, 1170–1178.

Fillingim, R.B., King, C.D., Ribeiro-Dasilva, M.C., Rahim-Williams, B., and Riley 3rd, J.L. (2009). Sex, gender, and pain: a review of recent clinical and experimental findings. *J. Pain* **10**, 447–485.

Flake, N.M., Bonebreak, D.B., and Gold, M.S. (2005). Estrogen and inflammation increase the excitability of rat temporomandibular joint afferent neurons. *J. Neurophysiol.* **93**, 1585–1597.

Forssell, H., Jaaskelainen, S., Tenovuo, O., and Hinkka, S. (2002). Sensory dysfunction in burning mouth syndrome. *Pain* **99**, 41–47.

Foryst-Ludwig, A., and Kintscher, U. (2010). Metabolic impact of estrogen signalling through ERalpha and ERbeta. *J. Steroid. Biochem. Mol. Biol.* **122**, 74–81.

Frenkel, B., Hong, A., Baniwal, S.K., Coetzee, G.A., Ohlsson, C., Khalid, O., and Gabet, Y. (2010). Regulation of adult bone turnover by sex steroids. *J. Cell Physiol.* **224**, 305–310.

Galal, N., El Beialy, W., Deyama, Y., Yoshimura, Y., Yoshikawa, T., Suzuki, K., and Totsuka, Y. (2008). Effect of estrogen on bone resorption and inflammation in the temporomandibular joint cellular elements. *Int. J. Mol. Med.* **21**, 785–790.

Ge, H.Y., Madeleine, P., and Arendt-Nielsen, L. (2004). Sex differences in temporal characteristics of descending inhibitory control: an evaluation using repeated bilateral experimental induction of muscle pain. *Pain* **110**, 72–78.

Geerling, J.C., Shin, J.W., Chimenti, P.C., and Loewy, A.D. (2010). Paraventricular hypothalamic nucleus: axonal projections to the brainstem. *J. Comp. Neurol.* **518**, 1460–1499.

Gesch, D., Bernhardt, O., Alte, D., Schwahn, C., Kocher, T., John, U., and Hensel, E. (2004). Prevalence of signs and symptoms of temporomandibular disorders in an urban and rural German population: results of a population-based study of health in Pomerania. *Quintessence Int.* **35**, 143–150.

Gillies, G.E., and McArthur, S. (2010). Estrogen actions in the brain and the basis for differential action in men and women: a case for sex-specific medicines. *Pharmacol. Rev.* **62**, 155–198.

Ginestal, E., and Matute, C. (1993). Gamma-aminobutyric acid-immunoreactive neurons in the rat trigeminal nuclei. *Histochemistry* **99**, 49–55.

Goncalves, D.A., Dal Fabbro, A.L., Campos, J.A., Bigal, M.E., and Speciali, J.G. (2010). Symptoms of temporomandibular disorders in the population: an epidemiological study. *J. Orofac. Pain* **24**, 270–278.

Groves, D.A., and Brown, V.J. (2005). Vagal nerve stimulation: a review of its applications and potential mechanisms that mediate its clinical effects. *Neurosci. Biobehav. Rev.* **29**, 493–500.

Gruber, C.J., Tschugguel, W., Schneeberger, C., and Huber, J.C. (2002). Production and actions of estrogens. *New Engl. J. Med.* **346**, 340–352.

Grundt, A., Grundt, C., Knoth, K., and Lemmer, B. (2010). Rhythmic supplementation of 17beta-estradiol according to the physiological estrous cycle: effect on blood pressure in female ovariectomized Rats. *Horm. Metab. Res.* **42**, 130–136.

Gwyn, D.G., Leslie, R.A., and Hopkins, D.A. (1985). Observations on the afferent and efferent organization of the vagus nerve and the innervation of the stomach in the squirrel monkey. *J. Comp. Neurol.* **239**, 163–175.

Hashem, G., Zhang, Q., Hayami, T., Chen, J., Wang, W., and Kapila, S. (2006). Relaxin and beta-estradiol modulate targeted matrix degradation in specific synovial joint fibrocartilages: progesterone prevents matrix loss. *Arthritis. Res. Ther.* **8**, R98.

Hathaway, C.B., Hu, J.W., and Bereiter, D.A. (1995). Distribution of Fos-like immunoreactivity in the caudal brainstem of the rat following noxious chemical stimulation of the temporomandibular joint. *J. Comp. Neurol* **356**, 444–456.

Heidrich, H. (2010). Functional vascular diseases: Raynaud's syndrome, acrocyanosis and erythromelalgia. *Vasa* **39**, 33–41.

Heinricher, M.M., Tavares, I., Leith, J.L., and Lumb, B.M. (2009). Descending control of nociception: Specificity, recruitment and plasticity. *Brain Res. Rev.* **60**, 214–225.

Henry, C.H., Tull, G.T., Whittum-Hudson, J.A., and Wolford, L.M. (2008). Analysis of estrogen binding sites of the posterior ligament of the human TMJ. *Oral Surg. Oral Med. Oral Pathol. Oral Radiol. Endod.* **105**, 698–701.

Herbison, A.E., Simonian, S.X., Thanky, N.R., and Bicknell, R.J. (2000). Oestrogen modulation of noradrenaline neurotransmission. *Novartis. Found Symp.* **230**(74-85); 85–93 discussion.

Hirata, H., Okamoto, K., and Bereiter, D.A. (2003). $GABA_A$ receptor activation modulates corneal unit activity in rostral and caudal portions of trigeminal subnucleus caudalis. *J. Neurophysiol.* **90**, 2837–2849.

Hollins, M., Harper, D., Gallagher, S., Owings, E.W., Lim, P.F., Miller, V., Siddiqi, M.Q., and Maixner, W. (2009). Perceived intensity and unpleasantness of cutaneous and auditory stimuli: an evaluation of the generalized hypervigilance hypothesis. *Pain* **141**, 215–221.

Hollins, M., Sigurdsson, A., Fillingim, L., and Goble, A.K. (1996). Vibrotactile threshold is elevated in temporomandibular disorders. *Pain* **67**, 89–96.

Hollins, M., Sigurdsson, A., and Morris, K.A. (2001). Local vibrotactile and pain sensitivities are negatively related in temporomandibular disorders. *J. Pain* **2**, 46–56.

Holtzman, D.A., Brooks, P.J., Pfaff, D.W., and Schwartz-Giblin, S. (1997). Preproenkephalin mRNA is regulated by an interaction between steroid hormones and nociceptive stimulation. *J. Neuroendocrinol.* **9**, 913–922.

Huang, G.J., LeResche, L., Critchlow, C.W., Martin, M.D., and Drangsholt MT,,Drangsholt MT. (2002). Risk factors for diagnostic subgroups of painful temporomandibular disorders (TMD). *J. Dent. Res.* **8**, 284–288.

Ishii, H., Niioka, T., and Izumi, H. (2009a). Circulating adrenaline released by sympathoadrenal activation elicits acute vasodilatation in the rat masseter muscle. *Arch. Oral Biol.* **54**, 486–494.

Ishii, H., Niioka, T., and Izumi, H. (2009b). Difference between male and female rats in cholinergic activity of parasympathetic vasodilatation in the masseter muscle. *Arch. Oral Biol.* **54**, 533–542.

Ishii, H., Niioka, T., and Izumi, H. (2010). Vagal visceral inputs to the nucleus of the solitary tract: involvement in a parasympathetic reflex vasodilator pathway in the rat masseter muscle. *Brain Res.* **1312**, 41–53.

Ishii, H., Niioka, T., Sudo, E., and Izumi, H. (2005). Evidence for parasympathetic vasodilator fibres in the rat masseter muscle. *J. Physiol.* **569**, 617–629.

Isong, U., Gansky, S.A., and Plesh, O. (2008). Temporomandibular joint and muscle disorder-type pain in U.S. adults: the National Health Interview Survey. *J. Orofac. Pain* **22**, 317–322.

Isselee, H., Laat, A.D., Mot, B.D., and Lysens, R. (2002). Pressure-pain threshold variation in temporomandibular disorder myalgia over the course of the menstrual cycle. *J. Orofac. Pain* **16**, 105–117.

Jacobsen, L.M., Eriksen, G.S., Pedersen, L.M., and Gjerstad, J. (2010). Catechol-O-methyltransferase (COMT) inhibition reduces spinal nociceptive activity. *Neurosci. Lett.* **473**, 212–215.

Jacquin, M.F., Semba, K., Egger, M.D., and Rhoades, R.W. (1983). Organization of HRP-labeled trigeminal mandibular primary afferent neurons in the rat. *J. Comp. Neurol.* **215**, 397–420.

Ji, R.R., Kohno, T., Moore, K.A., and Woolf, C.J. (2003). Central sensitization and LTP: do pain and memory share similar mechanisms? *Trends. Neurosci.* **26**, 696–705.

John, M.T., Miglioretti, D.L., LeResche, L., Von Korff, M., and Critchlow, C.W. (2003). Widespread pain as a risk factor for dysfunctional temporomandibular disorder pain. *Pain* **102**, 257–263.

Kang, S.C., Lee, D.G., Choi, J.H., Kim, S.T., Kim, Y.K., and Ahn, H.J. (2007). Association between estrogen receptor polymorphism and pain susceptibility in female temporomandibular joint osteoarthritis patients. *Int. J. Oral. Maxillofac. Surg.* **36**, 391–394.

Katusic, S., Williams, D.B., Beard, C.M., Bergstralh, E.J., and Kurland, L.T. (1991). Epidemiology and clinical features of idopathic trigeminal neuralgia and glossopharyngeal neuralgia: Similarities and differences, Rochester, Minnesota, 1945-1984. *Neuroepidemiology* **10**, 276–281.

Kawasaki, Y., Kohno, T., Zhuang, Z.Y., Brenner, G.J., Wang, H., Van Der Meer, C., Befort, K., Woolf, C.J., and Ji, R.R. (2004). Ionotropic and metabotropic receptors, protein kinase A, protein kinase C, and Src contribute to C-fiber-induced ERK activation and cAMP response element-binding protein phosphorylation in dorsal horn neurons, leading to central sensitization. *J. Neurosci.* **24**, 8310–8321.

Khasar, S.G., Dina, O.A., Green, P.G., and Levine, J.D. (2005). Estrogen regulates adrenal medullary function producing sexual dimorphism in nociceptive threshold and beta-adrenergic receptor-mediated hyperalgesia in the rat. *Eur. J. Neurosci.* **21**, 3379–3386.

Kido, M.A., Kiyoshima, T., Ibuki, T., Shimizu, S., Kondo, T., Terada, Y., and Tanaka, T. (1995). A topographical and ultrastructural study of sensory trigeminal nerve endings in the rat temporomandibular joint as demonstrated by anterograde transport of wheat germ agglutinin-horseradish peroxidase (WGA-HRP). *J. Dent. Res.* **74**, 1353–1359.

Kido, M.A., Kondo, T., Ayasaka, N., Terada, Y., and Tanaka, T. (1991). The peripheral distribution of trigeminal nerve fibres in the rat temporomandibular joint studied by an anterograde axonal transport method with wheat germ agglutinin-horseradish peroxidase. *Arch. Oral Biol.* **36**, 397–400.

Kido, M.A., Zhang, J.Q., Muroya, H., Yamaza, T., Terada, Y., and Tanaka, T. (2001). Topography and distribution of symapthetic nerve fibers in the rat temporomandibular joint: immunocytochemistry and ultrastructure. *Anat. Embryol.* **203**, 357–366.

King, C.D., Wong, F., Currie, T., Mauderli, A.P., Fillingim, R.B., and Riley 3rd, J.L. (2009). Deficiency in endogenous modulation of prolonged heat pain in patients with Irritable Bowel Syndrome and Temporomandibular Disorder. *Pain* **143**, 172–178.

Komiyama, O., Wang, K., Svensson, P., Arendt-Nielsen, L., and De Laat, A. (2005). Gender difference in masseteric exteroceptive suppression period and pain perception. *Clin. Neurophysiol.* **116**, 2599–2605.

Korszun, A., Young, E.A., Singer, K., Carlson, N.E., Brown, M.B., and Crofford, L. (2002). Basal circadian cortisol secretion in women with temporomandibular disorders. *J. Dent. Res.* **81**, 279–283.

Kramer, P.R., and Bellinger, L.L. (2009). The effects of cycling levels of 17{beta}-estradiol and progesterone on the magnitude of temporomandibular joint (TMJ)-induced nociception. *Endocrinology* **150**, 3680–3689.

Kreiner, M., Okeson, J.P., Michelis, V., Lujambio, M., and Isberg, A. (2007). Craniofacial pain as the sole symptom of cardiac ischemia: a prospective multicenter study. *J. Am. Dent. Assoc.* **138**, 74–79.

Kumada, M., Dampney, R.A.L., and Reis, D.J. (1977). The trigeminal depressor response: a novel vasodepressor response originating from the trigeminal system. *Brain Res.* **119**, 305–326.

Kurunczi, A., Hoyk, Z., Csakvari, E., Gyenes, A., and Parducz, A. (2009). 17beta-Estradiol-induced remodeling of GABAergic axo-somatic synapses on estrogen receptor expressing neurons in the anteroventral periventricular nucleus of adult female rats. *Neuroscience* **158**, 553–557.

Landi, N., Lombardi, I., Manfredini, D., Casarosa, E., Biondi, K., Gabbanini, M., and Bosco, M. (2005). Sexual hormone serum levels and temporomandibular disorders. A preliminary study. *Gynecol. Endocrinol.* **20**, 99–103.

LeDoux, V.A., and Woolley, C.S. (2005). Evidence that disinhibition is associated with a decrease in number of vesicles available for release at inhibitory synapses. *J. Neurosci.* **25**, 971–976.

LeResche, L. (1997). Epidemiology of temporomandibular disorders: implications for the investigation of etiological factors. *Crit. Rev. Oral Biol. Med.* **8**, 291–305.

LeResche, L., Mancl, L., Sherman, J.J., Gandara, B., and Dworkin, S.F. (2003). Changes in temporomandibular pain and other symptoms across the menstrual cycle. *Pain* **106**, 253–261.

LeResche, L., Mancl, L.A., Drangsholt, M.T., Saunders, K., and Korff, M.V. (2005a). Relationship of pain and symptoms to pubertal development in adolescents. *Pain* **118**, 201–209.

LeResche, L., Saunders, K., Korff, M.R.V., Barlow, W., and Dworkin, S.F. (1997). Use of exogenous hormones and risk of temporomandibular disorder pain. *Pain* **69**, 153–160.

LeResche, L., Sherman, J.J., Huggins, K., Saunders, K., Mancl, L.A., Lentz, G., and Dworkin SF,, Dworkin SF. (2005b). Musculoskeletal orofacial pain and other signs and symptoms of temporomandibular disorders during pregnancy: a prospective study. *J. Orofac. Pain* **19**, 193–201.

Levin, E.R. (2009). G protein-coupled receptor 30: estrogen receptor or collaborator? *Endocrinology* **150**, 1563–1565.

Li, B.Y., Qiao, G.F., Feng, B., Zhao, R.B., Lu, Y.J., and Schild, J.H. (2008). Electrophysiological and neuroanatomical evidence of sexual dimorphism in aortic baroreceptor and vagal afferents in rat. *Am. J. Physiol. Regul. Integr. Comp. Physiol.* **295**, R1301–1310.

Light, K.C., Bragdon, E.E., Grewen, K.M., Brownley, K.A., Girdler, S.S., and Maixner, W. (2009). Adrenergic dysregulation and pain with and without acute beta-blockade in women with fibromyalgia and temporomandibular disorder. *J. Pain.* **10**, 542–552.

Lipton, J.A., Ship, J.A., and Larach-Robinson, D. (1993). Estimated prevalence and distribution of reported orofacial pain in the United States. *J. Am. Dent. Assoc.* **124**, 115–121.

List, T., and Axelsson, S. (2010). Management of TMD: evidence from systematic reviews and meta-analyses. *J. Oral. Rehabil.* **37**, 430–451.

List, T., and Dworkin, S.F. (1996). Comparing TMD diagnoses, clinical findings at Swedish, US TMD centers using research diagnostic criteria for temporomandibular disorders. *J. Orofac. Pain.* **10**, 240–253.

List, T., Leijon, G., Helkimo, M., Oster, A., Dworkin, S.F., and Svensson, P. (2007). Clinical findings and psychosocial factors in patients with atypical odontalgia: a case-control study. *J. Orofac. Pain* **21**, 89–98.

List, T., Tegelberg, A., Haraldson, T., and Isacsson, G. (2001). Intra-articular morphine as analgesic in temporomandibular joint arthralgia/osteoarthritis. *Pain* **94**, 275–282.

Liuzzi, F.J., Scoville, S.A., and Bufton, S.M. (1999a). Long-term estrogen replacement coordinately decreases trkA and beta-PPT mRNA levels in dorsal root ganglion neurons. *Exp. Neurol.* **155**, 260–267.

Liuzzi, F.J., Scoville, S.A., and Bufton, S.M. (1999b). Effects of short-term estrogen replacement on trkA mRNA levels in axotomized dorsal root ganglion neurons. *Exp. Neurol.* **159**, 433–440.

Liverman, C.S., Brown, J.W., Sandhir, R., McCarson, K.E., and Berman, N.E. (2009). Role of the oestrogen receptors GPR30 and ERalpha in peripheral sensitization: relevance to trigeminal pain disorders in women. *Cephalalgia* **29**, 729–741.

Lovick, T.A. (2006). Plasticity of GABAA receptor subunit expression during the oestrous cycle of the rat: implications for premenstrual syndrome in women. *Exp. Physiol.* **91**, 655–660.

Lovick, T.A. (2008). GABA in the female brain – oestrous cycle-related changes in GABAergic function in the periaqueductal grey matter. *Pharmacol. Biochem. Behav.* **90**, 43–50.

Loyd, D.R., and Murphy, A.Z. (2009). The role of the periaqueductal gray in the modulation of pain in males and females: are the anatomy and physiology really that different? *Neural. Plast.*462879

Ma, W.L., Zhang, W.B., Xiong, K.H., and Guo, F. (2007). Visceral and orofacial somatic afferent fiber terminals converge onto the same neuron in paratrigeminal nucleus: An electron microscopic study in rats. *Auton. Neurosci.* **131**, 45–49.

Macfarlane, T.V., Blinkhorn, A.S., Davies, R.M., Kincey, J., and Worthington, H.V. (2002). Orofacial pain in the community: prevalence and associated impact. *Comm. Dent. Oral Epidemiol.* **30**, 52–60.

Maixner, W. (2009). Temporomandibular joint disorders. In: Mayer, E., Bushnell, M. (Eds.), *Functional pain syndromes: presentation and pathology. IASP Press, Seattle, pp. 55–69.*

Maixner, W., Fillingim, R., Booker, D., and Sigurdsson, A. (1995a). Sensitivity of patients with painful temporomandibular disorders to experimentally evoked pain. *Pain* **63**, 341–351.

Maixner, W., Fillingim, R., Kincaid, S., Sigurdsson, A., and Harris, M.B. (1997). Relationship between pain sensitivity and resting arterial blood pressure in patients with painful temporomandibular disorders. *Psychosom. Med.* **59**, 503–511.

Maixner, W., Fillingim, R., Sigurdsson, A., Kincaid, S., and Silva, S. (1998). Sensitivity of patients with temporomandibular disorders to experimentally evoked pain: evidence for altered temporal summation of pain. *Pain* **76**, 71–81.

Maixner, W., Sigurdsson, A., Fillingim, R.B., Lundeen, T., and Booker, D.K. (1995b). Regulation of acute and chronic orofacial pain. In: Fricton, J.R., Dubner, R. (Eds.), *Orofacial Pain and Temporomandibular Disorders*. Raven Press, New York, pp. 85–102.

Manfredini, D., Chiappe, G., and Bosco, M. (2006). Research diagnostic criteria for temporomandibular disorders (RDC/TMD) axis I diagnoses in an Italian patient population. *J. Oral Rehabil.* **33**, 551–558.

Mansour, A., Burke, S., Pavlic, R.J., Akil, H., and Watson, S.J. (1996). Immunohistochemical localization of the cloned kappa-1 receptor in the rat CNS and pituitary. *Neuroscience* **71**, 671–690.

Marfurt, C.F., and Rajchert, D.M. (1991). Trigeminal primary afferent projections to "non-trigeminal" areas of the rat central nervous system. *J. Comp. Neurol.* **303**, 489–511.

Mariotti, A., Rumpf, D., Malakhova, O., and Cooper, B. (2000). Gender-specific differences in temporomandibular retrodiscal tissues of the goat. *Eur. J. Oral Sci.* **108**, 461–463.

Markowska, A.L., and Savonenko, A.V. (2002). Effectiveness of estrogen replacement in restoration of cognitive function after long-term estrogen withdrawal in aging rats. *J. Neurosci.* **22**, 10985–10995.

McEwen, B.S. (2001). Estrogens effects on the brain: multiple sites and molecular mechanisms. *J. Appl. Physiol.* **91**, 2785–2801.

McMillan, A.S., and Blasberg, B. (1994). Pain-pressure threshold in painful jaw muscles following trigger point injection. *J. Orofac. Pain.* **8**, 384–390.

McNeill, D.L., Chandler, M.J., Fu, Q.G., and Foreman, R.D. (1991). Projection of nodose ganglion cells to the rat upper cervical spinal cord in the rat. *Brain Res. Bull.* **27**, 151–155.

Melzack, R. (2005). Evolution of the neuromatrix theory of pain. The Prithvi Raj Lecture: presented at the third World Congress of World Institute of Pain, Barcelona 2004. *Pain Pract.* **5**, 85–94.

Mense, S. (1993). Nociception from skeletal muscle in relation to clinical muscle pain. *Pain* **54**, 241–289.

Merchenthaler, I., Lane, M.V., Numan, S., and Dellovade, T.L. (2004). Distribution of estrogen receptor α and β in the mouse central nervous system: in vivo autoradiographic and immunocytochemical analyses. *J. Comp. Neurol.* **473**, 270–291.

Micevych, P.E., and Mermelstein, P.G. (2008). Membrane estrogen receptors acting through metabotropic glutamate receptors: an emerging mechanism of estrogen action in brain. *Mol. Neurobiol.* **38**, 66–77.

Michelotti, A., Farella, M., Stellato, A., Martina, R., and De Laat, A. (2008). Tactile and pain thresholds in patients with myofascial pain of the jaw muscles: a case-control study. *J. Orofac. Pain* **22**, 139–145.

Milam, S.B., Aufdemorte, T.B., Sheridan, P.J., Triplett, R.G., Sickels, J.E.V., and Holt, G.R. (1987). Sexual dimorphism in the distribution of estrogen receptors in the temporomandibular joint complex of the baboon. *Oral Surg. Oral Med. Pathol.* **64**, 527–532.

Millan, M.J. (2002). Descending control of pain. *Prog. Neurobiol.* **66**, 355–474.

Millan, M.J., Millan, M.H., Colpaert, F.C., and Herz, A. (1985). Chronic arthritis in the rat: differential changes in discrete brain pools of vasopressin as compared to oxytocin. *Neurosci. Lett.* **54**, 33–37.

Miller, V.M., and Duckles, S.P. (2008). Vascular actions of estrogens: functional implications. *Pharmacol. Rev.* **60**, 210–241.

Min, H.J., Lee, M.J., Kim, J.Y., Cho, S.W., Park, H.D., Lee, S.I., Kim, H.J., and Jung, H.S. (2007). Alteration of BMP-4 and Runx2 expression patterns in mouse temporomandibular joint after ovariectomy. *Oral Dis.* **13**, 220–227.

Mohn, C., Vassend, O., and Knardahl, S. (2008). Experimental pain sensitivity in women with temporomandibular disorders and pain-free controls: the relationship to orofacial muscular contraction and cardiovascular responses. *Clin. J. Pain* **24**, 343–352.

Morch, C.D., Hu, J.W., Arendt-Nielsen, L., and Sessle, B.J. (2007). Convergence of cutaneous, musculoskeletal, dural and visceral afferents onto nociceptive neurons in the first cervical dorsal horn. *Eur. J. Neurosci.* **26**, 142–154.

Morey, T.E., and Bjoraker, D.G. (1996). Asystole during temporomandibular joint arthrotomy. *Anesthesiology* **85**, 1488–1491.

Murphy, D.D., Cole, N.B., Greenberger, V., and Segal, M. (1998). Estradiol increases dendritic spine density by reducing GABA neurotransmission in hippocampal neurons. *J. Neurosci.* **18**, 2550–2559.

Myers, D.E. (2008). Vagus nerve pain referred to the craniofacial region. A case report and literature review with implications for referred cardiac pain. *Br. Dent. J.* **204**, 187–189.

Nag, S., and Mokha S.S.,,Mokha S.S.. (2004). Estrogen attenuates antinociception produced by stimulation of Kolliker-Fuse nucleus in the rat. *Eur. J. Neurosci.* **20**, 3203–3207.

Nakamura, N.H., Rosell, D.R., Akama, K.T., and McEwen, B.S. (2004). Estrogen and ovariectomy regulate mRNA and protein of glutamic acid decarboxylases and cation-chloride cotransporters in the adult rat hippocampus. *Neuroendocrinology* **80**, 308–323.

Nemeroff, C.B., Mayberg, H.S., Krahl, S.E., McNamara, J., Frazer, A., Henry, T.R., George, M.S., Charney, D.S., and Brannan, S.K. (2006). VNS therapy in treatment-resistant depression: clinical evidence and putative neurobiological mechanisms. *Neuropsychopharmacology* **31**, 1345–1355.

Nomura, S., and Mizuno, N. (1984). Central distribution of primary afferent fibers in the Arnold's nerve (the auricular branch of the vagus nerve): a transganglionic HRP study in the cat. *Brain Res.* **292**, 199–205.

Nozawa-Inoue, K., Amizuka, N., Ikeda, N., Suzuki, A., Kawano, Y., and Maeda, T. (2003). Synovial membrane in the temporomandibular joint–its morphology, function and development. *Arch. Histol. Cytol.* **66**, 289–306.

Ohrbach, R., and Dworkin, S.F. (1998). Five-year outcomes in TMD: relationship of changes in pain to changes in physical and psychological variables. *Pain* **74**, 315–326.

Okamoto, K., Bereiter, D.F., Thompson, R., Tashiro, A., and Bereiter, D.A. (2008). Estradiol replacement modifies c-fos expression at the spinomedullary junction evoked by temporomandibular joint stimulation in ovariectomized female rats. *Neuroscience* **156**, 729–736.

Okamoto, K., Hirata, H., Takeshita, S., and Bereiter, D.A. (2003). Response properties of TMJ neurons in superficial laminae at the spinomedullary junction of female rats vary over the estrous cycle. *J. Neurophysiol.* **89**, 1467–1477.

Papka, R.E., Srinivasan, B., Miller, K.E., and Hayashi, S. (1997). Localization of estrogen receptor protein and estrogen receptor messenger RNA in peripheral autonomic and sensory neurons. *Neuroscience* **79**, 1153–1163.

Papka, R.E., Storey-Workley, M., Shughrue, P.J., Merchenthaler, I., Collins,J.J., Usip, S., Saunders, P. T., and Shupnik, M. (2001). Estrogen receptor-α and -β immunoreactivity and mRNA in neurons of sensory and autonomic ganglia and spinal cord. *Cell Tissue Res.* **304**, 193–214.

Pfau, D.B., Rolke, R., Nickel, R., Treede, R.D., and Daublaender, M. (2009). Somatosensory profiles in subgroups of patients with myogenic temporomandibular disorders and Fibromyalgia Syndrome. *Pain* **147**, 72–83.

Pinto-Ribeiro, F., Ansah, O.B., Almeida, A., and Pertovaara, A. (2008). Influence of arthritis on descending modulation of nociception from the paraventricular nucleus of the hypothalamus. *Brain Res.* **1197**, 63–75.

Potts, J.T. (2006). Inhibitory neurotransmission in the nucleus tractus solitarii: implications for baroreflex resetting during exercise. *Exp. Physiol.* **91**, 59–72.

Puri, J., Hutchins, B., Bellinger, L.L., and Kramer, P.R. (2009). Estrogen and inflammation modulate estrogen receptor alpha expression in specific tissues of the temporomandibular joint. *Reprod. Biol. Endocrinol.* **7**, 155.

Puri, V., Cui, L., Liverman, C.S., Roby, K.F., Klein, R.M., Welch, K.M., and Berman, N.E. (2005a). Ovarian steroids regulate neuropeptides in the trigeminal ganglion. *Neuropeptides* **39**, 409–417.

Puri, V., Puri, S., Svojanovsky, S.R., Mathur, S., Macgregor, R.R., Klein, R.M., Welch, K.M., and Berman, N.E. (2005b). Effects of oestrogen on trigeminal ganglia in culture: implications for hormonal effects on migraine. *Cephalalgia* **26**, 33–42.

Qin, C., Chandler, M.J., Miller, K.E., and Foreman, R.D. (2001). Responses and afferent pathways of superficial and deeper C1-C2 spinal cells to intrapericardial algogenic chemicals in rats. *J. Neurophysiol.* **85**, 1522–1532.

Qiu, J., Bosch, M.A., Tobias, S.C., Krust, A., Graham, S.M., Murphy, S.J., Korach, K.S., Chambon, P., Scanlan, T.S., Ronnekleiv, O.K., and Kelly, M.J. (2006). A G-protein-coupled estrogen receptor is involved in hypothalamic control of energy homeostasis. *J. Neurosci.* **26**, 5649–5655.

Quartana, P.J., Buenaver, L.F., Edwards, R.R., Klick, B., Haythornthwaite, J.A., and Smith, M.T. (2010). Pain catastrophizing and salivary cortisol responses to laboratory pain testing in temporomandibular disorder and healthy participants. *J. Pain* **11**, 186–194.

Rammelsberg, P., LeResche, L., Dworkin, S., and Mancl, L. (2003). Longitudinal outcome of temporomandibular disorders: a 5-year epidemiologic study of muscle disorders defined by research diagnostic criteria for temporomandibular disorders. *J. Orofac. Pain* **17**, 9–20.

Randich, A., and Gebhart, G.F. (1992). Vagal afferent modulation of nociception. *Brain Res. Rev.* **17**, 77–99.

Rauhala, K., Oikarinen, K.S., Jarvelin, M.R., and Raustia, A.M. (2000). Facial pain and temporomandibular disorders: an epidemiological study of the Northern Finland 1966 birth cohort. *Cranio* **18**, 40–46.

Reid, K.I., Gracely, R.H., and Dubner, R.A. (1994). The influence of time, facial side, and location on pain-pressure thresholds in chronic myogenous temporomandibular disorder. *J. Orofacial Pain* **8**, 258–265.

Ribeiro-DaSilva, M.C., Peres Line, S.R., Leme Godoy dos Santos, M.C., Arthuri, M.T., Hou, W., Fillingim, R.B., and Rizzatti Barbosa, C.M. (2009). Estrogen receptor-alpha polymorphisms and predisposition to TMJ disorder. *J. Pain* **10**, 527–533.

Riley 3rd, J.L., Gilbert, G.H., and Heft, M.W. (2003). Socioeconomic and demographic disparities in symptoms of orofacial pain. *J. Public Health Dent.* **63**, 166–173.

Roepke, T.A., Qiu, J., Bosch, M.A., Ronnekleiv, O.K., and Kelly, M.J. (2009). Cross-talk between membrane-initiated and nuclear-initiated oestrogen signalling in the hypothalamus. *J. Neuroendocrinol.* **21**, 263–270.

Romaniello, A., Cruccu, G., Frisardi, G., Arendt-Nielsen, L., and Svensson, P. (2003). Assessment of nociceptive trigeminal pathways by laser-evoked potentials and laser silent periods in patients with painful temporomandibular disorders. *Pain* **103**, 31–39.

Rudick, C.N., and Woolley, C.S. (2001). Estrogen regulates functional inhibition of hippocampal CA1 pyramidal cells in the adult female rat. *J. Neurosci.* **21**, 6532–6543.

Rutkiewicz, T., Kononen, M., Suominen-Taipale, L., Nordblad, A., and Alanen, P. (2006). Occurrence of clinical signs of temporomandibular disorders in adult Finns. *J. Orofac. Pain* **20**, 208–217.

Sabban, E.L., Maharjan, S., Nostramo, R., and Serova, L.I. (2010). Divergent effects of estradiol on gene expression of catecholamine biosynthetic enzymes. *Physiol. Behav.* **99**, 163–168.

Sandkuhler, J. (2009). Models and mechanisms of hyperalgesia and allodynia. *Physiol. Rev.* **89**, 707–758.

Saper, C.B. (2002). The central autonomic nervous system: conscious visceral perception and autonomic pattern generation. *Annu. Rev. Neurosci.* **25**, 433–469.

Sarlani, E., Garrett, P.H., Grace, E.G., and Greenspan, J.D. (2007). Temporal summation of pain characterizes women but not men with temporomandibular disorders. *J. Orofac. Pain* **21**, 309–317.

Sarlani, E., Grace, E.G., Reynolds, M.A., and Greenspan, J.D. (2004). Sex differences in temporal summation of pain and aftersensations following repetitive noxious mechanical stimulation. *Pain* **109**, 115–123.

Sarlani, E., and Greenspan, J.D. (2003). Evidence for generalized hyperalgesia in temporomandibular disorders patients. *Pain* **102**, 221–226.

Sarlani, E., and Greenspan, J.D. (2005). Why look in the brain for answers to temporomandibular disorder pain? *Cells Tissues Organs* **180**, 69–75.

Sarlani, E., Schwartz, A.H., Greenspan, J.D., and Grace, E.G. (2003). Facial pain as first manifestation of lung cancer: a case of lung cancer-related cluster headache and a review of the literature. *J. Orofac. Pain* **17**, 262–267.

Sato, J., Segami, N., Kaneyama, K., Yoshimura, H., Fujimura, K., and Yoshitake, Y. (2004). Relationship of calcitonin gene-related peptide in synovial tissues and temporomandibular joint pain in humans. *Oral Surg. Oral Med. Oral Pathol. Oral Radiol. Endod.* **98**, 533–540.

Sato, J., Segami, N., Yoshitake, Y., Kaneyama, K., Abe, A., Yoshimura, H., and Fujimura, K. (2005). Expression of capsaicin receptor TRPV-1 in synovial tissues of patients with symptomatic internal derangement of the temporomandibular joint and joint pain. *Oral Surg. Oral Med. Oral Pathol. Oral Radiol. Endod.* **100**, 674–681.

Sato, J., Segami, N., Yoshitake, Y., Kaneyama, K., Yoshimura, H., Fujimura, K., and Kitagawa, Y. (2007). Specific expression of substance P in synovial tissues of patients with symptomatic, non-reducing internal derangement of the temporomandibular joint: comparison with clinical findings. *Br. J. Oral. Maxillofac. Surg.* **45**, 372–377.

Saxon, D.W., and Hopkins, D.A. (1998). Efferent and collateral organization of paratrigeminal nucleus projections: an anterograde and retrograde fluorescent tracer study in the rat. *J. Comp. Neurol.* **402**, 93–110.

Schaible, H.-G., and Grubb, B.D. (1993). Afferent and spinal mechanisms of joint pain. *Pain* **55**, 5–54.

Schaible, H.G., Ebersberger, A., and Von Banchet, G.S. (2002). Mechanisms of pain in arthritis. *Ann. N Y Acad. Sci.* **966**, 343–354.

Schaible, H.G., Richter, F., Ebersberger, A., Boettger, M.K., Vanegas, H., Natura, G., Vazquez, E., and Segond von Banchet, G. (2009). Joint pain. *Exp. Brain Res.* **196**, 153–162.

Schaller, B., Cornelius, J.F., Prabhakar, H., Koerbel, A., Gnanalingham, K., Sandu, N., Ottaviani, G., Filis, A., and Buchfelder, M. (2009). The trigemino-cardiac reflex: an update of the current knowledge. *J. Neurosurg. Anesthesiol.* **21**, 187–195.

Scharfman, H.E., Hintz, T.M., Gomez, J., Stormes, K.A., Barouk, S., Malthankar-Phatak, G.H., McCloskey, D.P., Luine, V.N., and Maclusky, N.J. (2007). Changes in hippocampal function of ovariectomized rats after sequential low doses of estradiol to simulate the preovulatory estrogen surge. *Eur. J. Neurosci.* **26**, 2595–2612.

Scharfman, H.E., and MacLusky, N.J. (2006). The influence of gonadal hormones on neuronal excitability, seizures, and epilepsy in the female. *Epilepsia* **47**, 1423–1440.

Scharfman, H.E., Mercurio, T.C., Goodman, J.H., Wilson, M.A., and MacLusky, N.J. (2003). Hippocampal excitability increases during the estrous cycle in the rat: a potential role for brain-derived neurotrophic factor. *J. Neurosci.* **23**, 11641–11652.

Schiffman, E.L., Truelove, E.L., Ohrbach, R., Anderson, G.C., John, M.T., List, T., and Look, J.O. (2010). The Research Diagnostic Criteria for Temporomandibular Disorders. I: overview and methodology for assessment of validity. *J. Orofac. Pain* **24**, 7–24.

Schorscher-Petcu, A., Dupre, A., and Tribollet, E. (2009). Distribution of vasopressin and oxytocin binding sites in the brain and upper spinal cord of the common marmoset. *Neurosci. Lett.* **461**, 217–222.

Schwartzman, R.J., Erwin, K.L., and Alexander, G.M. (2009). The natural history of complex regional pain syndrome. *Clin. J. Pain* **25**, 273–280.

Segall, S.K., Nackley, A.G., Diatchenko, L., Lariviere, W.R., Lu, X., Marron, J.S., Grabowski-Boase, L., Walker, J.R., Slade, G., Gauthier, J., Bailey, J.S., Steffy, B.M., Maynard, T.M., Tarantino, L. M., and Wiltshire, T. (2010). Comt1 genotype and expression predicts anxiety and nociceptive sensitivity in inbred strains of mice. *Genes Brain Behav.* **9**, 933–946.

Seo, K., Hu, J.W., Cairns, B.E., and Someya, G. (2001). Involvement of GABA(A) receptor in modulation of jaw muscle activity evoked by mustard oil application to the rat temporomandibular joint. *Brain Res.* **892**, 198–202.

Sherman, J.J., LeResche, L., Mancl, L.A., Huggins, K., Sage, J.C., and Dworkin, S.F. (2005). Cyclic effects on experimental pain response in women with temporomandibular disorders. *J. Orofac. Pain* **19**, 133–143.

Shi, H., Seeley, R.J., and Clegg, D.J. (2009). Sexual differences in the control of energy homeostasis. *Front. Neuroendocrinol.* **30**, 396–404.

Shigenaga, Y., Sera, M., Nishimori, T., Suemune, S., Nishimura, M., Yoshida, A., and Tsuru, K. (1988). The central projection of masticatory afferent fibers to the trigeminal sensory nuclear complex and upper cervical spinal cord. *J. Comp. Neurol.* **268**, 489–507.

Shughrue, P.J., Dellovade, T.L., and Merchenthaler, I. (2002). Estrogen modulates oxytocin gene expression in regions of the rat supraoptic and paraventricular nuclei that contain estrogen receptor-beta. *Prog. Brain Res.* **139**, 15–29.

Shughrue, P.J., Lane, M.V., and Merchenthaler, I. (1997). Comparative distribution of estrogen receptor-α and -β mRNA in the rat central nervous system. *J. Comp. Neurol.* **388**, 507–525.

Shughrue, P.J., and Merchenthaler, I. (2001). Distribution of estrogen receptor β immunoreactivity in the rat central nervous system. *J. Comp. Neurol.* **436**, 64–81.

Slade, G.D., Diatchenko, L., Bhalang, K., Sigurdsson, A., Fillingim, R.B., Belfer, I., Max, M.B., Goldman, D., and Maixner, W. (2007). Influence of psychological factors on risk of temporomandibular disorders. *J.Dent. Res.* **86**, 1120–1125.

Smith, C.C., Vedder, L.C., and McMahon, L.L. (2009). Estradiol and the relationship between dendritic spines, NR2B containing NMDA receptors, and the magnitude of long-term potentiation at hippocampal CA3-CA1 synapses. *Psychoneuroendocrinology* **34**(Suppl 1); S130–142.

Smith, Y.R., Stohler, C.S., Nichols, T.E., Bueller, J.A., Koeppe, R.A., and Zubieta, J.K. (2006). Pronociceptive and antinociceptive effects of estradiol through endogenous opioid neurotransmission in women. *J. Neurosci.* **26**, 5777–5785.

Sofroniew, M.V. (1983). Morphology of vasopressin and oxytocin neurones and their central and vascular projections. *Prog. Brain Res.* **60**, 101–114.

Spary, E.J., Maqbool, A., and Batten, T.F. (2010). Changes in oestrogen receptor alpha expression in the nucleus of the solitary tract of the rat over the oestrous cycle and following ovariectomy. *J. Neuroendocrinol.* **22**, 492–502.

Stohler, C.S., Kowalski, C.J., and Lund, J.P. (2001). Muscle pain inhibits cutaneous touch perception. *Pain* **92**, 327–333.

Straub, R.H. (2007). The complex role of estrogens in inflammation. *Endocr. Rev.* **28**, 521–574.

Sung, D., Dong, X., Ernberg, M., Kumar, U., and Cairns, B.E. (2008). Serotonin (5-HT) excites rat masticatory muscle afferent fibers through activation of peripheral 5-HT3 receptors. *Pain* **134**, 41–50.

Svensson, P. (2007). What can human experimental pain models teach us about clinical TMD? *Arch. Oral Biol.* **52**, 391–394.

Svensson, P., Arendt-Nielsen, L., Nielsen, H., and Larsen, J.K. (1995). Effect of chronic and experimental jaw muscle pain on pain-pressure thresholds and stimulus-response curves. *J. Orofac. Pain.* **9**, 347–356.

Svensson, P., and Graven-Nielsen, T. (2001). Craniofacial muscle pain: review of mechanisms and clinical manifestations. *J. Orofac. Pain* **15**, 117–145.

Svensson, P., List, T., and Hector, G. (2001). Analysis of stimulus-evoked pain in patients with myofascial temporomandibular pain disorders. *Pain* **92**, 399–409.

Svensson, P., Wang, M.W., Dong, X.D., Kumar, U., and Cairns, B.E. (2010). Human nerve growth factor sensitizes masseter muscle nociceptors in female rats. *Pain* **148**, 473–480.

Szego, E.M., Barabas, K., Balog, J., Szilagyi, N., Korach, K.S., Juhasz, G., and Abraham, I.M. (2006). Estrogen induces estrogen receptor alpha-dependent cAMP response element-binding protein phosphorylation via mitogen activated protein kinase pathway in basal forebrain cholinergic neurons in vivo. *J. Neurosci.* **26**, 4104–4110.

Takemura, M., Sugimoto, T., and Sakai, A. (1987). Topographic organization of central terminal region of different sensory branches of the rat mandibular nerve. *Exp. Neurol.* **96**, 540–557.

Tanko, L.B., Sondergaard, B.C., Oestergaard, S., Karsdal, M.A., and Christiansen, C. (2008). An update review of cellular mechanisms conferring the indirect and direct effects of estrogen on articular cartilage. *Climacteric* **11**, 4–16.

Tashiro, A., Okamoto, K., and Bereiter, D.A. (2008). Morphine modulation of temporomandibular joint-responsive units in superficial laminae at the spinomedullary junction in female rats depends on estrogen status. *Eur. J. Neurosci.* **28**, 2065–2074.

Tashiro, A., Okamoto, K., and Bereiter, D.A. (2009a). NMDA receptor blockade reduces temporomandibular joint-evoked activity of trigeminal subnucleus caudalis neurons in an estrogen-dependent manner. *Neuroscience* **164**, 1805–1812.

Tashiro, A., Okamoto, K., and Bereiter, D.A. (2009b). Chronic inflammation and estradiol interact through MAPK activation to affect TMJ nociceptive processing by trigeminal caudalis neurons. *Neuroscience* **164**, 1813–1820.

Tashiro, A., Okamoto, K., Milam, S.B., and Bereiter, D.A. (2007). Differential effects of estradiol on encoding properties of TMJ units in laminae I and V at the spinomedullary junction in female rats. *J. Neurophysiol.* **98**, 3242–3253.

Thor, K.B., and Helke, C.J. (1987). Serotonin- and substance P-containing projections to the nucleus tractus solitarii of the rat. *J. Comp. Neurol.* **265**, 275–293.

Torsney, C., and MacDermott, A.B. (2006). Disinhibition opens the gate to pathological pain signaling in superficial neurokinin 1 receptor-expressing neurons in rat spinal cord. *J. Neurosci.* **26**, 1833–1843.

Tracey, I., and Mantyh, P.W. (2007). The cerebral signature for pain perception and its modulation. *Neuron* **55**, 377–391.

Trafton, J.A., Abbadie, C., Marek, K., and Basbaum, A.I. (2000). Postsynaptic signaling via the m-opioid receptor: responses of dorsal horn neurons to exogenous opioids and noxious stimulation. *J. Neurosci.* **20**, 8578–8584.

Treede, R.D. (2003). Neurophysiological studies of pain pathways in peripheral and central nervous system disorders. *J. Neurol.* **250**, 1152–1161.

Turp, J.C., Kowalski, C.J., O'Leary, N., and Stohler, C.S. (1998). Pain maps from facial pain patients indicate a broad pain geography. *J. Dental Res.* **77**, 1465–1472.

Uddman, R., Grunditz, T., Kato, J., and Sundler, F. (1998). Distribution and origin of nerve fibers in the rat temporomandibular joint capsule. *Anat. Embryol.* **197**, 273–282.

Vanderhorst, V.G., Gustafsson, J.A., and Ulfhake, B. (2005). Estrogen receptor-alpha and -beta immunoreactive neurons in the brainstem and spinal cord of male and female mice: relationships to monoaminergic, cholinergic, and spinal projection systems. *J. Comp. Neurol.* **488**, 152–179.

Vanderhorst, V.G., Terasawa, E., and Ralston 3rd, H.J. (2009). Estrogen receptor-alpha immunoreactive neurons in the brainstem and spinal cord of the female rhesus monkey: species-specific characteristics. *Neuroscience* **158**, 798–810.

Vasudevan, N., and Pfaff, D.W. (2007). Membrane-initiated actions of estrogens in neuroendocrinology: emerging principles. *Endocr. Rev.* **28**, 1–19.

Wagner, E.J., Ronnekleiv, O.K., Bosch, M.A., and Kelly, M.J. (2001). Estrogen biphasically modifies hypothalamic GABAergic function concomitantly with negative and positive control of luteinizing hormone release. *J. Neurosci.* **21**, 2085–2093.

Wang, D., Wu, J.H., Dong, Y.X., and Li, Y. (2001). Synaptic connections between trigemino-parabrachial projection neurons and γ-aminobutyric acid- and glycine-immunoreactive terminals in the rat. *Brain Res.* **921**, 113–137.

Wang, G., Drake, C.T., Rozenblit, M., Zhou, P., Alves, S.E., Herrick, S.P., Hayashi, S., Warrier, S., Iadecola, C., and Milner, T.A. (2006). Evidence that estrogen directly and indirectly modulates C1 adrenergic bulbospinal neurons in the rostral ventrolateral medulla. *Brain Res.* **1094**, 163–178.

Wang, K., Svensson, P., Sessle, B.J., Cairns, B.E., and Arendt-Nielsen, L. (2010). Painful conditioning stimuli of the craniofacial region evokes diffuse noxious inhibitory controls in men and women. *J. Orofac. Pain* **24**, 255–261.

Wang, W., Hayami, T., and Kapila, S. (2009). Female hormone receptors are differentially expressed in mouse fibrocartilages. *Osteoarthritis Cartilage* **17**, 646–654.

Widenfalk, B., and Wiberg, M. (1990). Origin of sympathetic and sensory innervation of the temporomandibular joint. A retrograde axonal tracing study in the rat. *Neurosci. Lett.* **109**, 30–35.

Woolf, C.J., and Salter, M.W. (2000). Neuronal plasticity: increasing the gain in pain. *Science* **288**, 1765–1768.

Woolley, C.S. (1999). Effects of estrogen in the CNS. *Curr. Opinion Neurobiol.* **9**, 349–354.

Woolley, C.S. (2007). Acute effects of estrogen on neuronal physiology. *Annu. Rev. Pharmacol. Toxicol.* **47**, 657–680.

Woolley, C.S., Weiland, N.G., McEwen, B.S., and Schwartzkroin, P.A. (1997). Estradiol increases the sensitivity of hippocampal pyramidal cells to NMDA receptor-mediated synaptic input: correlation with dendritic spine density. *J. Neurosci.* **17**, 1848–1859.

Yamada, K., Nozawa-Inoue, K., Kawano, Y., Kohno, S., Amizuka, N., Iwanaga, T., and Maeda, T. (2003). Expression of estrogen receptor alpha (ERa) in the rat temporomandibular joint. *Anat. Rec. A* **274A**, 934–941.

Yamazaki, Y., Ren, K., Shimada, M., and Iwata, K. (2008). Modulation of paratrigeminal nociceptive neurons following temporomandibular joint inflammation in rats. *Exp. Neurol.* **214**, 209–218.

Yokoyama, T., Maeda, Y., Audette, K.M., and Sluka, K.A. (2007). Pregabalin reduces muscle and cutaneous hyperalgesia in two models of chronic muscle pain in rats. *J. Pain* **8**, 422–429.

Younger, J.W., Shen, Y.F., Goddard, G., and Mackey, S.C. (2010). Chronic myofascial temporomandibular pain is associated with neural abnormalities in the trigeminal and limbic systems. *Pain* **149**, 222–228.

Yu, S.B., Wang, M.Q., Li, Y.Q., Lv, X., Jiang, Y., Dong, G.Y., and Ma, Z.F. (2009). The effects of age and sex on the expression of oestrogen and its receptors in rat mandibular condylar cartilages. *Arch. Oral Biol.* **54**, 479–485.

Yunus, M.B. (2007). Fibromyalgia and overlapping disorders: the unifying concept of central sensitivity syndromes. *Semin. Arthritis Rheum.* **36**, 339–356.

Zhao, L., O'Neill, K., and Diaz Brinton, R. (2005). Selective estrogen receptor modulators (SERMs) for the brain: current status and remaining challenges for developing NeuroSERMs. *Brain Res. Brain Res. Rev.* **49**, 472–493.

Zubieta, J.K., Smith, Y.R., Bueller, J.A., Xu, Y., Kilbourn, M.R., Jewett, D.M., Meyer, C.R., Koeppe, R.A., and Stohler, C.S. (2002). mu-opioid receptor-mediated antinociceptive responses differ in men and women. *J. Neurosci.* **22**, 5100–5107.

MACROSCOPIC CONNECTION OF RAT INSULAR CORTEX: ANATOMICAL BASES UNDERLYING ITS PHYSIOLOGICAL FUNCTIONS

Masayuki Kobayashi[1,2,3]

[1]Department of Pharmacology, Nihon University School of Dentistry, 1-8-13 Kanda-Surugadai, Chiyoda-ku, Tokyo 101-8310, Japan
[2]Division of Oral and Craniomaxillofacial Research, Dental Research Center, Nihon University School of Dentistry, 1-8-13 Kanda-Surugadai, Chiyoda-ku, Tokyo 101-8310, Japan
[3]Functional Probe Research Laboratory, Molecular Imaging Research Program, RIKEN, 6-7-3 Minatojima-minamimachi, Chuo-ku, Kobe 650-0047, Japan

Abbreviations

AI	agranular insular cortex
BDA	biotinylated dextran amine
CGA	cortical gustatory area
DI	dysgranular insular cortex

INTERNATIONAL REVIEW OF NEUROBIOLOGY, VOL. 97
DOI: 10.1016/B978-0-12-385198-7.00011-4

DLO	dorsolateral orbital cortex
EPSPs	excitatory postsynaptic potentials
GI	granular insular cortex
HRP	horseradish peroxidase
IC	insular cortex
LTP	long-term potentiation
MCA	middle cerebral artery
MAPKs	mitogen-activated protein kinases
NADH	nicotinamide adenine dinucleotide
pERK1-2	phosphorylated extracellular signal-regulated kinase 1-2
SI	primary somatosensory area
SII	secondary somatosensory area
VPMpc	ventroposteromedial parvicellular thalamic nucleus
VPLpc	ventroposterolateral parvicellular thalamic nucleus
WGA-HRP	wheat germ agglutinin conjugated to horseradish peroxidase

I. Introduction

The insular cortex (IC) is a longitudinal strip, which occupies the dorsal bank of the rhinal fissure and extends ventrally to the piriform cortex and dorsally to the primary and secondary somatosensory areas (SI and SII, respectively) in rats (Saper, 1982; Fig. 1A left panel). Rostrally, the IC is continuous with the dorsolateral orbital cortex (DLO) and frontal cortex (FC), and caudal IC is adjacent to the temporal and perirhinal cortices. The IC has a unique cytoarchitecture; unlike other primary sensory cortices, such as visual, auditory and SI areas, a large part of the IC does not consist of typical 6-layer structure, which is composed of the superficial layer with less number of neurons (layer I), the layer with small pyramidal cells (layers II/III), the layer with densely packed spiny stellate cells (layer IV), the layer with large pyramidal cells (layer V) and the deepest layer with small pyramidal cells (layer VI). The IC is divided into three regions based on the layer structures: (1) agranular IC (AI), lacking a granular layer (layer IV), (2) dysgranular IC (DI), which involves an under-developed granular layer, and (3) granular IC (GI) with a granular layer (Cechetto and Saper, 1987). These subdivisions of IC lie on the dorsal bank of the rhinal sulcus in a ventro-dorsal order of the AI, DI and GI, though the GI does not exist in the rostral part of the IC (Shi and Cassell, 1998a and b). In other primary sensory cortices, layer IV plays critical roles in bridging sensory information from the thalamic nuclei to the cerebral cortex; layer IV

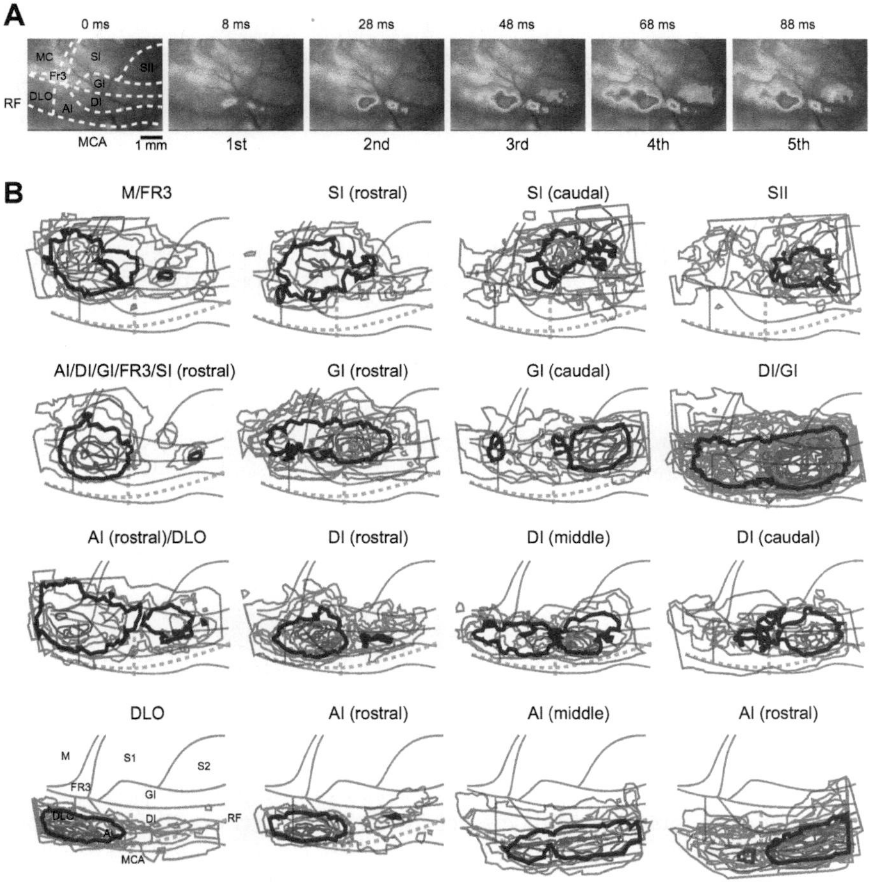

FIG. 1. Repetitive electrical stimulations of the insular cortex (IC) at 50 Hz demonstrated characteristic patterns of excitatory propagation depending on the stimulation sites. ***A,*** An example of excitatory propagation in response to the dysgranular insular cortex (DI) stimulation. Five electrical stimulation pulses were applied at 0, 20, 40, 60 and 80 ms. In the left panel, a template of each subdivision in the temporal and frontal cortices is superimposed on the lateral view of the cortex. ***B,*** Outlines of optical responses are superimposed on the template of each subdivision in the temporal and frontal cortices. Red and blue lines indicate outlines to the 1st and 5th stimulation, respectively. Thick black lines indicate the outlines of excitatory area in which 50% of animals exhibited significant excitation responding to 5th stimulation. Stimulation of the GI and other surrounding cortices such as the motor/primary sensory/secondary sensory cortices evoked round-shaped excitatory propagations, which often extended over the borders of adjacent areas, whereas excitation of the AI spread along the rostrocaudal axis parallel to the rhinal fissure. Red horizontal and vertical dotted lines indicate the rhinal fissure (RF) and middle cerebral artery (MCA), respectively. AI, agranular insular cortex; DLO, dorsolateral orbital cortex; Fr3, frontal cortex (area 3); GI, granular insular cortex; MC, motor cortex; SI, primary somatosensory cortex; SII, secondary somatosensory cortex. (Modified from Fujita *et al.*, 2010.). (For interpretation of the references to color in this figure legend, the reader is referred to the Web version of the chapter.).

receives projections from sensory thalamic nuclei, and is organized into columns, which represent a basis of functional processing in the cerebral cortex (Woolsey & Van der Loos, 1970; Gilbert, 1983; Petersen & Sakmann, 2001; Bender *et al.*, 2003). Therefore, these characteristic layer structures of the IC imply that mechanisms of information processing may be different in the IC, from those in typical primary sensory cortices.

Each subdivision of the IC is thought to mediate its own sensory information processing and has a functional heterogeneity as a whole. For example, the AI participates in nociceptive processing (Jasmin *et al.*, 2003) and autonomic responses (Cechetto and Saper, 1987), whereas the DI and GI are considered to play important roles in gustatory or visceral information processing (Yamamoto *et al.*, 1981; Yamamoto *et al.*, 1984; Yamamoto *et al.*, 1985; Cechetto and Saper, 1987). In addition to these sensations, orofacial movements and thermal sensation contribute to induction neural activity in the IC (Kosar *et al.*, 1986a). Among these sensations, gustation receives much attention and the mechanisms of gustatory information processing in the IC have been studied extensively by anatomical and electrophysiological approaches.

II. Anatomical and Physiological Features of the Insular Cortex

The IC exists in the ventral side of the adjacent cortical areas including the SI and SII. The characteristic difference between the IC and the other typical sensory cortex is that the additional structure, claustrum, exists between the white matter (external capsule) and layer VI of the GI. Previous anatomical studies have revealed that the claustrum connects with multiple brain areas, including the cerebral cortex (Carey and Neal, 1985; Li *et al.*, 1986; Shibuya and Yamamoto, 1998; Zhang *et al.*, 2001) and amygdala (Majak *et al.*, 2002). Functionally, the claustrum has been proposed to exert an important influence on the input to neocortex (Ptilo and Lassonde, 1981; Tsumoto and Suda, 1982; Sherk and LeVay, 1983), emotion (Majak *et al.*, 2002) and propagation of seizure activity from the temporal lobe (Majak *et al.*, 2002). However, little information is available on the anatomical and functional relationship between the claustrum and IC.

The IC is divided into three subdivisions (AI, DI and GI) based on the cytoarchitecture, which reflects connectional features of the thalamocortical projections. Therefore, the IC processes multisensory information, and each subdivision of the IC plays a functional role in a sensory information processing (Yamamoto *et al.*, 1981; Hanamori *et al.*, 1998; Ogawa and Wang, 2002). In addition to the afferents from multiple thalamic nuclei, the IC receives afferents from the limbic structures, and therefore, multisensory information that are processed in the IC, is likely to be integrated with limbic information. In the following sections, I summarize the physiological function of each subregion of the IC.

A. Agranular Insular Cortex

The rostral part of the IC, anterior to the genu of the corpus callosum, is subdivided into the dorsal and ventral AI (Krettek and Price, 1977). The rostral AI subdivision receives projections from the sub-medius and central lateral nuclei and the parvicellular part of the ventral posterior nucleus of the thalamus (Jasmin *et al.*, 2004). Additionally, the ventral part of the medial division of the mediodorsal nucleus, parafascicular and central medial nuclei project to the AI (Groenewegen, 1988; Ray and Price, 1992). An anterograde tracer injection in the rostral AI reveals the projections to the medial division of the mediodorsal thalamic nucleus, caudal AI and amygdaloid nuclei, including the lateral and basolateral nuclei (Shi and Cassell, 1998a). Jasmin *et al* (2003) have also shown that the rostral AI sends glutamatergic excitatory outputs to the amygdala and several nuclei in the brainstem, including the lateral parabrachial nucleus, locus coeruleus and nucleus raphe magnus. Behavioral and physiological studies have demonstrated that the rostral AI participates in nociceptive processing (Burkey *et al.*, 1996; Burkey *et al.*, 1999; Jasmin *et al.*, 2003). The rostral AI is likely to modulate activities of the spinal cord in a top-down manner via noradrenergic outputs from the locus coeruleus, which receive inhibitory GABAergic inputs from the lateral parabrachial nucleus and nucleus raphe magnus.

On the other hand, the caudal AI reciprocally connects to the medial mediodorsal thalamic nucleus, and sends dense projections to the rostrocaudal AI and adjacent DI (Ray and Price, 1992; Shi and Cassell, 1998a). Deep layers of the piriform cortex and endopiriform nucleus also receive dense projections from the caudal AI, suggesting its functional role in olfactory information processing (Shi and Cassell, 1998a).

Besides these projections, the AI neurons project to various amygdaloid nuclei, including the basomedial, central, lateral, basolateral posteromedial cortical nuclei (Ottersen, 1982; Allen *et al.*, 1991; Shi and Cassell, 1998a). The AI also receives dense projections from the lateral and basolateral amygdaloid nuclei. Furthermore, several other limbic structures, such as the medial prefrontal cortex and lateral hypothalamic area, send projections to the AI (Allen *et al.*, 1991).

B. Dysgranular Insular Cortex

The DI is located on the dorsal side of AI and the ventral side of GI. The DI has reciprocal connections with the ventroposteromedial parvicellular thalamic nucleus (VPMpc; Kosar *et al.*, 1986b; Cechetto and Saper, 1987; Allen *et al.*, 1991; Shi and Cassell, 1998a; Nakashima *et al.*, 2000), which mediates gustatory information via solitary and parabrachial nuclei in the brainstem (Cechetto and Saper, 1987; Karimnamazi and Travers, 1998; Bester *et al.*, 1999; Verhagen *et al.*, 2003). The DI receives direct inputs from the parabrachial nucleus in addition to the indirect inputs via VPMpc (Allen *et al.*, 1991). Axons arising from the VPMpc terminate in layers I/III/IV and superficial part of V. In contrast, neurons in layers VI and a part of superficial layer V project to the VPMpc (Allen *et al.*, 1991; Nakashima *et al.*, 2000).

The axons of DI neurons extend parallel to rhinal fissure and terminate throughout all the layers of the adjacent rostrocaudal DI (Shi and Cassell, 1998a). Their axon terminals are distributed throughout all layers of the DI. The AI and GI also receive relatively sparse projections from the DI. The caudal DI receives projections form the SII, suggesting that this region may play a role in somatosensory information processing (Shi and Cassell, 1998b).

Similar to the AI, the DI has reciprocal connections with the amygdala. The DI receives dense projections from the amygdala, including lateral, basorateral and central amygdaloid nuclei (Ottersen, 1982; Allen *et al.*, 1991; Shi and Cassel, 1998; Nakashima *et al.*, 2000). Amygdaloid axons are distributed throughout all layers of the DI, while layers II/III and V neurons in the DI project to the amygdala. The DI has reciprocal connections with the lateral hypothalamic area, but not with the medial prefrontal cortex (Allen *et al.*, 1991).

C. Granular Insular Cortex

The GI receives afferents from the ventroposterolateral parvicellular thalamic nucleus (VPLpc), which receives visceral information. For example, the parabrachial nucleus sends information regarding cardiorespiratory and cardiovascular function to the VPLpc (Allen *et al.*, 1991; Yasui *et al.*, 1991). In general, the primary sensory cortex, including the visual and somatosensory areas, shows a typical thalamo-cortical projection pattern; layer IV and VI receive dominant and sparse projection from the thalamic nuclei, respectively (Herkenham, 1980; Gibert 1983; Chmielowska *et al.*, 1989). In contrast, thalamic projections from the VPLpc to the GI terminate densely in layers III/IV/VI, and sparsely in other layers (Allen *et al.*, 1991; Nakashima *et al.*, 2000). The rostral GI receives axonal projection from the VPMpc with a similar laminar projection pattern as the VPLpc (Nakashima *et al.*, 2000). The GI neurons have reciprocal connections with the VPLpc and VPMpc; neurons in layer VI and deep part of layer V project to these thalamic nuclei (Allen *et al.*, 1991; Nakashima *et al.*, 2000). Functionally, GI neurons respond to gastric mechanoreceptor stimulation (Cechetto and Saper, 1987), though Ito (2002) reported that a part of the most ventral SI, rostral vagal area, also receives inputs from the vagal nerve. Yasui *et al.* (1991) have demonstrated that microstimulation of the rostral part of the posterior GI/DI increased arterial pressure, which is accompanied by tachycardia, whereas stimulation of the caudal part of the posterior GI/DI reduces arterial pressure, which is accompanied by bradycardia. These findings suggest that local circuits in the posterior GI/DI may independently regulate arterial pressure.

Studies using an anterograde tracer have demonstrated that the rostral and caudal GI are reciprocally connected, and they also send dense axonal projections to the rostral and caudal DI and to the ventral part of the SII (Shi and Cassell, 1998a and b). In contrast, the projection from the GI to SI is sparse, though the optical imaging showed a significant excitatory propagation from the GI to SI and SII (Fujita *et al.*, 2010). While a single electrical stimulation of the GI elicits excitation within the GI and DI, repetitive stimulation reveals a functional connection between the GI and the SI and SII (Fig. 1). This phenomenon is functionally reasonable because the GI and rostroventral part of the somatosensory cortex are thought to process similar sensory information, i.e. visceral sensation. The rostroventral part of the SI receives inputs from the vagal nerve (Ito, 2002), which mediate visceral information via solitary and parabrachial nuclei in the brainstem. Interestingly, the tongue region lies between the GI and rostroventral part of the SI, and this region processes tongue tactile, thermal, and taste information but not visceral information (Ito, 2002). Therefore, direct monosynaptic projections from the GI to the ventral SI as well as heterosynaptic cortico-cortical or cortico-thalamo-cortical projections may contribute to the excitatory propagation from the GI to SI. In contrast to the AI and DI, the GI has limited connections with the amygdaloid complex (Allen *et al.*, 1991; Shi and Cassell, 1998a), though the GI receives projections from the lateral hypothalamic area.

In the light of the sensory inputs and reciprocal connections between limbic structures, it is likely that the IC not only mediates sensory information from the thalamus to the higher cortical regions, but also integrates them with limbic information.

III. Where is the Gustatory Cortex?

A. Electrophysiological Approaches

Evoked field potential recording had been frequently used in the early stage of studies to identify the cortical gustatory area (CGA) in the cerebral cortex. Benjamin and his colleagues (Benjamin and Pfaffmann, 1955; Benjamin and

Akert, 1959) reported that dorsal part to the rhinal fissure is considered to be the CGA. Rostro-caudal level of the CGA was considered to be around the middle cerebral artery (MCA) in the DI/GI (Ganchrow and Erickson, 1972; Yamamoto and Kawamura, 1972; Yamamoto *et al.*, 1980). Although these evoked potential recordings provided a gross map of the CGA, precisely how these neurons respond to gustatory stimuli, remained unclear.

Yamamoto and his colleagues have pursued this issue by single unit recording from the IC (Yamamoto *et al.*, 1980; Yamamoto *et al.*, 1981; Yamamoto *et al.*, 1984; Yamamoto *et al.*, 1985; Yamamoto, 1987). The gustatory stimulation-sensitive neurons are distributed rostrocaudally around the dorsal part of the cross point between the rhinal fissure and MCA (Yamamoto *et al.*, 1981; Yamamoto *et al.*, 1985). This region overlaps with regions that are activated by the stimulation of the chorda tympani, lingual, glossopharyngeal, and palatal nerves (Yamamoto and Kawamura, 1979; Yamamoto *et al.*, 1980). In contrast to the properties of neurons in the pontine parabrachial nuclei (Ogawa *et al.*, 1982) and nucleus of the solitary tract (Ogawa and Hayama *et al.*, 1984), many gustatory neurons have wide receptive field (Yamamoto *et al.*, 1984), suggesting that gustatory information in the oropharyngeal region is integrated in the IC. In monkey IC, there are quite a few gustatory neurons that respond specifically to one of the four basic tastants: i.e. sucrose, NaCl, HCl, and quinine (Ito and Ogawa, 1994). In contrast, in the rat IC, most gustatory neurons show relatively broader sensitivity to four basic tastants (Yamamoto *et al.*, 1981).

B. Anatomical Approaches

Anterograde and retrograde tracers have anatomically confirmed the electrophysiological evidence that the IC receives gustatory information. The VPMpc, the sensory thalamic nucleus, which receives gustatory projection from the parabrachial nucleus in the brainstem (Cechetto and Saper, 1987; Karimnamazi and Travers, 1998; Bester *et al.*, 1999; Verhagen *et al.*, 2003), mediates peripheral gustatory information to the IC. Injection of horse radish peroxidase (HRP) into the subregion of DI/GI, which responds to stimulation of the anterior chorda tympani and ventral glossopharyngeal nerves, demonstrates that HRP-positive neurons are found in the VPMpc (Yamamoto *et al.*, 1980). Anatomical studies using HRP and wheat germ agglutinin-conjugate HRP (WGA-HRP), have confirmed the projection from the VPMpc to the CGA (Cechetto and Saper, 1987). Nakajima *et al.* (2000) illustrated that the reciprocal connections of the IC and VPMpc are similar to those between the thalamic nuclei and primary sensory cortices, such as visual and somatosensory cortex. According to their study, projections from the VPMpc to IC terminate in all layers, and layer VI neurons project back to the VPMpc.

Using immunohistochemistry for protein products of immedieate early genes, such as c-Fos, c-Jun, and Zif268, is another approach to functionally map the spatial distribution of neural activity in response to gustatory stimulation. Among these proteins of immediate early genes, c-Fos is one of the most widely used molecules to detect neural activity in the central nervous system. In the cerebral cortex, membrane depolarization results in Ca^{2+} influx via NMDA receptors and voltage-gated calcium channels, leading to the activation of downstream kinases, which increase the transcription of c-*fos* (Kaczmarek and Chaudhuri, 1997). Following transcription and translation, c-Fos protein forms a dimer with Jun and produces AP-1 transcription factor, which results in the production of neural plasticity-related proteins. In situ hybridization or immunohistochemistry of c-Fos and Fos protein synthesis would reveal a spatial distribution of activated neurons in the cerebral cortex. For example, by using immunocytochemistry, Koh *et al.* (2003) and Chen *et al.* (2004) demonstrated that gustatory stimulation induces c-Fos expression in all layers of the IC.

Recently, phosphorylated extracellular signal-regulated kinase 1-2 (pERK1-2) has been used to detect neurons that are activated by sensory stimulation (Boggio *et al.*, 2007; Takamura *et al.*, 2007; Alvarez *et al.*, 2009). ERK1-2, one of the mitogen-activated protein kinases (MAPKs), is thought to be phosphorylated by elevated neural activities. Alternatively, the activation of ERK1-2 may be related to neural plasticity because induction of long-term potentiation (LTP) in the IC as evoked by the stimulation of the basolateral amygdala requires the activation of ERK1-2 (Jones *et al.*, 1999). Berman *et al.* (1998) demonstrated that application of an unfamiliar taste induces phosphorylation of ERK1-2 in the IC. Therefore, the pERK1-2-immunopositive neurons that respond to gustatory stimulation are likely to constitute a neuronal group that is sensitive to gustatory stimulation and neuroplastic changes in response to a change of extracellular milieu. We have examined the spatial patterns of pERK-immunopositive IC neurons that are activated by gustatory stimulation in anesthetized and alert rats (Kobayashi *et al.*, 2010). The application of sucrose solution to the tongue of both anesthetized and alert rats increases the number of pERK-immunopositive neurons, especially around the intersection of the rhinal fissure and MCA, though the total number of these cells was much larger in alert rats (Fig. 2). Most of the pERK-immunopositive cells are layers II/III pyramidal cells, whereas there are few pERK-immunopositive neurons, expressing parvalbumin or somatostatin, which are GABAergic neuronal markers (Kawaguchi and Kubota, 1997). Taken together with the finding that naïve rats expressed more pERK-immunopositive cells than rats that had been exposed to sucrose solution for 1 week, our findings suggest that gustatory experience is likely to influence pERK-immunoreactivity in the IC.

Anatomical evidence supports the physiological findings that gustatory neurons exist around the intersection of the rhinal fissure and MCA in the IC.

However, the mechanisms by which these neurons interact with each other to process gustatory information still remain unknown. In order to approach this critical question, it is necessary to detect neuronal activities in the IC from macroscopic view with high spatial and temporal resolution.

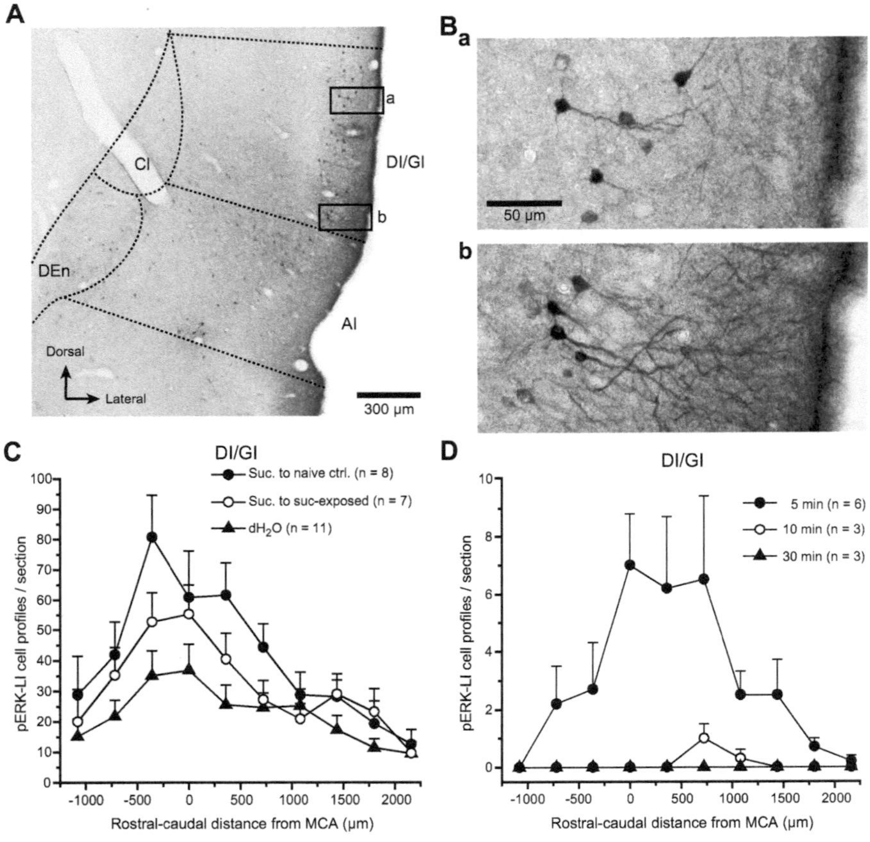

FIG. 2. Distribution pattern of phosphorylated extracellular signal-regulated kinase 1-2 (pERK) responding to 10% sucrose stimulation in the IC of alert or pentobarbital-anesthetized rats. ***A,*** Upper layers exhibit higher pERK-like immunoreactivity (pERK-LI) in the IC of alert rats. ***B,*** Expanded images of pERK-LI cells in the DI/GI in boxes of **A**. Note that most pERK-LI cells were pyramidal cells, with dense immunoreactivity in the somata and dendrites. ***C,*** Spatial profiles of pERK-LI cells in the DI/GI. Sucrose application to naïve controls induced a larger number of pERK-LI cell profiles in the DI/GI. The number of pERK-LI cell profile responding to sucrose stimulation in sucrose-exposed rats which were fed 10% sucrose solution for one week was significantly less than that in naïve rats. Note that the peak for pERK-LI cells existed around 0 μm, i.e. the intersection of the rhinal fissure and MCA. ***D,*** Spatiotemporal profiles of pERK-LI cells in the dysgranular/granular IC (DI/GI). Rats perfused 10 or 30 min after sucrose stimulation showed few pERK-LI cells in the DI/GI. In rats perfused 5 min after sucrose stimulation, the peak site of pERK-LI cells was around 0 μm. (Modified from Kobayashi *et al.*, 2010.).

IV. Optical Imaging Reveals Spatio-Temporal Properties of Excitation in the Gustatory Cortex

A. Limitation of the Conventional Anatomical and Electrophysiological Approaches

Anatomical approaches, using anterograde tracers, such as WGA and biotinylated dextran amine (BDA), have been used extensively to explore the spatial projection patterns from the IC to other areas, e.g. cortico-thalamic and cortico-amygdaloid connections. On the other hand, retrograde tracers like Fluorogold and HRP can reveal the source of projections to the IC as described above. These anatomical studies with tracers have demonstrated the spatial pattern of neural connection in the IC, but nevertheless, several critical questions remain unresolved. Even though the anatomical evidence for axonal projections has been found, the functional impact to synaptic transmission remains unknown. In addition, temporal profiles of excitation or inhibition via synapses are also open to question.

Electrophysiology is a potent method to address the questions raised above. For example, field potential recording has been used to examine the connections between the IC and other brain areas. The electrical stimulation of the peripheral gustatory nerves, i.e. chorda tympani and glossopharyngeal nerve, evoked field potentials in the IC (Yamamoto *et al.*, 1980). These electrophysiological studies have revealed not only the evidence of neural connections between the IC and other brain regions but also their physiological features, such as the magnitude and temporal profiles of the responses. However, there are several disadvantages in these methods. Limited spatial resolution is the first critical problem. Even though several studies have demonstrated the spatial distribution of excitation using single or multi-channel electrodes (Yamamoto, 1987; Nicolelis *et al.*, 1997), simultaneous recording from multiple sites provides only a gross map of the spatial patterns of neural activities. In addition, artifacts of electrical stimulation disturb evoked signals, which is an important consideration when recording from adjacent sites of stimulation. Therefore, unit or field potential recordings are not suitable for exploring the spatial pattern of excitation within the IC.

B. Optical Imaging of Intrinsic Signals

To overcome the limitations in these anatomical and electrophysiological approaches, a variety of optical imaging techniques have been developed to examine spatiotemporal distribution patterns of excitation in the cerebral cortex, e.g. imaging of intrinsic optical signal, intracellular calcium concentration, autofluorescence and fluorescence or absorbance of voltage-sensitive dyes.

Intrinsic optical signals arise from several sources, which are described below. First, as predicted by Roy and Sherrington (1890), neural activity is accompanied by changes in the local blood flow due to capillary recruitment, which in turn leads to changes in light absorption by hemoglobin. Another source of optical signal, the oximetric signal, is due to a rapid increase in deoxyhemoglobin concentration, resulting from an immediate need for oxygen by active neurons. Since deoxyhemoglobin has a different reflectance pattern than oxyhemoglobin, this concentration difference leads to a darkening of the cortex in the active area (Frostig *et al.*, 1990). A third intrinsic optical signal results from light scattering and birefringence that correlate with neural activity (Hill and Keynes, 1949; Cohen *et al.*, 1968). Intrinsic optical imaging enables us to explore functional architecture of the cerebral cortex (Grinvald *et al.*, 1986).

Autofluorescence of flavoprotein and nicotinamide adenine dinucleotide (NADH) have also been used to detect neural activities in the cerebral cortex (Shibuki *et al.*, 2003; Husson *et al.*, 2007). Neural excitation induces Ca^{2+} influx via voltage-gated Ca^{2+} channels and activation of Na^{+}-K^{+} ATPase, which in turn increases cytoplasmic ADP. Intracellular ADP and Ca^{2+} increases lead to mitochondrial depolarization and activation of glycolysis and mitochondrial metabolism, which cause oxidation of mitochondrial respiratory components, including flavoprotein and NADH. Finally, the oxidation of flavoprotein and NADH results in an increase in flavoprotein fluorescence and a decrease in NADH fluorescence (Reinert *et al.*, 2004), which can be used as markers for neural activity and metabolic state.

Although these imaging techniques enable us to examine the spatial distribution of neural activities on a large-scale, the temporal resolution of their signals is not adequate enough to assess the temporal pattern of neural activity, that accompanies excitatory postsynaptic potentials (EPSPs) and action potentials. The earliest intrinsic responses can be detected at several hundred milliseconds after the stimulus onset and persist for seconds. Such temporal resolution cannot assess the distributed pattern of activity that accompanies EPSPs and action potentials. In addition to the temporal limitation, there are potential inaccuracies between these intrinsic signals and neural activities, including the EPSPs and action potentials.

C. Optical Imaging with Voltage-Sensitive Dyes

Optical imaging with a voltage-sensitive dye has adequate spatial and temporal resolution to explore neural excitation in the cerebral cortex based on the following reasons. First, optical imaging with a voltage-sensitive dye directly measures the linearly-correlated membrane potential changes, ranging from ~-20 to + 110 mV, at the level of a single cortical neuron. Such temporal resolution is comparable to electrophysiological measurements (Tominaga *et al.*, 2000; Takashima *et al.*, 2001; Petersen *et al.*, 2003; Berger *et al.*, 2007). On a larger scale, such as *in vivo* preparations, the optical signals reflect the spatiotemporal pattern of subthreshold changes of membrane potential (Petersen and Sakmann, 2001; Berger *et al.*, 2007). Second, simultaneous measurements of the optical signal in multiple regions can reveal the spatiotemporal correlation of neural activities. Third, pharmacological manipulation, by applying drugs to the surface of preparations, enables us to examine the contributions of specific neurotransmitters and receptors to information processing, including neural excitability and synaptic transmissions.

Optical imaging with a voltage-sensitive dye has several disadvantages. The duration of recording is limited due to bleaching of the dye. Optical recordings using *in vivo* preparations only image superficial layers (0-~300 μm from the surface; Fujita *et al.*, 2010). Furthermore, the smaller responses in optical imaging, as compared to the electrophysiological data, require repeated measurements to average data and improve signal-to-noise ratio. Recent improvements in voltage-sensitive dyes and hardware, such as photodiodes and imaging devices, lessen these disadvantages. Therefore, we considered this technique suitable for visualizing excitatory propagation in response to electrical stimulation, which elicited neural responses in the millisecond range in the cerebral cortex.

V. Functional Dynamics of Excitatory Propagation in the Insular Cortex

A. Gustatory Cortex Revealed by Optical Imaging

Several optical imaging studies have elucidated the spatial pattern of IC-activated regions that is induced by gustatory stimulation. By measuring intrinsic optical signals, Accolla *et al.* (2007, 2008) demonstrated that dorsal region of the rhinal fissure around the MCA is activated by gustatory stimulation. They also reported that four basic tastants (sucrose, NaCl, quinine and citric acid) share patterns of activation, based on similarity in tastant hedonic values. An optical imaging study using a voltage-sensitive dye, RH-1691, demonstrated that a similar region of the IC to Accolla's report (2007) is activated by gustatory stimulation, and such activation occurs after SI activation and lasts longer than in SI (Kobayashi *et al.*, 2010). These studies support the previous electrophysiological and anatomical results as described above and extend them to more a precise spatial pattern of CGA. Interestingly, this CGA activation is accompanied by the activation of more caudal parts of the DI/GI (Kobayashi *et al.*, 2010), suggesting a functional connection between the rostral and caudal DI/GI during gustatory information processing.

B. Spatiotemporal Patterns of Excitatory Propagation in the Insular Cortex

To explore the functional connectivity in the IC, an electrical stimulation of 5 train pulses was applied to various sites and optical responses were recorded using a voltage-sensitive dye (Fujita *et al.*, 2010). Train pulse stimulation of the DI rostrally or caudally adjacent to the MCA induces a characteristic excitatory propagation. A train of stimulation at 50 Hz induced an additive effect in the area of excitatory propagation. Excitation spreads along the rostrocaudal axis parallel to the rhinal fissure and frequently propagates into the dorsolateral orbital cortex (DLO) as shown in Fig. 1. This flattened excitatory propagation pattern is observed more intensely in the AI, whereas the GI stimulation shows less flattening than the DI. In contrast, stimulating the border between the IC and adjacent cortices, including the ventral part of the SI/SII/FrC, tends to induce excitatory propagation with a less flattened pattern.

Taken together with the anatomical evidence that there are dense cortico-cortical connections in the IC as described above (Shi and Cassell, 1998a, b), the characteristic pattern of excitatory propagation is likely to be mediated by cortico-cortical connections. Application of DNQX, a non-NMDA receptor antagonist, strongly diminishes excitatory propagation except for around the stimulation site, suggesting that glutamatergic synaptic transmission induces IC excitatory propagation. This is supported by the findings that microinjection of lidocaine, a voltage-sensitive Na^+ channel blocker, into the IC or incision of the surface of the IC inhibits excitatory propagation in the remote site (Fujita *et al.*, 2010).

The characteristic excitatory propagation pattern is likely to play a role in information processing within the IC. Considering the physiological functions during feeding behavior, such as detecting orofacial movements, thermal sensation and gustation, this information should be processed together in the higher brain region. The findings of the dorso-ventrally-restricted excitatory propagation by optical imaging imply a possible neural mechanism, underlying the integration of multi-modal sensory information processing in the IC.

VI. Future Direction

The characteristic features of excitatory propagation in the IC are thought to play critical roles in integrating sensory information, including gustation with emotion. This hypothesis should be explored at cellular level. For instance, examining the anatomical and electrophysiological properties of synapses from the thalamic nuclei and limbic structures to IC neurons will address the essential question of how gustatory inputs via VPMpc are modulated by limbic inputs.

In addition to the IC's roles in processing gustatory information, clinical studies in patients with epilepsy have demonstrated involvement of the IC in epileptogenesis (Isnard *et al.*, 2000, 2004; Ryvlin *et al.*, 2006; Dobesberger *et al.*, 2008; Nguyen *et al.*, 2009), which may be related to dense reciprocal projections between the IC, and limbic structures. We have demonstrated that pilocarpine-treated post-status epilepticus rats show facilitated excitation in response to caudal AI stimulation (Chen *et al.*, 2010). Finally, the mechanisms of inhibition of excitatory propagation in the IC should also be addressed.

Acknowledgments

I thank Drs. Satoshi Fujita and Izumi Toyoda for critical reading of the manuscript. This work was supported by KAKENHI 20592188; Grant for the Promotion of Multi-disciplinary Research Projects entitled "Translational Research Network on Orofacial Neurological Disorders" from the Japanese Ministry of Education, Culture, Sports, Science, and Technology; The Promotion and Mutual Aid Corporation for Private School of Japan; and Nihon University Joint Research Grant.

References

Accolla, R., and Carleton, A. (2008). Internal body state influences topographical plasticity of sensory representations in the rat gustatory cortex. *Proc. Natl. Acad. Sci. U.S.A.* **105**, 4010–4015.

Accolla, R., Bathellier, B., Petersen, C.C., and Carleton, A. (2007). Differential spatial representation of taste modalities in the rat gustatory cortex. *J. Neurosci.* **27**, 1396–1404.

Allen, G.V., Saper, C.B., Hurley, K.M., and Cechetto, D.F. (1991). Organization of visceral and limbic connections in the insular cortex of the rat. *J. Comp. Neurol.* **311**, 11–16.

Alvarez, P., Dieb, W., Hafidi, A., Voisin, D.L., and Dallel, R. (2009). Insular cortex representation of dynamic mechanical allodynia in trigeminal neuropathic rats. *Neurobiol. Dis.* **33**, 89–95.

Bender, K.J., Rangel, J., and Feldman, D.E. (2003). Development of columnar topography in the excitatory layer 4 to layer 2 / 3 projection in rat barrel cortex. *J. Neurosci.* **23**, 8759–8770.

Benjamin, R.M., and Pfaffmann, C. (1955). Cortical localization of taste in albino rat. *J. Neurophysiol.* **18**, 56–64.

Benjamin, R.M., and Akert, K. (1959). Cortical and thalamic areas involved in taste discrimination in the albino rat. *J. Comp. Neurol.* **111**, 231–259.

Berger, T., Borgdorff, A., Crochet, S., Neubauer, F.B., Lefort, S., Fauvet, B., Ferezou, I., Carleton, A., Lüscher, H.R., and Petersen, C.C. (2007). Combined voltage and calcium epifluorescence imaging *in vitro* and *in vivo* reveals subthreshold and suprathreshold dynamics of mouse barrel cortex. *J. Neurophysiol.* **97**, 3751–3762.

Berman, D.E., Hazvi, S., Rosenblum, K., Seger, R., and Dudai, Y. (1998). Specific and differential activation of mitogen-activated protein kinase cascades by unfamiliar taste in the insular cortex of the behaving rat. *J. Neurosci.* **18**, 10037–10044.

Bester, H., Bourgeais, L., Villanueva, L., Besson, J.M., and Bernard, J.F. (1999). Differential projections to the intralaminar and gustatory thalamus from the parabrachial area: a PHA-L study in the rat. *J. Comp. Neurol.* **405**, 421–449.

Boggio, E.M., Putignano, E., Sassoè-Pognetto, M., Pizzorusso, T., and Giustetto, M. (2007). Visual stimulation activates ERK in synaptic and somatic compartments of rat cortical neurons with parallel kinetics. *PLoS One* **2**, e604.

Burkey, A.R., Carstens, E., and Jasmin, L. (1999). Dopamine reuptake inhibition in the rostral agranular insular cortex produces antinociception. *J. Neurosci.* **19**, 4169–4179.

Burkey, A.R., Carstens, E., Wenniger, J.J., Tang, J., and Jasmin, L. (1996). An opioidergic cortical antinociception triggering site in the agranular insular cortex of the rat that contributes to morphine antinociception. *J. Neurosci.* **16**, 6612–6623.

Carey, R.G., and Neal, T.L. (1985). The rat claustrum: afferent and efferent connections with visual cortex. *Brain Res.* **329**, 185–193.

Cechetto, D.F., and Saper, C.B. (1987). Evidence for a viscerotopic sensory representation in the cortex and thalamus in the rat. *J. Comp. Neurol.* **262**, 27–45.

Chen, S., Fujita, S., Koshikawa, N., and Kobayashi, M. (2010). Pilocarpine-induced status epilepticus causes acute interneuron loss and hyper-excitatory propagation in rat insular cortex. *Neuroscience* **166**, 341–353.

Chen, J., Lin, W., Wang, W., Shao, F., Yang, J., Wang, B., Kuang, F., Duan, X., and Ju, G. (2004). Enhancement of antibody production and expression of c-Fos in the insular cortex in response to a conditioned stimulus after a single-trial learning paradigm. *Behav. Brain Res.* **154**, 557–565.

Chmielowska, J., Carvell, G.E., and Simons, D.J. (1989). Spatial organization of thalamocortical and corticothalamic projection systems in the rat SmI barrel cortex. *J. Comp. Neurol.* **285**, 325–338.

Cohen, L.B., Keynes, R.D., and Hille, B. (1968). Light scattering and birefringence changes during nerve activity. *Nature* **218**, 438–441.

Dobesberger, J., Ortler, M., Unterberger, I., Walser, G., Falkenstetter, T., Bodner, T., Benke, T., Bale, R., Fiegele, T., Donnemiller, E., Gotwald, T., and Trinka, E. (2008). Successful surgical treatment of insular epilepsy with nocturnal hypermotor seizures. *Epilepsia* **49**, 159–162.

Frostig, R.D., Lieke, E.E., Ts'o, D.Y., and Grinvald, A. (1990). Cortical functional architecture and local coupling between neuronal activity and the microcirculation revealed by *in vivo* high-resolution optical imaging of intrinsic signals. *Proc. Natl. Acad. Sci. U.S.A.* **87**, 6082–6086.

Fujita, S., Adachi, K., Koshikawa, N., and Kobayashi, M. (2010). Spatiotemporal dynamics of excitation in rat insular cortex: intrinsic corticocortical circuit regulates caudal-rostro excitatory propagation from the insular to frontal cortex. *Neuroscience* **165**, 278–292.

Ganchrow, D., and Erickson, R.P. (1972). Thalamocortical relations in gustation. *Brain Res.* **36**, 298–305.

Gilbert, C.D. (1983). Microcircuitry of the visual cortex. *Annu. Rev. Neurosci.* **6**, 217–247.

Grinvald, A., Lieke, E., Frostig, R.D., Gilbert, C.D., and Wiesel, T.N. (1986). Functional architecture of cortex revealed by optical imaging of intrinsic signals. *Nature* **324**, 361–364.

Groenewegen, H.J. (1988). Organization of the afferent connections of the mediodorsal thalamic nucleus in the rat, related to the mediodorsal-prefrontal topography. *Neuroscience* **24**, 379–431.

Hanamori, T., Kunitake, T., Kato, K., and Kannan, H. (1998). Responses of neurons in the insular cortex to gustatory, visceral, and nociceptive stimuli in rats. *J. Neurophysiol.* **79**, 2535–2545.

Herkenham, M. (1980). Laminar organization of thalamic projections to the rat neocortex. *Science* **207**, 532–535.

Hill, D.K., and Keynes, R.D. (1949). Opacity changes in stimulated nerve. *J. Physiol.* **108**, 278–281.

Husson, T.R., Mallik, A.K., Zhang, J.X., and Issa, N.P. (2007). Functional imaging of primary visual cortex using flavoprotein autofluorescence. *J. Neurosci.* **27**, 8665–8675.

Isnard, J., Guénot, M., Ostrowsky, K., Sindou, M., and Mauguière, F. (2000). The role of the insular cortex in temporal lobe epilepsy. *Ann. Neurol.* **48**, 614–623.

Isnard, J., Guénot, M., Sindou, M., and Mauguière, F. (2004). Clinical manifestations of insular lobe seizures: a stereo-electroencephalographic study. *Epilepsia* **45**, 1079–1090.

Ito, S. (2002). Visceral region in the rat primary somatosensory cortex identified by vagal evoked potential. *J. Comp. Neurol.* **444**, 10–24.

Ito, S., and Ogawa, H. (1994). Neural activities in the fronto-opercular cortex of macaque monkeys during tasting and mastication. *Jpn. J. Physiol.* **44**, 141–156.

Jasmin, L., Rabkin, S.D., Granato, A., Boudah, A., and Ohara, P.T. (2003). Analgesia and hyperalgesia from GABA-mediated modulation of the cerebral cortex. *Nature* **424**, 316–320.

Jasmin, L., Burkey, A.R., Granato, A., and Ohara, P.T. (2004). Rostral agranular insular cortex and pain areas of the central nervous system: a tract-tracing study in the rat. *J. Comp. Neurol.* **468**, 425–440, Erratum in: *J. Comp. Neurol.* **480**, 330.

Jones, M.W., French, P.J., Bliss, T.V., and Rosenblum, K. (1999). Molecular mechanisms of long-term potentiation in the insular cortex *in vivo*. *J. Neurosci.* **19**, RC36.

Kaczmarek, L., and Chaudhuri, A. (1997). Sensory regulation of immediate-early gene expression in mammalian visual cortex: implications for functional mapping and neural plasticity. *Brain Res. Rev.* **23**, 237–256.

Kawaguchi, Y., and Kubota, Y. (1997). GABAergic cell subtypes and their synaptic connections in rat frontal cortex. *Cereb. Cortex* **7**, 476–486.

Karimnamazi, H., and Travers, J.B. (1998). Differential projections from gustatory responsive regions of the parabrachial nucleus to the medulla and forebrain. *Brain Res.* **813**, 283–302.

Kobayashi, M., Fujita, S., Takei, H., Song, L., Chen, S., Suzuki, I., Yoshida, A., Iwata, K., and Koshikawa, N. (2010). Functional mapping of gustatory neurons in the insular cortex revealed by pERK-immunohistochemistry and *in vivo* optical imaging. *Synapse* **64**, 323–334.

Koh, M.T., Wilkins, E.E., and Bernstein, I.L. (2003). Novel tastes elevate c-fos expression in the central amygdala and insular cortex: implication for taste aversion learning. *Behav. Neurosci.* **117**, 1416–1422.

Kosar, E., Grill, H.J., and Norgren, R. (1986 a) Gustatory cortex in the rat. I. Physiological properties and cytoarchitecture. *Brain Res.* **379**, 329–341.

Kosar, E., Grill, H.J., and Norgren, R. (1986 b) Gustatory cortex in the rat. II. Thalamocortical projections. *Brain Res.* **379**, 342–352.

Krettek, J.E., and Price, J.L. (1977). The cortical projections of the mediodorsal nucleus and adjacent thalamic nuclei in the rat. *J. Comp. Neurol.* **171**, 157–191.

Li, Z.K., Takada, M., and Hattori, T. (1986). Topographic organization and collateralization of claustrocortical projections in the rat. *Brain Res. Bull.* **17**, 529–532.

Majak, K., Pikkarainen, M., Kemppainen, S., Jolkkonen, E., and Pitkänen, A. (2002). Projections from the amygdaloid complex to the claustrum and the endopiriform nucleus: a Phaseolus vulgaris leucoagglutinin study in the rat. *J. Comp. Neurol.* **451**, 236–249.

Nakashima, M., Uemura, M., Yasui, K., Ozaki, H.S., Tabata, S., and Taen, A. (2000). An anterograde and retrograde tract-tracing study on the projections from the thalamic gustatory area in the rat:

distribution of neurons projecting to the insular cortex and amygdaloid complex. *Neurosci. Res.* **36**, 297–309.

Nguyen, D.K., Nguyen, D.B., Malak, R., Leroux, J.M., Carmant, L., Saint-Hilaire, J.M., Giard, N., Cossette, P., and Bouthillier, A. (2009). Revisiting the role of the insula in refractory partial epilepsy. *Epilepsia* **50**, 510–520.

Nicolelis, M.A., Ghazanfar, A.A., Faggin, B.M., Votaw, S., and Oliveira, L.M. (1997). Reconstructing the engram: simultaneous, multisite, many single neuron recordings. *Neuron* **18**, 529–537.

Ogawa, H., Hayama, T., and Ito, S. (1982). Convergence of input from tongue and palate to the parabrachial nucleus neurons of rats. *Neurosci Lett.* **28**, 9–14.

Ogawa, H., and Hayama, T. (1984). Receptive fields of solitario-parabrachial relay neurons responsive to natural stimulation of the oral cavity in rats. *Exp. Brain Res.* **54**, 359–366.

Ogawa, H., and Wang, X.D. (2002). Neurons in the cortical taste area receive nociceptive inputs from the whole body as well as the oral cavity in the rat. *Neurosci. Lett.* **322**, 87–90.

Ottersen, O.P. (1982). Connections of the amygdala of the rat. IV: Corticoamygdaloid and intraamygdaloid connections as studied with axonal transport of horseradish peroxidase. *J. Comp. Neurol.* **205**, 30–48.

Petersen, C.C., Grinvald, A., and Sakmann, B. (2003). Spatiotemporal dynamics of sensory responses in layer 2/3 of rat barrel cortex measured *in vivo* by voltage-sensitive dye imaging combined with whole-cell voltage recordings and neuron reconstructions. *J. Neurosci.* **23**, 1298–1309 Erratum in: *J. Neurosci.* **24**, 1 p following 906.

Petersen, C.C., and Sakmann, B. (2001). Functionally independent columns of rat somatosensory barrel cortex revealed with voltage-sensitive dye imaging. *J. Neurosci.* **21**, 8435–8446.

Ptito, M., and Lassonde, M.C. (1981). Effects of claustral stimulation on the properties of visual cortex neurons in the cat. *Exp. Neurol.* **73**, 315–320.

Ray, J.P., and Price, J.L. (1992). The organization of the thalamocortical connections of the mediodorsal thalamic nucleus in the rat, related to the ventral forebrain-prefrontal cortex topography. *J. Comp. Neurol.* **323**, 167–197.

Reinert, K.C., Dunbar, R.L., Gao, W., Chen, G., and Ebner, T.J. (2004). Flavoprotein autofluorescence imaging of neuronal activation in the cerebellar cortex *in vivo*. *J. Neurophysiol.* **92**, 199–211.

Roy, C.S., and Sherrington, C.S. (1890). On the regulation of the blood-supply of the brain. *J. Physiol.* **11**, 85–158.

Ryvlin, P., Minotti, L., Demarquay, G., Hirsch, E., Arzimanoglou, A., Hoffman, D., Guénot, M., Picard, F., Rheims, S., and Kahane, P. (2006). Nocturnal hypermotor seizures, suggesting frontal lobe epilepsy, can originate in the insula. *Epilepsia* **47**, 755–765.

Saper, C.B. (1982). Convergence of autonomic and limbic connections in the insular cortex of the rat. *J. Comp. Neurol.* **210**, 163–173.

Sherk, H., and LeVay, S. (1983). Contribution of the cortico-claustral loop to receptive field properties in area 17 of the cat. *J. Neurosci.* **3**, 2121–2127.

Shi, C.J., and Cassell, M.D. (1998 a) Cortical, thalamic, and amygdaloid connections of the anterior and posterior insular cortices. *J. Comp. Neurol.* **399**, 440–468.

Shi, C.J., and Cassell, M.D. (1998 b) Cascade projections from somatosensory cortex to the rat basolateral amygdala via the parietal insular cortex. *J. Comp. Neurol.* **399**, 469–491.

Shibuki, K., Hishida, R., Murakami, H., Kudoh, M., Kawaguchi, T., Watanabe, M., Watanabe, S., Kouuchi, T., and Tanaka, R. (2003). Dynamic imaging of somatosensory cortical activity in the rat visualized by flavoprotein autofluorescence. *J. Physiol.* **549**, 919–927.

Shibuya, H., and Yamamoto, T. (1998). Electrophysiological and morphological features of rat claustral neurons: an intracellular staining study. *Neuroscience* **85**, 1037–1049.

Takamura, H., Ichisaka, S., Hayashi, C., Maki, H., and Hata, Y. (2007). Monocular deprivation enhances the nuclear signalling of extracellular signal-regulated kinase in the developing visual cortex. *Eur. J. Neurosci.* **26**, 2884–2898.

Takashima, I., Kajiwara, R., and Iijima, T. (2001). Voltage-sensitive dye versus intrinsic signal optical imaging: comparison of optically determined functional maps from rat barrel cortex. *Neuroreport* **12**, 2889–2894.

Tominaga, T., Tominaga, Y., Yamada, H., Matsumoto, G., and Ichikawa, M. (2000). Quantification of optical signals with electrophysiological signals in neural activities of Di-4-ANEPPS stained rat hippocampal slices. *J. Neurosci. Methods* **102**, 11–23.

Tsumoto, T., and Suda, K. (1982). Effects of stimulation of the dorsocaudal claustrum on activities of striate cortex neurons in the cat. *Brain Res.* **240**, 345–349.

Verhagen, J.V., Giza, B.K., and Scott, T.R. (2003). Responses to taste stimulation in the ventroposteromedial nucleus of the thalamus in rats. *J. Neurophysiol.* **89**, 265–275.

Woolsey, T.A., and Van der Loos, H. (1970). The structural organization of layer IV in the somatosensory region (SI) of mouse cerebral cortex. The description of a cortical field composed of discrete cytoarchitectonic units. *Brain Res.* **17**, 205–242.

Yamamoto, T. (1987). Cortical organization in gustatory perception. *Ann. N.Y. Acad. Sci.* **510**, 49–54.

Yamamoto, T., and Kawamura, Y. (1972). Summated cerebral responses to taste stimuli in rat. *Physiol. Behav.* **9**, 789–793.

Yamamoto, T., Matsuo, R., and Kawamura, Y. (1980). Localization of cortical gustatory area in rats and its role in taste discrimination. *J. Neurophysiol.* **44**, 440–455.

Yamamoto, T., Yuyama, N., Kato, T., and Kawamura, Y. (1984). Gustatory responses of cortical neurons in rats. I. Response characteristics. *J. Neurophysiol.* **51**, 616–635.

Yamamoto, T., Yuyama, N., and Kawamura, Y. (1981). Cortical neurons responding to tactile, thermal and taste stimulations of the rat's tongue. *Brain Res.* **221**, 202–206.

Yamamoto, T., Yuyama, N., Kato, T., and Kawamura, Y. (1985). Gustatory responses of cortical neurons in rats. II. Information processing of taste quality. *J. Neurophysiol.* **53**, 1356–1369.

Yasui, Y., Breder, C.D., Saper, C.B., and Cechetto, D.F. (1991). Autonomic responses and efferent pathways from the insular cortex in the rat. *J. Comp. Neurol.* **303**, 355–374.

Zhang, X., Hannesson, D.K., Saucier, D.M., Wallace, A.E., Howland, J., and Corcoran, M.E. (2001). Susceptibility to kindling and neuronal connections of the anterior claustrum. *J. Neurosci.* **21**, 3674–3687.

THE BALANCE BETWEEN EXCITATION AND INHIBITION AND FUNCTIONAL SENSORY PROCESSING IN THE SOMATOSENSORY CORTEX

Zhi Zhang and Qian-Quan Sun

Department of Zoology and Physiology, University of Wyoming, Laramie, WY 82071

I. An Overview of Somatosensory (barrel) Cortex with Focus on Sensory Processing at Local Circuits

In the sensory cortical areas, neurons that respond to similar stimuli are clustered together in vertical cortical columns (Albright *et al.*, 1984; Fujita *et al.*, 1992; Hafting *et al.*, 2005). Cortical columns are typically arranged into somatotopic maps, so that columns with similar response properties are close to each other along the cortical surface (Hubel and Wiesel, 1962; Blasdel and Salama, 1986; Bonhoeffer and Grinvald, 1991; Issa *et al.*, 2000). Rodent primary somatosensory (SI) cortex contains a rich and diverse neuronal organization in which the local circuits are characterized by a high degree of connectional specificity. The SI cortex can be divided along its depth into anatomically defined layers, from a superficial layer 1 (L1) to a deep layer 6 (L6). A barrel column is defined as the entire thickness of the cortex (from L1 to L6) and laterally bounded by the extent of the layer 4 (L4) barrel (Woolsey and Van der Loos, 1970). The L4 SI cortex reveals a well-defined isomorphic representation of the mystacial whisker pad (Woolsey and Van der Loos, 1970; Welker, 1971; Land and Simons, 1985): each mystacial whisker is represented in L4 by a "barrel," and the neighboring barrels are

INTERNATIONAL REVIEW OF NEUROBIOLOGY, VOL. 97
DOI: 10.1016/B978-0-12-385198-7.00012-6

separated by narrower zones called "septa." Each barrel is selectively activated by the corresponding whisker on the contralateral whisker pad, and responds only weakly to inputs from surrounding whiskers (Welker, 1971; Welker, 1976; Simons, 1978; Armstrong-James and Fox, 1987; Armstrong-James *et al.*, 1991; Fox, 1994; Moore and Nelson, 1998; Zhu and Connors, 1999). The L4 barrels receive dense inputs exclusively from the thalamic ventro posterior medial (VPM) nucleus (Killackey, 1973; Killackey and Leshin, 1975; Koralek *et al.*, 1988; Chmielowska *et al.*, 1989; Lu and Lin, 1993) and are the first stage of cortical processing for sensory input. Each L4 barrel is composed of a central region of high density neuropil, containing the clustered VPM axonal arborizations, surrounded by a cell-dense wall of L4 neurons that orient their dendritic and axonal arborizations into one specific barrel (Woolsey *et al.*, 1975).

Layer 2/3 (L2/3) pyramidal neurons receive strong columnar input from L4, the major ascending projection in the cortex. L2/3 neurons exhibit robust experience dependent plasticity (Diamond *et al.*, 1994; Feldman, 2000b; Stern *et al.*, 2001; Allen *et al.*, 2003; Shepherd *et al.*, 2003; Foeller and Feldman, 2004) and are the key components in some of the earliest stages of intracortical processing (Armstrong-James *et al.*, 1992; Ahissar *et al.*, 2000; Brecht *et al.*, 2003). Neurons in L5a receive strong input from posterior medial nucleus (POm, "paralemniscal" pathway) and project to L2 (Bureau *et al.*, 2006).

Neurons in SI cortex have diverse response properties (Porter *et al.*, 2001; Bruno and Simons, 2002; Petersen *et al.*, 2003b; Schubert *et al.*, 2003; Staiger *et al.*, 2004). The local neuronal connections and interactions vary systematically with laminar and columnar locations (Shepherd and Svoboda, 2005; Shepherd *et al.*, 2005; Schubert *et al.*, 2006). Excitatory neurons in L4 dominate synaptic connectivity within a barrel column (Lefort *et al.*, 2009; Brecht *et al.*, 2003; Petersen, 2003; Broser *et al.*, 2008a; Dittgen *et al.*, 2004) and transfer received tactile information to neurons located in all other cortical layers. In addition, the reciprocal connectivity between L2/3 and L5a is also prominent neocortical signaling pathways in the barrel column (Bureau *et al.*, 2006; Lefort *et al.*, 2009). Certain subclasses of fast-spiking interneurons in L4 receive massive thalamic inputs, which results in a fast-rising inhibitory activity that provides feed-forward inhibition (Gabernet *et al.*, 2005; Sun *et al.*, 2006; Cruikshank *et al.*, 2007). The recruitment of local inhibition within L4 defines "a brief window of opportunity," in which cortical L4 cells can actually respond to thalamic excitation (Pinto *et al.*, 2000; Moore and Nelson, 1998; Zhu and Connors, 1999). The exact timing of excitation relative to inhibition is crucial in determining the direction selectivity of SI cortex neurons (Wilent and Contreras, 2005). *In vivo* recordings from mouse SI cortex neurons start shedding light on how these neocortical microcircuits operate functionally during different behavior states (Crochet and Petersen, 2006; Poulet and Petersen, 2008; Gentet *et al.*, 2010).

The maturation of neuronal circuits is strongly dependent on experience and activity (Katz and Shatz, 1996). Previous work indicates that somatosensory maps are highly malleable both during brain development (Van der Loos and Woolsey, 1973; Simons and Land, 1987) and in the adult animal (Buonomano and Merzenich, 1998), which offers an excellent model system to investigate experience-dependent changes in cortical development (Fox, 1992). A recent study shows that in the early developmental stage, postnatal days 6-11 (P6-11), sensory experience can induce target-specific plasticity at thalamocortical inputs onto both inhibitory and excitatory neurons in L4 of the barrel cortex (Chittajallu and Isaac, 2010). In the following sections of this review, we will focus on the E-I balance and homeostatic plasticity in the barrel cortical circuits and cellular mechanisms underlying homeostatic plasticity.

II. E-I Balance and Homeostatic Plasticity in the Somatosensory (barrel) Cortical Circuits

The neurons in mature neocortex form highly complex connectivity, which contains horizontal and vertical connections traveling within and between the cortical layers (Szentagothai, 1978; Douglas and Martin, 2004). The response of any individual neuron is determined by the influence of both excitatory (glutamatergic) and inhibitory (GABAergic and glycinergic) synaptic inputs that originated in dynamic local recurrent networks (DeFelipe *et al.*, 2002; Binzegger *et al.*, 2004). A delicate balance between excitation and inhibition (E-I balance) that a cell receives is maintained within a narrow window to avoid runaway excitation or quiescence, in response to alterations in neuronal activity (Shadlen and Newsome, 1994; Salinas and Sejnowski, 2000; Turrigiano and Nelson, 2004; Wehr and Zador, 2003; Wilent and Contreras, 2004; Wehr and Zador, 2005; Pouille *et al.*, 2009), and give rise to balanced network stability (Marino *et al.*, 2005) or amplification (Carvalho and Buonomano, 2009; Murphy and Miller, 2009). In sensory cortices, a balance between feedback or feedforward inhibition and recurrent excitation reduces the randomness of cortical operation and increases temporal precision (Monier *et al.*, 2003; Wehr and Zador, 2003; Cruikshank *et al.*, 2007; Pouille *et al.*, 2009).

The functional E-I balance in single cortical neurons has been widely investigated in neocortex. For example, in the prefrontal cortex, persistent network activity during "up" states is maintained by dynamically and tightly balanced excitatory and inhibitory synaptic inputs (Shu *et al.*, 2003; Haider *et al.*, 2006). In the cat primary visual cortex, excitatory and inhibitory conductances evoked by visual sensory inputs are exquisitely balanced in neurons at all locations within the orientation map (Marino *et al.*, 2005). In the rat primary auditory cortex, excitatory and inhibitory conductances exhibit a strong linear correlation (Wehr and Zador, 2003; Zhang *et al.*, 2003; Tan *et al.*, 2004). It was also shown that the number of excitatory and inhibitory synapses across individual dendrites maintains a constant ratio *in vitro* (Liu, 2004).

In adults, the tightly regulated E-I balance is achieved by homeostatic control of the strength and weight of synaptic transmission in response to external stimuli (Marder and Goaillard, 2006; Rich and Wenner, 2007; Turrigiano, 2007). This homeostatic regulation is bidirectional. For example, the glutamatergic system is up-scaled after prolonged pharmacological inactivation of the ionotropic glutamate receptors or tetrodo toxin (TTX)- sensitive sodium channels. This homeostatic mechanism prevents neuronal quiescence as long as neurons are silenced (Ramakers *et al.*, 1990; Ramakers *et al.*, 1994). In contrast, pharmacological blockade of $GABA_A$ receptors induce a down-scaled firing rate that prevents runaway excitation as long as $GABA_A$ receptors are blocked (Corner and Ramakers, 1992). Sensory deprivation causes a clear down-regulation of hyperpolarization-activated cyclic nucleotide gated (HCN) channels in the barrel cortex, which result in the increase in dendritic excitability and burst firing (Berger *et al.*, 2003; Breton and Stuart, 2009). This represents a homeostatic mechanism to increase activity in the barrel cortex in response to reduced sensory input.

An altered E-I balance postulates a disturbance in homeostatic control resulting from either insufficient or excessive compensatory mechanisms in response to the changes in network activity. Deregulation of the E-I balance has been involved in a number of nervous system disorders reviewed by Eichler and Meier (2008), such as epilepsy (Gale, 1992; Bradford, 1995; Thompson *et al.*, 1996; Olsen and Avoli, 1997; Cobos *et al.*, 2005), schizophrenia (Lewis *et al.*, 2003; Kehrer *et al.*, 2008), autism (Jamain *et al.*, 2003; Laumonnier *et al.*, 2004) and acoustic trauma (Scholl and Wehr, 2008). Despite the importance of the functional E-I balance, little is known about how this important feature of neural circuits arises during development.

During early postnatal stages (P<10) the inhibitory postsynaptic response to electrical stimulation is absent or rare (Komatsu and Iwakiri, 1991; Luhmann and Prince, 1991; Agmon and Connors, 1992; Burgard and Hablitz, 1993), and often manifests as long-lasting polysynaptic barrages (Agmon *et al.*, 1996). In rodents, however, the total number of GABAergic synapses (Blue and Parnavelas, 1983; Miller, 1986; Micheva and Beaulieu, 1997; Kobayashi *et al.*, 2008) and the magnitude of the evoked GABAergic responses (Morales *et al.*, 2002; Kobayashi *et al.*, 2008) increase during development. Recent work in visual cortex (Morales *et al.*, 2002; Chattopadhyaya *et al.*, 2004; Chandrasekaran *et al.*, 2005) and barrel cortex (Jiao *et al.*, 2006; Chittajallu and Isaac, 2010) demonstrate that this process is experience-dependent. In contrast, excitatory synaptic response already exists in the neonatal neocortical neurons (Kriegstein *et al.*, 1987; Agmon and O'Dowd, 1992; Burgard and Hablitz, 1993; Kim *et al.*, 1995). However, the transmitter release probability of excitatory neurons (Frick *et al.*, 2007; Feldmeyer and Radnikow, 2009) and the amplitude of excitatory postsynaptic potentials (Reyes and Sakmann, 1999; Oswald and Reyes, 2008) decrease during development, which may result from dramatic changes in the intrinsic and synaptic properties of neurons (Oswald *et al.*, 2009).

How the E-I ratio in barrel cortex changes during development? Using a method that allows the decomposition of the response of pyramidal neuron into its excitatory and inhibitory components (Borg-Graham *et al.*, 1998; Monier *et al.*, 2003; Wehr and Zador, 2003; Le *et al.*, 2006; Shu *et al.*, 2003; Higley and Contreras, 2007b; Cruikshank *et al.*, 2007), we directly measured the E-I ratio in principal neurons from four major layers of barrel cortex at four critical postnatal ages (P8, P18, P30 and P60). Our results indicate that there is a significant developmental decrease in the E-I ratio, which occurred after P8 and almost finished at P18. The decrease in E-I ratio is due to a disproportional significant increase of the inhibitory, but not excitatory conductance. Furthermore, our own data using Western blot (WB) measurement of inhibitory proteins and direct measurement of monosynaptic evoked IPSCs also support the idea that a "mismatch" in the strength of local E and I occurs during postnatal development, which gives rise to a decreased E/I ratio. In addition, we found that the E-I balance was tightly regulated and remained highly constant across all major layers of barrel cortex at given developmental stages (Zhang *et al.*, 2011). Another recent study shows that the E/I ratio is slightly larger in L5 barrel cortex and the layer-specific E/I ratio is the underlying mechanism for cortical domains to exploit horizontal projections to compete for cortical space (Adesnik and Scanziani, 2010).

What are the physiological implications of decreased E-I ratio during development? At the earlier developmental stage, the high excitability of excitatory neurons has advantage in response to low-input currents (Oswald and Reyes, 2008), which may be beneficial to the formation of neural network and synaptic plasticity. In mature neuronal network, the reduction in intrinsic excitability of pyramidal neurons may enhance temporal fidelity by somatic feed-forward inhibition (Pouille and Scanziani, 2001). It is well known that GABAergic circuits control the engagement of activity dependent synaptic modification by controlling excitation (Kirkwood and Bear, 1994; Hensch *et al.*, 1998). The delay in maturation of inhibition can define a critical period for activity dependent plasticity to occur in early development (Knudsen and Knudsen, 1990; Huang *et al.*, 1999).

III. Cellular Mechanisms Underlying Balanced Function in Somatosensory (barrel) Cortex

A. How do the Excitatory and Inhibitory Synapses Change During Postnatal Development?

What are the cellular and molecular mechanisms underlying the decrease in the E-I balance in barrel cortex? The E-I balance in adult cortical neurons may be established from developmental and experience-dependent co-regulation of developing glutamatergic and GABAergic synapses (Desai *et al.*, 2002; Turrigiano and Nelson, 2004). Earlier in development the dramatic changes in the number, distribution and subtype of $GABA_A$ receptors (Luhmann and Prince, 1991; Chattopadhyaya *et al.*, 2004) and glutamate receptors (Mierau *et al.*, 2004; Bannister *et al.*, 2005; Brill and Huguenard, 2008; Oswald and Reyes, 2008), profoundly alter the synaptic transmission.

1. Changes in Excitatory Synapses during Postnatal Development.

During postnatal development, there is an increase of synaptic AMPA receptors, accompanied by a decrease in synaptic kainate receptors (Kidd and Isaac, 1999; Bannister *et al.*, 2005). The developmental shift from kainate to AMPA receptor-mediated transmission in the barrel cortex is likely to alter the information processing properties of the thalamocortical input to L4 dramatically (Bannister *et al.*, 2005). What are the physiological implications of the switch from kainite to AMPA receptor? In the early development, the summation of inputs promotes the development and plasticity of neurons. The kainate receptor induces EPSPs with long decay that favor long temporal summation of inputs, which may be important for developmental plasticity (Daw *et al.*, 2006). In mature somatosensory cortex, however, timing precision is critical for information processing (Celikel *et al.*, 2004; Foffani *et al.*, 2004; Ghazanfar *et al.*, 2000; Panzeri *et al.*, 2001). The switch from kainate receptor-mediated slow transmission to AMPA receptor-mediated fast transmission will favor precise coincidence detection that is important for mature information processing (Bannister *et al.*, 2005). In addition, during postnatal development the switch of AMPA receptor to GluR2-expressing subunits in excitatory neurons reduces neuronal excitotoxicity (Kumar *et al.*, 2002; Brill and Huguenard, 2008).

The NMDA receptors play a central role in activity dependent regulation of dendrite development [reviewed in (Constantine-Paton *et al.*, 1990; Cline, 2001; Wong and Ghosh, 2002; Newpher and Ehlers, 2008)], learning and developmental plasticity [see reviews (Perez-Otano and Ehlers, 2005; Rebola *et al.*, 2010)]. NMDA receptors have unique physiological properties: the voltage dependent magnesium block at resting membrane potential and calcium permeability, which have made them strong candidate for Hebbian plasticity, such as long-term potentiation (LTP) and long-term depression (LTD) (Paulsen and Sejnowski, 2000; Bi and Poo, 1998; Malenka and Nicoll, 1999; Zhang and Bodznick, 2010). Previous studies in barrel cortex have shown both timing-dependent LTP (t-LTP) and timing-dependent LTD (t-LTD) require activation of NMDA receptors (Feldman, 2000b; Froemke *et al.*, 2005; Bender *et al.*, 2006).

NMDA receptors are heteromers that are composed of multiple glycine-binding $\zeta 1$ (NR1) subunits and at least one type of $\varepsilon 1$–4 (NR2 A-D) subunit that determines the receptor's distinct functional, kinetic, pharmacological, and intracellular signaling properties (Cull-Candy *et al.*, 2001). In the neocortex, there is a change in NMDA receptor subunit composition in excitatory neurons from mostly NR1/NR2B heteromers at neonatal age (~P7) to mixed NR1-NR2A&B-containing receptors at older ages (Watanabe *et al.*, 1992; Monyer *et al.*, 1994; Sheng *et al.*, 1994), which is indicated by decreases in decay times, and in the sensitivity to the NR2B subunit-selective antagonist, ifenprodil (Liu *et al.*, 2004b; Mierau *et al.*, 2004). Compared to NR2A, NR2B mediated EPSCs exhibit a 3- to 4-fold slower decay time course (Flint *et al.*, 1997; Vicini *et al.*, 1998), which results in a larger Ca^{2+} influx [reviewed in (Cull-Candy and Leszkiewicz, 2004)]. An increase in the NR2A content during development shortens NMDA receptor mediated EPSC (Carmignoto and Vicini, 1992), which causes less sufficient Ca^{2+} entry for LTP induction and is responsible for the end of the critical period in the visual and barrel cortices.

The switch from NR2B to NR2A is experience dependent. In the visual cortex, dark rearing extends NR2B expression and the critical period for ocular dominance plasticity (ODP) (Philpot *et al.*, 2001; Quinlan *et al.*, 1999). In barrel cortex, the switch from NR2B to NR2A correlates well with the end of the L4 critical period for LTP and for experience-dependent plasticity at the end of the first postnatal week (Barth and Malenka, 2001; Lu *et al.*, 2001). In newborn rats, blockage of NMDA receptors over the barrel cortex extended the duration of the critical period, following whisker lesions on different postnatal days (Schlaggar *et al.*, 1993). However, recent studies, particularly studies on cortex-specific NR1 knockout mice, have shown that when the cortical NMDA receptors are genetically impaired, whisker lesion-induced plasticity and its developmental duration does not change (Datwani *et al.*, 2002). In addition, NR2A knock-out mice exhibit similar critical period and experience dependent plasticity of the anatomical barrel map (Lu *et al.*, 2001). Another study found that the change in both, subtypes and kinetics of NMDA receptors coincides with the onset rather than the end of the critical period (Roberts and Ramoa, 1999). Thus, a simple switch from NR2B to NR2A alone is not responsible for the end of the critical period. The role of the NMDA receptor subunit switch is still unclear.

Distinct subpopulations of NMDA receptors at different developmental stages and in different brain regions raise the attractive hypothesis that different receptor subtypes play different roles in brain function (Cull-Candy and Leszkiewicz, 2004). It has been shown that the NR2A subunits are required for the induction of LTP, and NR2B subunits are required for the induction of LTD in the hippocampus (Liu *et al.*, 2004a), perirhinal cortex (Massey *et al.*, 2004), visual cortex (Sjostrom *et al.*, 2003). However, other studies indicate that both NR2A and NR2B subunits are involved in the induction of LTP in the hippocampus (Berberich *et al.*, 2005), and in the induction of LTD in the anterior cingulate cortex (Toyoda *et al.*, 2005). Moreover, it has been reported that the NR2A subunit is not required for LTP in the dorsolateral bed nucleus of the stria terminalis (Weitlauf *et al.*, 2005), and that the NR2B subunit is not required for LTD in the hippocampus (Morishita *et al.*, 2007).

2. *Changes in Inhibitory Synapses during Postnatal Development.*

In the normal functioning brain, the inhibitory synaptic strength is also developmentally regulated similar to the excitatory synapses. Approximately 10-20% neurons in the neocortex are GABAergic interneurons (Cauli *et al.*, 1997; Kawaguchi and Kubota, 1997; Gupta *et al.*, 2000; DeFelipe, 2002). GABAergic interneurons can be broadly classified into several groups based on different criteria, such as action potential firing properties, somato-dendritic architecture and axonal ramification pattern, neurochemical content, voltage and ligand-gated conductances as well as plastic changes in the excitatory synaptic transmission [for reviews see (Freund and Buzsaki, 1996; McBain and Fisahn, 2001)].

Specific classes of GABAergic synapses preferentially target to subcellular compartments of principal neurons (i.e., dendrite, spines, soma, and axon initial segment) (Somogyi *et al.*, 1998) and contribute to the differential regulations of pyramidal neurons. Perisomatic inhibitory neurons controlling the firing of principal cells, dendritic inhibitory interneurons regulating dendritic electrogenesis, synaptic input and Ca^{2+} signalling (Miles *et al.*, 1996; Tamas *et al.*, 1997; Tamas *et al.*, 2003), and GABAergic cells specifically innervating other inhibitory interneurons (Miles *et al.*, 1996; Somogyi and Klausberger, 2005). In the rat barrel cortex, inhibitory GABA synapses contact mainly to dendritic shafts (54%) and spines (39%), but also cell bodies (7%) (Micheva and Beaulieu, 1996). In this way, the GABA system is not only able to fine-tune the gain of a particular excitatory input, by targeting distal dendrites and spines, but is also able to efficiently control the general responsiveness of neurons through proximal synaptic contacts. Relatively small changes in the GABA circuitry can lead to both profound and specific changes in the function of the cortex, which make the GABA system an ideal candidate for cortical plasticity.

GABAergic interneurons evoke chloride-mediated, inhibitory postsynaptic potentials [IPSPs; (Houser *et al.*, 1983; Beaulieu *et al.*, 1992); for a review see (Soltesz and Staley, 2006)]. A major facet of GABAergic transmission is the intimate link between $GABA_A$ receptor function and ion homeostasis (Mody, 2005). $GABA_A$ receptors are pentamers that are composed of subunits from several related sequence classes (Unwin, 1989). In the rodent, 13 subunit genes have been identified and subdivided into α, β, γ and δ classes [reviewed by (Olsen and Tobin, 1990; Seeburg *et al.*, 1990; Luddens and Wisden, 1991; Wisden and Seeburg, 1992)]. The change in the expression of $GABA_A$ receptor subunit gene (Laurie *et al.*, 1992) and regional differences in subunit gene expression (Laurie *et al.*, 1992; Wisden *et al.*, 1992) could account for the change in the pharmacological properties of $GABA_A$ receptors during development (Chisholm *et al.*, 1983; Meier *et al.*, 1987; Reichelt *et al.*, 1991), and the pharmacological diversity of GABA receptors in the adult rat CNS (Unnerstall *et al.*, 1981; Young, III *et al.*, 1981; Niddam *et al.*, 1987; Olsen *et al.*, 1990).

$GABA_A$ receptors are primarily permeable to Cl^-. Cl^- gradients are determined by two specific potassium-chloride co-transporters such as NKCC1 and KCC2. The expression of NKCC1 and KCC2 are developmentally regulated (Rivera *et al.*, 2005), which can render the reversal potential of Cl^- more negative (Rivera *et al.*, 2005; Farrant and Kaila, 2007; Fiumelli and Woodin, 2007). These co-transporters can also undergo rapid changes in expression and function under pathological conditions, leading to chronic dysregulation of GABAergic inhibition (Price *et al.*, 2005). In both cerebellar and cortical neurons, the activation of neonatal $GABA_A$receptors increases intracellular calcium concentration (Connor *et al.*, 1987; Yuste and Katz, 1991), which may have resulted from membrane depolarization and activation of voltage-sensitive calcium channels [(Ben-Ari *et al.*, 1989); reviewed by (Cherubini *et al.*, 1991)]. $GABA_A$ receptors are possible mediators of plastic changes in sensory cortex in early postnatal development (Fagiolini *et al.*, 2004; Jiao *et al.*, 2006; Hensch and Fagiolini, 2005).

Despite the importance of NMDA receptors in GABAergic interneurons, little is known regarding the changes in the NMDA receptor subunit composition in interneurons during development. Therefore, it is crucial to investigate the changes in NMDA receptors in GABAergic cells during critical period. It is difficult to study the GABAergic cells with most widely used techniques (e.g. western blot, in situ hybridization) in analyzing receptor molecular composition. This is because the interneurons occupy only 10-20% of total neurons within the neocortex (Cauli *et al.*, 1997; Kawaguchi and Kubota, 1997; Gupta *et al.*, 2000; DeFelipe, 2002); these techniques could not provide quantitative information regarding receptors involved in synaptic transmission in this small group of cells. By using whole-cell patch clamp recording from GAD67 GFP-positive neurons, we demonstrate the change in NR2A/NR2B ratio in L2/3 interneurons during critical period development (P12-14). Our data demonstrate that there is a significant increase of the peak amplitude of NMDA receptor-mediated EPSCs ($EPSCs_{NMDAR}$), accompanying with significant decrease in the coefficient of variation (CV) of the peak amplitude, τ_{decay} and half-width of $EPSCs_{NMDAR}$ in the neurons from post-critical period group.Our pharmacological data indicate that there is a postnatal developmental shift in NR2 composition towards more NR2A and less NR2B mediated $EPSCs_{NMDAR}$ in the post critical period. These developmental changes occurred within a 2-day narrow window of critical period and were similar between fast-spiking (FS) and regular spiking (RSNP) interneurons (Zhang and Sun, 2011).

B. How does the E-I Balance Change upon Acute or Prolonged Sensory Deprivation or Stimulation?

Cortical reorganization in response to alteration in sensory experience may be mediated both through excitatory and inhibitory connections. The strength and short-term dynamics of existing synapses are experience-dependent (Finnerty *et al.*, 1999). In the barrel cortex, tactile experience drives robust plasticity (Blake *et al.*, 2002; Fox and Wong, 2005; Butz *et al.*, 2009), which can be induced from birth to adulthood. Different layers of the barrel cortex exhibit different time windows for sensitivity to sensory manipulation (Fox, 1992; Fox, 2002). Depending on the timing and the experimental paradigms, manipulation of sensory activity can induce layer-, cell-type-, and synapse-specific long-lasting physiological alterations in barrel cortex (Shoykhet *et al.*, 2005; Lee *et al.*, 2007). For example, sensory deprivation induced by whisker trimming or plucking in the first postnatal week, causes changes in the structure of barrel cortex (Van der Loos and Woolsey, 1973; Woolsey and Wann, 1976; Micheva and Beaulieu, 1995; Fox and Wong, 2005; Briner *et al.*, 2010) and in synaptic plasticity at thalamocortical synapses (Crair and Malenka, 1995; Isaac *et al.*, 1997; Feldman *et al.*, 1998). The receptive field properties can be changed by sensory experience throughout development (Fox, 1992; Diamond *et al.*, 1993) in a layer specific manner (Diamond *et al.*, 1994; Glazewski and Fox, 1996; Stern *et al.*, 2001; Polley *et al.*, 2004).

1. *Hebbian Form Plasticity*

Trimming or plucking a subset of whiskers will induce Hebbian-form plasticity. Neural responses to deprived whiskers will rapidly decrease and cause the weakening and shrinking of the representation of deprived whiskers within the map. In contrast, the responses to spared whiskers will increase slowly, and lead to the strengthening and expanding of the representation of spared whiskers within the map (Fox, 1992; Diamond *et al.*, 1993; Glazewski and Fox, 1996). The dynamic relocation of cortical processing space from deprived inputs toward spared inputs will optimize sensory processing (Feldman and Brecht, 2005). The depression of deprived whisker input is restricted to the first 2 months of postnatal age and disappears in older animals (Glazewski and Fox, 1996; Skibinska *et al.*, 2000). Whereas, potentiation of spared whisker input in L2/3 of the barrel cortex is present in adult animals (Glazewski *et al.*, 1996; Glazewski *et al.*, 1998). Meanwhile, repeated activation of a specific sensory input (without deprivation) potentiates neural responses to that input, which is usually most robust in young animals (Diamond *et al.*, 1993; Dan and Poo, 2006; Frenkel *et al.*, 2006; Keuroghlian and Knudsen, 2007).

It has been postulated that LTP and LTD are the mechanisms underlying this Hebbian form of plasticity. LTP has been proposed to underlie strengthening of spared inputs during deprivation-induced plasticity (Glazewski *et al.*, 1999; Clem and Barth, 2006) and use-dependent strengthening of sensory responses in juveniles (Crair and Malenka, 1995; Feldman *et al.*, 1999; Jiang *et al.*, 2007). LTP can be expressed presynaptically and postsynaptically. The postsynaptic LTP is mostly NMDA receptor-dependent. The activation of postsynaptic NMDA receptors induces calcium influx, which in turn activates CaMKII. The activation of CaMKII drives specific AMPA receptor phosphorylation, and insertion of GluR1-containing AMPA receptors into synaptic membranes (Malinow and Malenka, 2002). During early development, the postsynaptic NMDA receptor-dependent LTP is strongly implicated in activity and use-dependent strengthening of cortical synapses (Bear *et al.*, 1990; Rema *et al.*, 1998; Roberts *et al.*, 1998). The presynaptic LTP is induced by an increase in release probability mediated by retrograde nitric oxide (NO) signaling (Hardingham *et al.*, 2003; Hardingham and Fox, 2006), which alters short-term synaptic dynamics (Markram and Tsodyks, 1996; Buonomano, 1999; Eder *et al.*, 2002). The LTD is a major mechanism for depression of responses to deprived sensory inputs in barrel cortex. The LTD can be NMDA receptor-dependent (Bender *et al.*, 2006) or cannabinoid type 1 (CB1)-dependent (Adermark *et al.*, 2009), expressed as a decrease in the presynaptic release probability (Allen *et al.*, 2003; Bender *et al.*, 2006). The induction of LTD is age-dependent (Kemp and Bashir, 2001). Sensory deprivation drives LTD in barrel cortex primarily in young animals (<2 months), not in adults (Sawtell *et al.*, 2003; Fox and Wong, 2005; Sato and Stryker, 2008). There are also functional and structural changes to sensory deprivation, such as the decreases in the probability of synaptic connections (Cheetham *et al.*, 2007), and the reduction in the horizontal axonal projections extending toward deprived columns (Broser *et al.*, 2008b).

2. *Homeostatic Plasticity*

In addition to Hebbian plasticity, homeostatic regulation of cortical activity in response to substantial sensory overuse or deprivation is a distinct non-Hebbian form of plasticity. Homeostatic plasticity drives compensatory changes that will at least partially restore cortical activity to a set point level, and keep neuronal or network activity within a functional range (Miller, 1996; Marder and Prinz, 2002; Turrigiano and Nelson, 2004; Feldman, 2009). For example, excitatory synapse strength increases (or decreases) in response to experimentally decreasing (or increasing) network activity over hours to days. In contrast, decreased activity causes a reduction in inhibitory synapse strength at some inhibitory synapses (Turrigiano and Nelson, 2004). Homeostatic regulation of synaptic strength in response to prolonged changes in activity is called synaptic scaling (Wierenga *et al.*, 2005). Change in the synaptic strength can be due to the changes in presynaptic release probability (Bacci *et al.*, 2001; Thiagarajan *et al.*, 2002), change in postsynaptic receptor accumulation (Lissin *et al.*, 1998; O'Brien *et al.*, 1998; Wierenga *et al.*, 2005) and responsiveness (O'Brien *et al.*, 1998; Turrigiano *et al.*, 1998), as well as the functional synaptic connectivity between pairs of neurons (Nakayama *et al.*, 2005; Samsonovich and Ascoli, 2006; Wilson *et al.*, 2007). Intrinsic excitability (Brager and Johnston, 2007; Echegoyen *et al.*, 2007; Pratt and Aizenman, 2007; Azdad *et al.*, 2009), NMDA receptor content at synapses (Kanold *et al.*, 2009; Lee *et al.*, 2010), and E-I balance (De *et al.*, 2005; Le *et al.*, 2006; Maffei and Turrigiano, 2008) are also homeostatically regulated. In barrel cortex sensory activation drives homeostatic changes in L4 inhibitory circuits and in glutamate transport by astrocytes (Genoud *et al.*, 2006).

3. *Other Changes in Local Circuit Properties after Sensory Manipulation*

After the first postnatal week, L4 barrel cortex becomes relatively inert to changes, whereas layer 2/3 barrel cortex continues to undergo experience-dependent plasticity (Fox, 1992). Sensory deprivation can change layer 2/3 pyramidal neurons properties, such as change in spine motility (Lendvai *et al.*, 2000) and in the basal dendritic branching pattern (Maravall *et al.*, 2004), increase in back-propagation action potential-evoked calcium influx (Krieger, 2009), change in short-term synaptic dynamics (Finnerty *et al.*, 1999; Finnerty and Connors, 2000) and in LTP (Allen *et al.*, 2003), redistribution of the L4 sensory input (Shepherd *et al.*, 2003) and distortion of the receptive field map (Stern *et al.*, 2001). In addition, sensory deprivation increases the dendritic excitability of cortical L5 pyramidal neurons by down-regulated dendritic HCN channels (Breton and Stuart, 2009).

Pyramidal neurons in the superficial cortical layers form long-range horizontally projecting axons, which undergo a process of sprouting and synaptogenesis that parallels the functional reorganization of the cortex following altered sensory experience (Kaas *et al.*, 1990; Darian-Smith and Gilbert, 1994; Yamahachi *et al.*, 2009). For example, trimming the whiskers decreases the density of L2/3 axons projecting between the spared and the deprived barrel columns (Broser *et al.*, 2008a; Krieger, 2009), and increases the synaptic connectivity between the spared and neighboring spared columns (Diamond *et al.*, 1993; Lebedev *et al.*, 2000; Petersen *et al.*, 2003a; Wallace and Sakmann, 2008).

While the role of these excitatory cells in cortical reorganization has received most attention, inhibition is also known to regulate plasticity during the critical period in early postnatal development [for reviews see (Feldman, 2000a; Hensch and Fagiolini, 2005)]. Synaptic inhibition is involved in sensory processing in L4 of the rodent barrel cortex (White and Rock, 1981). Both feedforward and feedback inhibition from local inhibitory neurons regulates the integration of thalamic and intracortical sensory inputs (Thomson *et al.*, 1996; Agmon and Connors, 1992). In our study, we chronically blocked the NR2A subunits from P7 to P25 to decrease the excitatory synaptic inputs mediated by NMDA receptors. We found that the density of parvalbumin (PV)-positive interneurons in layer 2/3 and L4 barrel cortex was reduced after the chronic blockage of NR2A. In addition, by measuring the evoked IPSCs and spontaneous IPSCs in L4 spiny cells, we have demonstrated that the perisomatic inhibition, which was mainly mediated by PV-positive fast spiking interneurons, was impaired after blocking NR2A activity, which may be due to a homeostatic adjustment of E-I balance (Zhang and Sun, 2011).

C. How does Cellular E-I Balance Contribute Balanced Function during Sensory Processing?

The central nervous system is composed of neurons that have the exceptional ability to compensate for perturbations and therefore make homeostatic responses to reestablish a proper balance of excitation and inhibition (Marder and Goaillard, 2006; Rich and Wenner, 2007; Turrigiano, 2007). Computational models have assumed that the influence of excitatory and inhibitory neurons must be proportionally and well balanced in active cortical networks to ensure the normal sensory processing (van and Sompolinsky, 1996; Shadlen and Newsome, 1998; Salinas and Sejnowski, 2000; Litvak *et al.*, 2003). An *in vivo* study has confirmed that excitatory and inhibitory inputs remain dynamically balanced in active local networks in the intact neocortex (Haider *et al.*, 2006). The changes in neuronal excitability will induce compensatory changes in inhibitory circuits. In the mammalian trigeminal somatosensory system, the spatiotemporal patterns of sensory inputs are integrated at multiple levels and well adapted for appropriate detection and discrimination of peripheral stimuli (Fanselow and Nicolelis, 1999; Moore, 2004; Castro-Alamancos, 2002; Higley and Contreras, 2007b; Varga *et al.*, 2002). For example, repetitive stimulation leads to a balanced reduction in the timing and magnitude of thalamocortical and corticocortical excitatory and inhibitory synaptic relays (Chung *et al.*, 2002; Higley and Contreras, 2007a; Higley and Contreras, 2007b), to match the neuronal sensitivity to the particular input conditions (Higley and Contreras, 2006).

Insufficient or excessive compensatory mechanisms in response to a change in network activity will lead to disturbance in homeostatic plasticity. Deregulation of the E-I balance has been associated with a variety of human neurological disorders. Increased E-I ratios of synaptic input accompany the phenomenology of epilepsy (Gale, 1992; Bradford, 1995; Olsen and Avoli, 1997). For example glutamate receptor agonists, in particular kainate, can induce strong epileptogenic effects (Ben-Ari *et al.*, 1980; Sperk, 1994). Considerable changes in the function of interneurons and their control over pyramidal cells have been demonstrated in epileptic tissue (Cossart *et al.*, 2005; Ratte and Lacaille, 2006). Decreased E-I ratios of synaptic input are associated with mental retardation (Todd *et al.*, 2003; Laumonnier *et al.*, 2004) and Rett Syndrome (Dani *et al.*, 2005). The E-I ratio can be increased (Rubenstein and Merzenich, 2003;Ramocki and Zoghbi, 2008) or decreased (Jamain *et al.*, 2003; Feng *et al.*, 2006; Durand *et al.*, 2007; Tabuchi *et al.*, 2007) in autism, which may result from the disruption of E-I balance during critical periods of development (Rubenstein and Merzenich, 2003; Tabuchi *et al.*, 2007; Ramocki and Zoghbi, 2008). For example, in *Fmr1* knockout mice, the excitatory drive onto fast spiking interneurons, decreased approximately to 50% and the excitatory neurons became intrinsically more excitable (Gibson *et al.*, 2008). Overall, these changes would be expected to lead to an increase in E-I ratio. The mutation of neuroligin-3, on the other hand, increases inhibitory synaptic transmission and decreases the E-I ratio in autism (Tabuchi *et al.*, 2007).

The imbalanced E/I ratios are closely associated with the abnormal sensory processing in neurological diseases. For example, autistic individuals exhibit a range of perceptual processing abnormalities, such as hypersensitive to auditory and tactile stimuli (Rubenstein and Merzenich, 2003). An increased E/I ratio can lead to a prolonged neocortical circuit activity, elicited by thalamic stimulation in the *Fmr1* knockout mice, which may be involved in sensory stimulus hypersensitivity, epilepsy, and cognitive impairment (Hagerman and Hagerman, 2002; Gibson *et al.*, 2008). A decrease E/I ratio resulted from the mutation of neuroligin-3 may be responsible for the impaired social interactions in human autism spectrum disorders (ASDs) (Tabuchi *et al.*, 2007). In Rett Syndrom, a decreased E/I ratio resulted from the abnormal methyl CpG-binding protein (*MECP2*) gene may be associated with mental retardation, autistic behavior, and loss of previously acquired skills in human disorders (Dani *et al.*, 2005).

IV. Conclusions

The brain works appropriately only when the E-I ratio is properly balanced. Although multiple interrelations between homeostatic glutamatergic and GABAergic mechanisms have been investigated, little is known about the cellular and molecular mechanisms underlying homeostatic plasticity. Also, although rapid progresses has been made in understanding sensory manipulation induced plasticity of glutamatergic or GABAergic synapses, our knowledge regarding adaptive changes in E-I balance of the central nervous system in response to sensory deprivation is very limited. Little work has been done to understand the E-I balance disturbances in many nervous system disorders. Therefore, we desperately need to investigate such interrelation between the excitatory and inhibitory systems in the brain, which will certainly shed light on the understanding of the computation algorithms of brain circuits as well as the treatment of nervous system disorders resulting from a deregulated E-I balance.

References

Adermark, L., Talani, G., and Lovinger, D.M. (2009). Endocannabinoid-dependent plasticity at GABAergic and glutamatergic synapses in the striatum is regulated by synaptic activity. *Eur. J. Neurosci.* **29**, 32–41.

Adesnik, H., and Scanziani, M. (2010). Lateral competition for cortical space by layer-specific horizontal circuits. *Nature* **464**, 1155–1160.

Agmon, A., and Connors, B.W. (1992). Correlation between intrinsic firing patterns and thalamocortical synaptic responses of neurons in mouse barrel cortex. *J. Neurosci.* **12**, 319–329.

Agmon, A., Hollrigel, G., and O'Dowd, D.K. (1996). Functional GABAergic synaptic connection in neonatal mouse barrel cortex. *J. Neurosci.* **16**, 4684–4695.

Agmon, A., and O'Dowd, D.K. (1992). NMDA receptor-mediated currents are prominent in the thalamocortical synaptic response before maturation of inhibition. *J. Neurophysiol.* **68**, 345–349.

Ahissar, E., Sosnik, R., and Haidarliu, S. (2000). Transformation from temporal to rate coding in a somatosensory thalamocortical pathway. *Nature* **406**, 302–306.

Albright, T.D., Desimone, R., and Gross, C.G. (1984). Columnar organization of directionally selective cells in visual area MT of the macaque. *J. Neurophysiol.* **51**, 16–31.

Allen, C.B., Celikel, T., and Feldman, D. (2003). Long-term depression induced by sensory deprivation during cortical map plasticity *in vivo*. *Nat. Neurosci.* **6**, 291–299.

Armstrong-James, M., Callahan, C.A., and Friedman, M. (1991). Thalamo-cortical processing of vibrissal information in the rat I. Intracortical origins of surround but not centre-receptive fields of layer IV neurones in the rat S1 barrel field cortex. *J. Comp. Neurol.* **303**, 193–210.

Armstrong-James, M., and Fox, K. (1987). Spatiotemporal convergence and divergence in the rat S1 "barrel" cortex. *J. Comp. Neurol.* **263**, 265–281.

Armstrong-James, M., Fox, K., and Das-Gupta, A. (1992). Flow of excitation within rat barrel cortex on striking a single vibrissa. *J. Neurophysiol.* **68**, 1345–1358.

Azdad, K., Chavez, M., Don, B.P., Wetzelaer, P., Marescau, B., De Deyn, P.P., Gall, D., and Schiffmann, S.N. (2009). Homeostatic plasticity of striatal neurons intrinsic excitability following dopamine depletion. *PLoS One* **4**, e6908.

Bacci, A., Coco, S., Pravettoni, E., Schenk, U., Armano, S., Frassoni, C., Verderio, C., De, C.P., and Matteoli, M. (2001). Chronic blockade of glutamate receptors enhances presynaptic release and downregulates the interaction between synaptophysin-synaptobrevin-vesicle-associated membrane protein 2. *J. Neurosci.* **21**, 6588–6596.

Bannister, N.J., Benke, T.A., Mellor, J., Scott, H., Gurdal, E., Crabtree, J.W., and Isaac, J.T. (2005). Developmental changes in AMPA and kainate receptor-mediated quantal transmission at thalamocortical synapses in the barrel cortex. *J. Neurosci.* **25**, 5259–5271.

Barth, A.L., and Malenka, R.C. (2001). NMDAR EPSC kinetics do not regulate the critical period for LTP at thalamocortical synapses. *Nat. Neurosci.* **4**, 235–236.

Bear, M.F., Kleinschmidt, A., Gu, Q.A., and Singer, W. (1990). Disruption of experience-dependent synaptic modifications in striate cortex by infusion of an NMDA receptor antagonist. *J. Neurosci.* **10**, 909–925.

Beaulieu, C., Kisvarday, Z., Somogyi, P., Cynader, M., and Cowey, A. (1992). Quantitative distribution of GABA-immunopositive and -immunonegative neurons and synapses in the monkey striate cortex (area 17). *Cereb. Cortex* **2**, 295–309.

Ben-Ari, Y., Cherubini, E., Corradetti, R., and Gaiarsa, J.L. (1989). Giant synaptic potentials in immature rat CA3 hippocampal neurones. *J. Physiol.* **416**, 303–325.

Ben-Ari, Y., Tremblay, E., Ottersen, O.P., and Meldrum, B.S. (1980). The role of epileptic activity in hippocampal and "remote" cerebral lesions induced by kainic acid. *Brain Res.* **191**, 79–97.

Bender, V.A., Bender, K.J., Brasier, D.J., and Feldman, D.E. (2006). Two coincidence detectors for spike timing-dependent plasticity in somatosensory cortex. *J. Neurosci.* **26**, 4166–4177.

Berberich, S., Punnakkal, P., Jensen, V., Pawlak, V., Seeburg, P.H., Hvalby, O., and Kohr, G. (2005). Lack of NMDA receptor subtype selectivity for hippocampal long-term potentiation. *J. Neurosci.* **25**, 6907–6910.

Berger, T., Senn, W., and Luscher, H.R. (2003). Hyperpolarization-activated current Ih disconnects somatic and dendritic spike initiation zones in layer V pyramidal neurons. *J. Neurophysiol.* **90**, 2428–2437.

Bi, G.Q., and Poo, M.M. (1998). Synaptic modifications in cultured hippocampal neurons: dependence on spike timing, synaptic strength, and postsynaptic cell type. *J. Neurosci.* **18**, 10464–10472.

Binzegger, T., Douglas, R.J., and Martin, K.A. (2004). A quantitative map of the circuit of cat primary visual cortex. *J. Neurosci.* **24**, 8441–8453.

Blake, D.T., Byl, N.N., and Merzenich, M.M. (2002). Representation of the hand in the cerebral cortex. *Behav. Brain Res.* **135**, 179–184.

Blasdel, G.G., and Salama, G. (1986). Voltage-sensitive dyes reveal a modular organization in monkey striate cortex. *Nature* **321**, 579–585.

Blue, M.E., and Parnavelas, J.G. (1983). The formation and maturation of synapses in the visual cortex of the rat I. Qualitative analysis. *J. Neurocytol.* **12**, 599–616.

Bonhoeffer, T., and Grinvald, A. (1991). Iso-orientation domains in cat visual cortex are arranged in pinwheel-like patterns. *Nature* **353**, 429–431.

Borg-Graham, L.J., Monier, C., and Fregnac, Y. (1998). Visual input evokes transient and strong shunting inhibition in visual cortical neurons. *Nature* **393**, 369–373.

Bradford, H.F. (1995). Glutamate GABA and epilepsy. *Prog. Neurobiol.* **47**, 477–511.

Brager, D.H., and Johnston, D. (2007). Plasticity of intrinsic excitability during long-term depression is mediated through mGluR-dependent changes in I(h) in hippocampal CA1 pyramidal neurons. *J. Neurosci.* **27**, 13926–13937.

Brecht, M., Roth, A., and Sakmann, B. (2003). Dynamic receptive fields of reconstructed pyramidal cells in layers 3 and 2 of rat somatosensory barrel cortex. *J. Physiol.* **553**, 243–265.

Breton, J.D., and Stuart, G.J. (2009). Loss of sensory input increases the intrinsic excitability of layer 5 pyramidal neurons in rat barrel cortex. *J. Physiol.* **587**, 5107–5119.

Brill, J., and Huguenard, J.R. (2008). Sequential changes in AMPA receptor targeting in the developing neocortical excitatory circuit. *J. Neurosci.* **28**, 13918–13928.

Briner, A., De, R.M., Dayer, A., Muller, D., Kiss, J.Z., and Vutskits, L. (2010). Bilateral whisker trimming during early postnatal life impairs dendritic spine development in the mouse somatosensory barrel cortex. *J. Comp. Neurol.* **518**, 1711–1723.

Broser, P., Grinevich, V., Osten, P., Sakmann, B., and Wallace, D.J. (2008a). Critical period plasticity of axonal arbors of layer 2/3 pyramidal neurons in rat somatosensory cortex: layer-specific reduction of projections into deprived cortical columns. *Cereb. Cortex.* **18**, 1588–1603.

Broser, P.J., Erdogan, S., Grinevich, V., Osten, P., Sakmann, B., and Wallace, D.J. (2008b). Automated axon length quantification for populations of labelled neurons. *J. Neurosci. Methods* **169**, 43–54.

Bruno, R.M., and Simons, D.J. (2002). Feedforward mechanisms of excitatory and inhibitory cortical receptive fields. *J. Neurosci.* **22**, 10966–10975.

Buonomano, D.V. (1999). Distinct functional types of associative long-term potentiation in neocortical and hippocampal pyramidal neurons. *J. Neurosci.* **19**, 6748–6754.

Buonomano, D.V., and Merzenich, M.M. (1998). Cortical plasticity: from synapses to maps. *Annu. Rev. Neurosci.* **21**, 149–186.

Bureau, I., von Saint, P.F., and Svoboda, K. (2006). Interdigitated paralemniscal and lemniscal pathways in the mouse barrel cortex. *PLoS Biol.* **4**, e382.

Burgard, E.C., and Hablitz, J.J. (1993). NMDA receptor-mediated components of miniature excitatory synaptic currents in developing rat neocortex. *J. Neurophysiol.* **70**, 1841–1852.

Butz, M., Worgotter, F., and van, O.A. (2009). Activity-dependent structural plasticity. *Brain Res. Rev.* **60**, 287–305.

Carmignoto, G., and Vicini, S. (1992). Activity-dependent decrease in NMDA receptor responses during development of the visual cortex. *Science* **258**, 1007–1011.

Carvalho, T.P., and Buonomano, D.V. (2009). Differential effects of excitatory and inhibitory plasticity on synaptically driven neuronal input-output functions. *Neuron.* **61**, 774–785.

Castro-Alamancos, M.A. (2002). Different temporal processing of sensory inputs in the rat thalamus during quiescent and information processing states *in vivo*. *J. Physiol.* **539**, 567–578.

Cauli, B., Audinat, E., Lambolez, B., Angulo, M.C., Ropert, N., Tsuzuki, K., Hestrin, S., and Rossier, J. (1997). Molecular and physiological diversity of cortical nonpyramidal cells. *J. Neurosci.* **17**, 3894–3906.

Celikel, T., Szostak, V.A., and Feldman, D.E. (2004). Modulation of spike timing by sensory deprivation during induction of cortical map plasticity. *Nat. Neurosci.* **7**, 534–541.

Chandrasekaran, A.R., Plas, D.T., Gonzalez, E., and Crair, M.C. (2005). Evidence for an instructive role of retinal activity in retinotopic map refinement in the superior colliculus of the mouse. *J. Neurosci.* **25**, 6929–6938.

Chattopadhyaya, B., Di, C.G., Higashiyama, H., Knott, G.W., Kuhlman, S.J., Welker, E., and Huang, Z.J. (2004). Experience and activity-dependent maturation of perisomatic GABAergic innervation in primary visual cortex during a postnatal critical period. *J. Neurosci.* **24**, 9598–9611.

Cheetham, C.E., Hammond, M.S., Edwards, C.E., and Finnerty, G.T. (2007). Sensory experience alters cortical connectivity and synaptic function site specifically. *J. Neurosci.* **27**, 3456–3465.

Cherubini, E., Gaiarsa, J.L., and Ben-Ari, Y. (1991). GABA: an excitatory transmitter in early postnatal life. *Trends Neurosci.* **14**, 515–519.

Chisholm, J., Kellogg, C., and Lippa, A. (1983). Development of benzodiazepine binding subtypes in three regions of rat brain. *Brain Res.* **267**, 388–391.

Chittajallu, R., and Isaac, J.T. (2010). Emergence of cortical inhibition by coordinated sensory-driven plasticity at distinct synaptic loci. *Nat. Neurosci.* **13**, 1240–1248.

Chmielowska, J., Carvell, G.E., and Simons, D.J. (1989). Spatial organization of thalamocortical and corticothalamic projection systems in the rat SmI barrel cortex. *J. Comp. Neurol.* **285**, 325–338.

Chung, S., Li, X., and Nelson, S.B. (2002). Short-term depression at thalamocortical synapses contributes to rapid adaptation of cortical sensory responses *in vivo*. *Neuron.* **34**, 437–446.

Clem, R.L., and Barth, A. (2006). Pathway-specific trafficking of native AMPARs by *in vivo* experience. *Neuron.* **49**, 663–670.

Cline, H.T. (2001). Dendritic arbor development and synaptogenesis. *Curr. Opin. Neurobiol.* **11**, 118–126.

Cobos, I., Calcagnotto, M.E., Vilaythong, A.J., Thwin, M.T., Noebels, J.L., Baraban, S.C., and Rubenstein, J.L. (2005). Mice lacking Dlx1 show subtype-specific loss of interneurons, reduced inhibition and epilepsy. *Nat. Neurosci.* **8**, 1059–1068.

Connor, J.A., Tseng, H.Y., and Hockberger, P.E. (1987). Depolarization- and transmitter-induced changes in intracellular Ca2+ of rat cerebellar granule cells in explant cultures. *J. Neurosci.* **7**, 1384–1400.

Constantine-Paton, M., Cline, H.T., and Debski, E. (1990). Patterned activity, synaptic convergence, and the NMDA receptor in developing visual pathways. *Annu. Rev. Neurosci.* **13**, 129–154.

Corner, M.A., and Ramakers, G.J. (1992). Spontaneous firing as an epigenetic factor in brain development–physiological consequences of chronic tetrodotoxin and picrotoxin exposure on cultured rat neocortex neurons. *Brain Res. Dev.* **65**, 57–64.

Cossart, R., Bernard, C., and Ben-Ari, Y. (2005). Multiple facets of GABAergic neurons and synapses: multiple fates of GABA signalling in epilepsies. *Trends Neurosci.* **28**, 108–115.

Crair, M.C., and Malenka, R.C. (1995). A critical period for long-term potentiation at thalamocortical synapses. *Nature* **375**, 325–328.

Crochet, S., and Petersen, C.C. (2006). Correlating whisker behavior with membrane potential in barrel cortex of awake mice. *Nat. Neurosci.* **9**, 608–610.

Cruikshank, S.J., Lewis, T.J., and Connors, B.W. (2007). Synaptic basis for intense thalamocortical activation of feedforward inhibitory cells in neocortex. *Nat. Neurosci.* **10**, 462–468.

Cull-Candy, S., Brickley, S., and Farrant, M. (2001). NMDA receptor subunits: diversity, development and disease. *Curr. Opin. Neurobiol.* **11**, 327–335.

Cull-Candy, S.G., and Leszkiewicz, D.N. (2004). Role of distinct NMDA receptor subtypes at central synapses. *Sci. STKE.* **2004**, re16.

Dan, Y., and Poo, M.M. (2006). Spike timing-dependent plasticity: from synapse to perception. *Physiol. Rev.* **86**, 1033–1048.

Dani, V.S., Chang, Q., Maffei, A., Turrigiano, G.G., Jaenisch, R., and Nelson, S.B. (2005). Reduced cortical activity due to a shift in the balance between excitation and inhibition in a mouse model of Rett syndrome. *Proc. Natl. Acad. Sci. USA* **102**, 12560–12565.

Darian-Smith, C., and Gilbert, C.D. (1994). Axonal sprouting accompanies functional reorganization in adult cat striate cortex. *Nature* **368**, 737–740.

Datwani, A., Iwasato, T., Itohara, S., and Erzurumlu, R.S. (2002). Lesion-induced thalamocortical axonal plasticity in the S1 cortex is independent of NMDA receptor function in excitatory cortical neurons. *J. Neurosci.* **22**, 9171–9175.

Daw, M.I., Bannister, N.V., and Isaac, J.T. (2006). Rapid, activity-dependent plasticity in timing precision in neonatal barrel cortex. *J. Neurosci.* **26**, 4178–4187.

De, G.S., Schafer, M.K., Defamie, N., Chen, C., Ricci, A., Weihe, E., Varoqui, H., and Erickson, J.D. (2005). Homeostatic scaling of vesicular glutamate and GABA transporter expression in rat neocortical circuits. *J. Neurosci.* **25**, 7121–7133.

DeFelipe, J. (2002). Cortical interneurons: from Cajal to 2001. *Prog. Brain Res.* **136**, 215–238.

DeFelipe, J., Arellano, J.I., Merchan-Perez, A., Gonzalez-Albo, M.C., Walton, K., and Llinas, R. (2002). Spaceflight induces changes in the synaptic circuitry of the postnatal developing neocortex. *Cereb. Cortex.* **12**, 883–891.

Desai, N.S., Cudmore, R.H., Nelson, S.B., and Turrigiano, G.G. (2002). Critical periods for experience-dependent synaptic scaling in visual cortex. *Nat. Neurosci.* **5**, 783–789.

Diamond, M.E., Huang, W., and Ebner, F.F. (1994). Laminar comparison of somatosensory cortical plasticity. *Science* **265**, 1885–1888.

Diamond, M.E., Armstrong-James, M., and Ebner, F.F. (1993). Experience-dependent plasticity in adult rat barrel cortex. *Proc. Natl. Acad. Sci. USA* **90**, 2082–2086.

Dittgen, T., Nimmerjahn, A., Komai, S., Licznerski, P., Waters, J., Margrie, T.W., Helmchen, F., Denk, W., Brecht, M., and Osten, P. (2004). Lentivirus-based genetic manipulations of cortical neurons and their optical and electrophysiological monitoring *in vivo*. *Proc. Natl. Acad. Sci. USA* **101**, 18206–18211.

Douglas, R.J., and Martin, K.A. (2004). Neuronal circuits of the neocortex. *Annu. Rev. Neurosci.* **27**, 419–451.

Durand, C.M *et al.*, (2007). Mutations in the gene encoding the synaptic scaffolding protein SHANK3 are associated with autism spectrum disorders. *Nat. Genet.* **39**, 25–27.

Echegoyen, J., Neu, A., Graber, K.D., and Soltesz, I. (2007). Homeostatic plasticity studied using in vivo hippocampal activity-blockade: synaptic scaling, intrinsic plasticity and age-dependence. *PLoS One* **2**, e700.

Eder, M., Zieglgansberger, W., and Dodt, H.U. (2002). Neocortical long-term potentiation and long-term depression: site of expression investigated by infrared-guided laser stimulation. *J. Neurosci.* **22**, 7558–7568.

Eichler, S.A., and Meier, J.C. (2008). E-I balance and human diseases - from molecules to networking. *Front Mol. Neurosci.* **1**, 2.

Fagiolini, M., Fritschy, J.M., Low, K., Mohler, H., Rudolph, U., and Hensch, T.K. (2004). Specific GABAA circuits for visual cortical plasticity. *Science* **303**, 1681–1683.

Fanselow, E.E., and Nicolelis, M.A. (1999). Behavioral modulation of tactile responses in the rat somatosensory system. *J. Neurosci.* **19**, 7603–7616.

Farrant, M., and Kaila, K. (2007). The cellular, molecular and ionic basis of GABA(A) receptor signalling. *Prog. Brain Res.* **160**, 59–87.

Feldman, D.E. (2000a). Inhibition and plasticity. *Nat. Neurosci.* **3**, 303–304.

Feldman, D.E. (2000b). Timing-based LTP and LTD at vertical inputs to layer II/III pyramidal cells in rat barrel cortex. *Neuron.* **27**, 45–56.

Feldman, D.E. (2009). Synaptic mechanisms for plasticity in neocortex. *Annu. Rev. Neurosci.* **32**, 33–55.

Feldman, D.E., and Brecht, M. (2005). Map plasticity in somatosensory cortex. *Science* **310**, 810–815.

Feldman, D.E., Nicoll, R.A., and Malenka, R.C. (1999). Synaptic plasticity at thalamocortical synapses in developing rat somatosensory cortex: LTP LTD, and silent synapses. *J. Neurobiol.* **41**, 92–101.

Feldman, D.E., Nicoll, R.A., Malenka, R.C., and Isaac, J.T. (1998). Long-term depression at thalamocortical synapses in developing rat somatosensory cortex. *Neuron.* **21**, 347–357.

Feldmeyer, D., and Radnikow, G. (2009). Developmental alterations in the functional properties of excitatory neocortical synapses. *J. Physiol.* **587**, 1889–1896.

Feng, J., Schroer, R., Yan, J., Song, W., Yang, C., Bockholt, A., Cook Jr., E.H., Skinner, C., Schwartz, C.E., and Sommer, S.S. (2006). High frequency of neurexin 1beta signal peptide structural variants in patients with autism. *Neurosci. Lett.* **409**, 10–13.

Finnerty, G.T., and Connors, B.W. (2000). Sensory deprivation without competition yields modest alterations of short-term synaptic dynamics. *Proc. Natl. Acad. Sci. USA* **97**, 12864–12868.

Finnerty, G.T., Roberts, L.S., and Connors, B.W. (1999). Sensory experience modifies the short-term dynamics of neocortical synapses. *Nature* **400**, 367–371.

Fiumelli, H., and Woodin, M.A. (2007). Role of activity-dependent regulation of neuronal chloride homeostasis in development. *Curr. Opin. Neurobiol* **17**, 81–86.

Flint, A.C., Maisch, U.S., Weishaupt, J.H., Kriegstein, A.R., and Monyer, H. (1997). NR2A subunit expression shortens NMDA receptor synaptic currents in developing neocortex. *J. Neurosci.* **17**, 2469–2476.

Foeller, E., and Feldman, D.E. (2004). Synaptic basis for developmental plasticity in somatosensory cortex. *Curr. Opin. Neurobiol.* **14**, 89–95.

Foffani, G., Tutunculer, B., and Moxon, K.A. (2004). Role of spike timing in the forelimb somatosensory cortex of the rat. *J. Neurosci.* **24**, 7266–7271.

Fox, K. (1994). The cortical component of experience-dependent synaptic plasticity in the rat barrel cortex. *J. Neurosci.* **14**, 7665–7679.

Fox, K. (1992). A critical period for experience-dependent synaptic plasticity in rat barrel cortex. *J. Neurosci.* **12**, 1826–1838.

Fox, K. (2002). Anatomical pathways and molecular mechanisms for plasticity in the barrel cortex. *Neuroscience* **111**, 799–814.

Fox, K., and Wong, R.O. (2005). A comparison of experience-dependent plasticity in the visual and somatosensory systems. *Neuron.* **48**, 465–477.

Frenkel, M.Y., Sawtell, N.B., Diogo, A.C., Yoon, B., Neve, R.L., and Bear, M.F. (2006). Instructive effect of visual experience in mouse visual cortex. *Neuron.* **51**, 339–349.

Freund, T.F., and Buzsaki, G. (1996). Interneurons of the hippocampus. *Hippocampus* **6**, 347–470.

Frick, A., Feldmeyer, D., and Sakmann, B. (2007). Postnatal development of synaptic transmission in local networks of L5A pyramidal neurons in rat somatosensory cortex. *J. Physiol.* **585**, 103–116.

Froemke, R.C., Poo, M.M., and Dan, Y. (2005). Spike-timing-dependent synaptic plasticity depends on dendritic location. *Nature* **434**, 221–225.

Fujita, I., Tanaka, K., Ito, M., and Cheng, K. (1992). Columns for visual features of objects in monkey inferotemporal cortex. *Nature* **360**, 343–346.

Gabernet, L., Jadhav, S.P., Feldman, D.E., Carandini, M., and Scanziani, M. (2005). Somatosensory integration controlled by dynamic thalamocortical feed-forward inhibition. *Neuron.* **48**, 315–327.

Gale, K. (1992). GABA and epilepsy: basic concepts from preclinical research. *Epilepsia 33 Suppl* **5**, S3–12.

Genoud, C., Quairiaux, C., Steiner, P., Hirling, H., Welker, E., and Knott, G.W. (2006). Plasticity of astrocytic coverage and glutamate transporter expression in adult mouse cortex. *PLoS Biol.* **4**, e343.

Gentet, L.J., Avermann, M., Matyas, F., Staiger, J.F., and Petersen, C.C. (2010). Membrane potential dynamics of GABAergic neurons in the barrel cortex of behaving mice. *Neuron.* **65**, 422–435.

Ghazanfar, A.A., Stambaugh, C.R., and Nicolelis, M.A. (2000). Encoding of tactile stimulus location by somatosensory thalamocortical ensembles. *J. Neurosci.* **20**, 3761–3775.

Gibson, J.R., Bartley, A.F., Hays, S.A., and Huber, K.M. (2008). Imbalance of neocortical excitation and inhibition and altered UP states reflect network hyperexcitability in the mouse model of fragile X syndrome. *J. Neurophysiol.* **100**, 2615–2626.

Glazewski, S., Barth, A.L., Wallace, H., McKenna, M., Silva, A., and Fox, K. (1999). Impaired experience-dependent plasticity in barrel cortex of mice lacking the alpha and delta isoforms of CREB. *Cereb Cortex* **9**, 249–256.

Glazewski, S., Chen, C.M., Silva, A., and Fox, K. (1996). Requirement for alpha-CaMKII in experience-dependent plasticity of the barrel cortex. *Science* **272**, 421–423.

Glazewski, S., and Fox, K. (1996). Time course of experience-dependent synaptic potentiation and depression in barrel cortex of adolescent rats. *J. Neurophysiol.* **75**, 1714–1729.

Glazewski, S., McKenna, M., Jacquin, M., and Fox, K. (1998). Experience-dependent depression of vibrissae responses in adolescent rat barrel cortex. *Eur. J. Neurosci.* **10**, 2107–2116.

Gupta, A., Wang, Y., and Markram, H. (2000). Organizing principles for a diversity of GABAergic interneurons and synapses in the neocortex. *Science* **287**, 273–278.

Hafting, T., Fyhn, M., Molden, S., Moser, M.B., and Moser, E.I. (2005). Microstructure of a spatial map in the entorhinal cortex. *Nature* **436**, 801–806.

Hagerman, R.J., and Hagerman, P.J. (2002). The fragile X premutation: into the phenotypic fold. *Curr. Opin. Genet. Dev.* **12**, 278–283.

Haider, B., Duque, A., Hasenstaub, A.R., and McCormick, D.A. (2006). Neocortical network activity *in vivo* is generated through a dynamic balance of excitation and inhibition. *J. Neurosci.* **26**, 4535–4545.

Hardingham, N., and Fox, K. (2006). The role of nitric oxide and GluR1 in presynaptic and postsynaptic components of neocortical potentiation. *J. Neurosci.* **26**, 7395–7404.

Hardingham, N., Glazewski, S., Pakhotin, P., Mizuno, K., Chapman, P.F., Giese, K.P., and Fox, K. (2003). Neocortical long-term potentiation and experience-dependent synaptic plasticity require alpha-calcium/calmodulin-dependent protein kinase II autophosphorylation. *J. Neurosci.* **23**, 4428–4436.

Hensch, T.K., and Fagiolini, M. (2005). Excitatory-inhibitory balance and critical period plasticity in developing visual cortex. *Prog. Brain Res.* **147**, 115–124.

Hensch, T.K., Fagiolini, M., Mataga, N., Stryker, M.P., Baekkeskov, S., and Kash, S.F. (1998). Local GABA circuit control of experience-dependent plasticity in developing visual cortex. *Science* **282**, 1504–1508.

Higley, M.J., and Contreras, D. (2006). Balanced excitation and inhibition determine spike timing during frequency adaptation. *J. Neurosci.* **26**, 448–457.

Higley, M.J., and Contreras, D. (2007a). Cellular mechanisms of suppressive interactions between somatosensory responses *in vivo*. *J. Neurophysiol.* **97**, 647–658.

Higley, M.J., and Contreras, D. (2007b). Frequency adaptation modulates spatial integration of sensory responses in the rat whisker system. *J. Neurophysiol.* **97**, 3819–3824.

Houser, C.R., Hendry, S.H., Jones, E.G., and Vaughn, J.E. (1983). Morphological diversity of immunocytochemically identified GABA neurons in the monkey sensory-motor cortex. *J. Neurocytol.* **12**, 617–638.

Huang, Z.J., Kirkwood, A., Pizzorusso, T., Porciatti, V., Morales, B., Bear, M.F., Maffei, L., and Tonegawa, S. (1999). BDNF regulates the maturation of inhibition and the critical period of plasticity in mouse visual cortex. *Cell* **98**, 739–755.

Hubel, D.H., and Wiesel, T.N. (1962). Receptive fields, binocular interaction and functional architecture in the cat's visual cortex. *J. Physiol.* **160**, 106–154.

Isaac, J.T., Crair, M.C., Nicoll, R.A., and Malenka, R.C. (1997). Silent synapses during development of thalamocortical inputs. *Neuron.* **18**, 269–280.

Issa, N.P., Trepel, C., and Stryker, M.P. (2000). Spatial frequency maps in cat visual cortex. *J. Neurosci.* **20**, 8504–8514.

Jamain, S., Quach, H., Betancur, C., Rastam, M., Colineaux, C., Gillberg, I.C., Soderstrom, H., Giros, B., Leboyer, M., Gillberg, C., and Bourgeron, T. (2003). Mutations of the X-linked genes encoding neuroligins NLGN3 and NLGN4 are associated with autism. *Nat. Genet.* **34**, 27–29.

Jiang, B., Trevino, M., and Kirkwood, A. (2007). Sequential development of long-term potentiation and depression in different layers of the mouse visual cortex. *J. Neurosci.* **27**, 9648–9652.

Jiao, Y., Zhang, C., Yanagawa, Y., and Sun, Q.Q. (2006). Major effects of sensory experiences on the neocortical inhibitory circuits. *J. Neurosci.* **26**, 8691–8701.

Kaas, J.H., Krubitzer, L.A., Chino, Y.M., Langston, A.L., Polley, E.H., and Blair, N. (1990). Reorganization of retinotopic cortical maps in adult mammals after lesions of the retina. *Science* **248**, 229–231.

Kanold, P.O., Kim, Y.A., GrandPre, T., and Shatz, C.J. (2009). Co-regulation of ocular dominance plasticity and NMDA receptor subunit expression in glutamic acid decarboxylase-65 knock-out mice. *J. Physiol.* **587**, 2857–2867.

Katz, L.C., and Shatz, C.J. (1996). Synaptic activity and the construction of cortical circuits. *Science* **274**, 1133–1138.

Kawaguchi, Y., and Kubota, Y. (1997). GABAergic cell subtypes and their synaptic connections in rat frontal cortex. *Cereb. Cortex* **7**, 476–486.

Kehrer, C., Maziashvili, N., Dugladze, T., and Gloveli, T. (2008). Altered Excitatory-Inhibitory Balance in the NMDA-Hypofunction Model of Schizophrenia. *Front Mol. Neurosci.* **1**, 6.

Kemp, N., and Bashir, Z.I. (2001). Long-term depression: a cascade of induction and expression mechanisms. *Prog. Neurobiol* **65**, 339–365.

Keuroghlian, A.S., and Knudsen, E.I. (2007). Adaptive auditory plasticity in developing and adult animals. *Prog. Neurobiol.* **82**, 109–121.

Kidd, F.L., and Isaac, J.T. (1999). Developmental and activity-dependent regulation of kainate receptors at thalamocortical synapses. *Nature* **400**, 569–573.

Killackey, H.P. (1973). Anatomical evidence for cortical subdivisions based on vertically discrete thalamic projections from the ventral posterior nucleus to cortical barrels in the rat. *Brain Res.* **51**, 326–331.

Killackey, H.P., and Leshin, S. (1975). The organization of specific thalamocortical projections to the posteromedial barrel subfield of the rat somatic sensory cortex. *Brain Res.* **86**, 469–472.

Kim, H.G., Fox, K., and Connors, B.W. (1995). Properties of excitatory synaptic events in neurons of primary somatosensory cortex of neonatal rats. *Cereb. Cortex.* **5**, 148–157.

Kirkwood, A., and Bear, M.F. (1994). Hebbian synapses in visual cortex. *J. Neurosci.* **14**, 1634–1645.

Knudsen, E.I., and Knudsen, P.F. (1990). Sensitive and critical periods for visual calibration of sound localization by barn owls. *J. Neurosci.* **10**, 222–232.

Kobayashi, M., Hamada, T., Kogo, M., Yanagawa, Y., Obata, K., and Kang, Y. (2008). Developmental profile of GABAA-mediated synaptic transmission in pyramidal cells of the somatosensory cortex. *Eur. J. Neurosci.* **28**, 849–861.

Komatsu, Y., and Iwakiri, M. (1991). Postnatal development of neuronal connections in cat visual cortex studied by intracellular recording in slice preparation. *Brain Res.* **540**, 14–24.

Koralek, K.A., Jensen, K.F., and Killackey, H.P. (1988). Evidence for two complementary patterns of thalamic input to the rat somatosensory cortex. *Brain Res.* **463**, 346–351.

Krieger, P. (2009). Experience-dependent increase in spine calcium evoked by backpropagating action potentials in layer 2/3 pyramidal neurons in rat somatosensory cortex. *Eur. J. Neurosci.* **30**, 1870–1877.

Kriegstein, A.R., Suppes, T., and Prince, D.A. (1987). Cellular and synaptic physiology and epileptogenesis of developing rat neocortical neurons *in vivo*. *Brain Res.* **431**, 161–171.

Kumar, S.S., Bacci, A., Kharazia, V., and Huguenard, J.R. (2002). A developmental switch of AMPA receptor subunits in neocortical pyramidal neurons. *J. Neurosci.* **22**, 3005–3015.

Land, P.W., and Simons, D.J. (1985). Metabolic and structural correlates of the vibrissae representation in the thalamus of the adult rat. *Neurosci. Lett.* **60**, 319–324.

Laumonnier, F., Bonnet-Brilhault, F., Gomot, M., Blanc, R., David, A., Moizard, M.P., Raynaud, M., Ronce, N., Lemonnier, E., Calvas, P., Laudier, B., Chelly, J., Fryns, J.P., Ropers, H.H., Hamel, B. C., Andres, C., Barthelemy, C., Moraine, C., and Briault, S. (2004). X-linked mental retardation and autism are associated with a mutation in the NLGN4 gene, a member of the neuroligin family. *Am. J. Hum. Genet.* **74**, 552–557.

Laurie, D.J., Wisden, W., and Seeburg, P.H. (1992). The distribution of thirteen GABAA receptor subunit mRNAs in the rat brain III Embryonic and postnatal development. *J. Neurosci.* **12**, 4151–4172.

Le, R.N., Amar, M., Baux, G., and Fossier, P. (2006). Homeostatic control of the excitation-inhibition balance in cortical layer 5 pyramidal neurons. *Eur. J. Neurosci.* **24**, 3507–3518.

Lebedev, M.A., Mirabella, G., Erchova, I., and Diamond, M.E. (2000). Experience-dependent plasticity of rat barrel cortex: redistribution of activity across barrel-columns. *Cereb. Cortex.* **10**, 23–31.

Lee, M.C., Yasuda, R., and Ehlers, M.D. (2010). Metaplasticity at single glutamatergic synapses. *Neuron* **66**, 859–870.

Lee, S.H., Land, P.W., and Simons, D.J. (2007). Layer- and cell-type-specific effects of neonatal whisker-trimming in adult rat barrel cortex. *J. Neurophysiol* **97**, 4380–4385.

Lefort, S., Tomm, C., Floyd Sarria, J.C., and Petersen, C.C. (2009). The excitatory neuronal network of the C2 barrel column in mouse primary somatosensory cortex. *Neuron* **61**, 301–316.

Lendvai, B., Stern, E.A., Chen, B., and Svoboda, K. (2000). Experience-dependent plasticity of dendritic spines in the developing rat barrel cortex *in vivo*. *Nature* **404**, 876–881.

Lewis, D.A., Glantz, L.A., Pierri, J.N., and Sweet, R.A. (2003). Altered cortical glutamate neurotransmission in schizophrenia: evidence from morphological studies of pyramidal neurons. *Ann. NY Acad. Sci.* **1003**, 102–112.

Lissin, D.V., Gomperts, S.N., Carroll, R.C., Christine, C.W., Kalman, D., Kitamura, M., Hardy, S., Nicoll, R.A., Malenka, R.C., and von, Z.M. (1998). Activity differentially regulates the surface expression of synaptic AMPA and NMDA glutamate receptors. *Proc. Natl. Acad. Sci. USA* **95**, 7097–7102.

Litvak, V., Sompolinsky, H., Segev, I., and Abeles, M. (2003). On the transmission of rate code in long feedforward networks with excitatory-inhibitory balance. *J. Neurosci.* **23**, 3006–3015.

Liu, G. (2004). Local structural balance and functional interaction of excitatory and inhibitory synapses in hippocampal dendrites. *Nat. Neurosci.* **7**, 373–379.

Liu, L., Wong, T.P., Pozza, M.F., Lingenhoehl, K., Wang, Y., Sheng, M., Auberson, Y.P., and Wang, Y.T. (2004a). Role of NMDA receptor subtypes in governing the direction of hippocampal synaptic plasticity. *Science* **304**, 1021–1024.

Liu, X.B., Murray, K.D., and Jones, E.G. (2004 b) Switching of NMDA receptor 2A and 2B subunits at thalamic and cortical synapses during early postnatal development. *J. Neurosci.* **24**, 8885–8895.

Lu, H.C., Gonzalez, E., and Crair, M.C. (2001). Barrel cortex critical period plasticity is independent of changes in NMDA receptor subunit composition. *Neuron* **32**, 619–634.

Lu, S.M., and Lin, R.C. (1993). Thalamic afferents of the rat barrel cortex: a light- and electron-microscopic study using Phaseolus vulgaris leucoagglutinin as an anterograde tracer. *Somatosens Mot. Res.* **10**, 1–16.

Luddens, H., and Wisden, W. (1991). Function and pharmacology of multiple GABAA receptor subunits. *Trends Pharmacol. Sci.* **12**, 49–51.

Luhmann, H.J., and Prince, D.A. (1991). Postnatal maturation of the GABAergic system in rat neocortex. *J. Neurophysiol.* **65**, 247–263.

Maffei, A., and Turrigiano, G.G. (2008). Multiple modes of network homeostasis in visual cortical layer 2/3. *J. Neurosci.* **28**, 4377–4384.

Malenka, R.C., and Nicoll, R.A. (1999). Long-term potentiation–a decade of progress? *Science* **285**, 1870–1874.

Malinow, R., and Malenka, R.C. (2002). AMPA receptor trafficking and synaptic plasticity. *Annu. Rev. Neurosci.* **25**, 103–126.

Maravall, M., Koh, I.Y., Lindquist, W.B., and Svoboda, K. (2004). Experience-dependent changes in basal dendritic branching of layer 2/3 pyramidal neurons during a critical period for developmental plasticity in rat barrel cortex. *Cereb. Cortex.* **14**, 655–664.

Marder, E., and Goaillard, J.M. (2006). Variability, compensation and homeostasis in neuron and network function. *Nat. Rev. Neurosci.* **7**, 563–574.

Marder, E., and Prinz, A.A. (2002). Modeling stability in neuron and network function: the role of activity in homeostasis. *Bioessays.* **24**, 1145–1154.

Marino, J., Schummers, J., Lyon, D.C., Schwabe, L., Beck, O., Wiesing, P., Obermayer, K., and Sur, M. (2005). Invariant computations in local cortical networks with balanced excitation and inhibition. *Nat. Neurosci.* **8**, 194–201.

Markram, H., and Tsodyks, M. (1996). Redistribution of synaptic efficacy between neocortical pyramidal neurons. *Nature* **382**, 807–810.

Massey, P.V., Johnson, B.E., Moult, P.R., Auberson, Y.P., Brown, M.W., Molnar, E., Collingridge, G. L., and Bashir, Z.I. (2004). Differential roles of NR2A and NR2B-containing NMDA receptors in cortical long-term potentiation and long-term depression. *J. Neurosci.* **24**, 7821–7828.

McBain, C.J., and Fisahn, A. (2001). Interneurons unbound. *Nat. Rev. Neurosci.* **2**, 11–23.

Meier, E., Jorgensen, O.S., and Schousboe, A. (1987). Effect of repeated treatment with a gamma-aminobutyric acid receptor agonist on postnatal neural development in rats. *J. Neurochem.* **49**, 1462–1470.

Micheva, K.D., and Beaulieu, C. (1995). Neonatal sensory deprivation induces selective changes in the quantitative distribution of GABA-immunoreactive neurons in the rat barrel field cortex. *J. Comp. Neurol.* **361**, 574–584.

Micheva, K.D., and Beaulieu, C. (1996). Quantitative aspects of synaptogenesis in the rat barrel field cortex with special reference to GABA circuitry. *J. Comp. Neurol.* **373**, 340–354.

Micheva, K.D., and Beaulieu, C. (1997). Development and plasticity of the inhibitory neocortical circuitry with an emphasis on the rodent barrel field cortex: a review. *J. Physiol. Pharmacol.* **75**, 470–478.

Mierau, S.B., Meredith, R.M., Upton, A.L., and Paulsen, O. (2004). Dissociation of experience-dependent and -independent changes in excitatory synaptic transmission during development of barrel cortex. *Proc. Natl. Acad. Sci. USA* **101**, 15518–15523.

Miles, R., Toth, K., Gulyas, A.I., Hajos, N., and Freund, T.F. (1996). Differences between somatic and dendritic inhibition in the hippocampus. *Neuron.* **16**, 815–823.

Miller, K.D. (1996). Synaptic economics: competition and cooperation in synaptic plasticity. *Neuron.* **17**, 371–374.

Miller, M.W. (1986). Maturation of rat visual cortex III. Postnatal morphogenesis and synaptogenesis of local circuit neurons. *Brain Res.* **390**, 271–285.

Mody, . (2005). Aspects of the homeostaic plasticity of GABAA receptor-mediated inhibition. *J. Physiol.* **562**, 37–46.

Monier, C., Chavane, F., Baudot, P., Graham, L.J., and Fregnac, Y. (2003). Orientation and direction selectivity of synaptic inputs in visual cortical neurons: a diversity of combinations produces spike tuning. *Neuron.* **37**, 663–680.

Monyer, H., Burnashev, N., Laurie, D.J., Sakmann, B., and Seeburg, P.H. (1994). Developmental and regional expression in the rat brain and functional properties of four NMDA receptors. *Neuron.* **12**, 529–540.

Moore, C.I. (2004). Frequency-dependent processing in the vibrissa sensory system. *J. Neurophysiol.* **91**, 2390–2399.

Moore, C.I., and Nelson, S.B. (1998). Spatio-temporal subthreshold receptive fields in the vibrissa representation of rat primary somatosensory cortex. *J. Neurophysiol.* **80**, 2882–2892.

Morales, B., Choi, S.Y., and Kirkwood, A. (2002). Dark rearing alters the development of GABAergic transmission in visual cortex. *J. Neurosci.* **22**, 8084–8090.

Morishita, W., Lu, W., Smith, G.B., Nicoll, R.A., Bear, M.F., and Malenka, R.C. (2007). Activation of NR2B-containing NMDA receptors is not required for NMDA receptor-dependent long-term depression. *Neuropharmacology* **52**, 71–76.

Murphy, B.K., and Miller, K.D. (2009). Balanced amplification: a new mechanism of selective amplification of neural activity patterns. *Neuron.* **61**, 635–648.

Nakayama, K., Kiyosue, K., and Taguchi, T. (2005). Diminished neuronal activity increases neuron-neuron connectivity underlying silent synapse formation and the rapid conversion of silent to functional synapses. *J. Neurosci.* **25**, 4040–4051.

Newpher, T.M., and Ehlers, M.D. (2008). Glutamate receptor dynamics in dendritic microdomains. *Neuron.* **58**, 472–497.

Niddam, R., Dubois, A., Scatton, B., Arbilla, S., and Langer, S.Z. (1987). Autoradiographic localization of [3H]zolpidem binding sites in the rat CNS: comparison with the distribution of [3H]flunitrazepam binding sites. *J. Neurochem.* **49**, 890–899.

O'Brien, R.J., Kamboj, S., Ehlers, M.D., Rosen, K.R., Fischbach, G.D., and Huganir, R.L. (1998). Activity-dependent modulation of synaptic AMPA receptor accumulation. *Neuron.* **21**, 1067–1078.

Olsen, R.W., and Avoli, M. (1997). GABA and epileptogenesis. *Epilepsia.* **38**, 399–407.

Olsen, R.W., Bureau, M., Khrestchatisky, M., MacLennan, A.J., Chiang, M.Y., Tobin, A.J., Xu, W., Jackson, M., Sternini, C., and Brecha, N. (1990). Isolation of pharmacologically distinct GABA-benzodiazepine receptors by protein chemistry and molecular cloning. *Adv. Biochem. Psychopharmacol* **46**, 35–49.

Olsen, R.W., and Tobin, A.J. (1990). Molecular biology of GABAA receptors. *FASEB J.* **4**, 1469–1480.

Oswald, A.M., Doiron, B., Rinzel, J., and Reyes, A.D. (2009). Spatial profile and differential recruitment of GABAB modulate oscillatory activity in auditory cortex. *J. Neurosci.* **29**, 10321–10334.

Oswald, A.M., and Reyes, A.D. (2008). Maturation of intrinsic and synaptic properties of layer 2/3 pyramidal neurons in mouse auditory cortex. *J. Neurophysiol.* **99**, 2998–3008.

Panzeri, S., Petersen, R.S., Schultz, S.R., Lebedev, M., and Diamond, M.E. (2001). The role of spike timing in the coding of stimulus location in rat somatosensory cortex. *Neuron.* **29**, 769–777.

Paulsen, O., and Sejnowski, T.J. (2000). Natural patterns of activity and long-term synaptic plasticity. *Curr. Opin. Neurobiol.* **10**, 172–179.

Perez-Otano, I., and Ehlers, M.D. (2005). Homeostatic plasticity and NMDA receptor trafficking. *Trends Neurosci.* **28**, 229–238.

Petersen, C.C. (2003). The barrel cortex–integrating molecular, cellular and systems physiology. *Pflugers Arch.* **447**, 126–134.

Petersen, C.C., Grinvald, A., and Sakmann, B. (2003a). Spatiotemporal dynamics of sensory responses in layer 2/3 of rat barrel cortex measured *in vivo* by voltage-sensitive dye imaging combined with whole-cell voltage recordings and neuron reconstructions. *J. Neurosci.* **23**, 1298–1309.

Petersen, C.C., Hahn, T.T., Mehta, M., Grinvald, A., and Sakmann, B. (2003b). Interaction of sensory responses with spontaneous depolarization in layer 2/3 barrel cortex. *Proc. Natl. Acad. Sci. USA* **100**, 13638–13643.

Philpot, B.D., Sekhar, A.K., Shouval, H.Z., and Bear, M.F. (2001). Visual experience and deprivation bidirectionally modify the composition and function of NMDA receptors in visual cortex. *Neuron.* **29**, 157–169.

Pinto, D.J., Brumberg, J.C., and Simons, D.J. (2000). Circuit dynamics and coding strategies in rodent somatosensory cortex. *J. Neurophysiol* **83**, 1158–1166.

Polley, D.B., Kvasnak, E., and Frostig, R.D. (2004). Naturalistic experience transforms sensory maps in the adult cortex of caged animals. *Nature.* **429**, 67–71.

Porter, J.T., Johnson, C.K., and Agmon, A. (2001). Diverse types of interneurons generate thalamus-evoked feedforward inhibition in the mouse barrel cortex. *J. Neurosci.* **21**, 2699–2710.

Pouille, F., Marin-Burgin, A., Adesnik, H., Atallah, B.V., and Scanziani, M. (2009). Input normalization by global feedforward inhibition expands cortical dynamic range. *Nat. Neurosci.* **12**, 1577–1585.

Pouille, F., and Scanziani, M. (2001). Enforcement of temporal fidelity in pyramidal cells by somatic feed-forward inhibition. *Science* **293**, 1159–1163.

Poulet, J.F., and Petersen, C.C. (2008). Internal brain state regulates membrane potential synchrony in barrel cortex of behaving mice. *Nature* **454**, 881–885.

Pratt, K.G., and Aizenman, C.D. (2007). Homeostatic regulation of intrinsic excitability and synaptic transmission in a developing visual circuit. *J. Neurosci.* **27**, 8268–8277.

Price, C.J., Cauli, B., Kovacs, E.R., Kulik, A., Lambolez, B., Shigemoto, R., and Capogna, M. (2005). Neurogliaform neurons form a novel inhibitory network in the hippocampal CA1 area. *J. Neurosci.* **25**, 6775–6786.

Quinlan, E.M., Olstein, D.H., and Bear, M.F. (1999). Bidirectional, experience-dependent regulation of N-methyl-D-aspartate receptor subunit composition in the rat visual cortex during postnatal development. *Proc. Natl. Acad. Sci. USA* **96**, 12876–12880.

Ramakers, G.J., Corner, M.A., and Habets, A.M. (1990). Development in the absence of spontaneous bioelectric activity results in increased stereotyped burst firing in cultures of dissociated cerebral cortex. *Exp. Brain. Res.* **79**, 157–166.

Ramakers, G.J., van, G.H., Feenstra, M.G., Corner, M.A., and Boer, G.J. (1994). Activity-dependent plasticity of inhibitory and excitatory amino acid transmitter systems in cultured rat cerebral cortex. *Int. J. Dev. Neurosci.* **12**, 611–621.

Ramocki, M.B., and Zoghbi, H.Y. (2008). Failure of neuronal homeostasis results in common neuropsychiatric phenotypes. *Nature* **455**, 912–918.

Ratte, S., and Lacaille, J.C. (2006). Selective degeneration and synaptic reorganization of hippocampal interneurons in a chronic model of temporal lobe epilepsy. *Adv. Neurol.* **97**, 69–76.

Rebola, N., Srikumar, B.N., and Mulle, C. (2010). Activity-dependent synaptic plasticity of NMDA receptors. *J. Physiol.* **588**, 93–99.

Reichelt, R., Hofmann, D., Fodisch, H.J., Mohler, H., Knapp, M., and Hebebrand, J. (1991). Ontogeny of the benzodiazepine receptor in human brain: fluorographic, immunochemical, and reversible binding studies. *J. Neurochem.* **57**, 1128–1135.

Rema, V., Armstrong-James, M., and Ebner, F.F. (1998). Experience-dependent plasticity of adult rat S1 cortex requires local NMDA receptor activation. *J. Neurosci.* **18**, 10196–10206.

Reyes, A., and Sakmann, B. (1999). Developmental switch in the short-term modification of unitary EPSPs evoked in layer 2/3 and layer 5 pyramidal neurons of rat neocortex. *J. Neurosci.* **19**, 3827–3835.

Rich, M.M., and Wenner, P. (2007). Sensing and expressing homeostatic synaptic plasticity. *Trends Neurosci.* **30**, 119–125.

Rivera, C., Voipio, J., and Kaila, K. (2005). Two developmental switches in GABAergic signalling: the K+-Cl- cotransporter KCC2 and carbonic anhydrase CAVII. *J. Physiol.* **562**, 27–36.

Roberts, E.B., Meredith, M.A., and Ramoa, A.S. (1998). Suppression of NMDA receptor function using antisense DNA block ocular dominance plasticity while preserving visual responses. *J. Neurophysiol.* **80**, 1021–1032.

Roberts, E.B., and Ramoa, A.S. (1999). Enhanced NR2A subunit expression and decreased NMDA receptor decay time at the onset of ocular dominance plasticity in the ferret. *J. Neurophysiol.* **81**, 2587–2591.

Rubenstein, J.L., and Merzenich, M.M. (2003). Model of autism: increased ratio of excitation/inhibition in key neural systems. *Genes Brain Behav.* **2**, 255–267.

Salinas, E., and Sejnowski, T.J. (2000). Impact of correlated synaptic input on output firing rate and variability in simple neuronal models. *J. Neurosci.* **20**, 6193–6209.

Samsonovich, A.V., and Ascoli, G.A. (2006). Morphological homeostasis in cortical dendrites. *Proc. Natl. Acad. Sci. USA* **103**, 1569–1574.

Sato, M., and Stryker, M.P. (2008). Distinctive features of adult ocular dominance plasticity. *J. Neurosci.* **28**, 10278–10286.

Sawtell, N.B., Frenkel, M.Y., Philpot, B.D., Nakazawa, K., Tonegawa, S., and Bear, M.F. (2003). NMDA receptor-dependent ocular dominance plasticity in adult visual cortex. *Neuron.* **38**, 977–985.

Schlaggar, B.L., Fox, K., and O'Leary, D.D. (1993). Postsynaptic control of plasticity in developing somatosensory cortex. *Nature* **364**, 623–626.

Scholl, B., and Wehr, M. (2008). Disruption of balanced cortical excitation and inhibition by acoustic trauma. *J. Neurophysiol.* **100**, 646–656.

Schubert, D., Kotter, R., Luhmann, H.J., and Staiger, J.F. (2006). Morphology, electrophysiology and functional input connectivity of pyramidal neurons characterizes a genuine layer va in the primary somatosensory cortex. *Cereb. Cortex.* **16**, 223–236.

Schubert, D., Kotter, R., Zilles, K., Luhmann, H.J., and Staiger, J.F. (2003). Cell type-specific circuits of cortical layer IV spiny neurons. *J. Neurosci.* **23**, 2961–2970.

Seeburg, P.H., Wisden, W., Verdoorn, T.A., Pritchett, D.B., Werner, P., Herb, A., Luddens, H., Sprengel, R., and Sakmann, B. (1990). The GABAA receptor family: molecular and functional diversity. *Cold Spring Harb. Symp. Quant. Biol.* **55**, 29–40.

Shadlen, M.N., and Newsome, W.T. (1998). The variable discharge of cortical neurons: implications for connectivity, computation, and information coding. *J. Neurosci.* **18**, 3870–3896.

Shadlen, M.N., and Newsome, W.T. (1994). Noise, neural codes and cortical organization. *Curr. Opin. Neurobiol* **4**, 569–579.

Sheng, M., Cummings, J., Roldan, L.A., Jan, Y.N., and Jan, L.Y. (1994). Changing subunit composition of heteromeric NMDA receptors during development of rat cortex. *Nature* **368**, 144–147.

Shepherd, G.M., Pologruto, T.A., and Svoboda, K. (2003). Circuit analysis of experience-dependent plasticity in the developing rat barrel cortex. *Neuron.* **38**, 277–289.

Shepherd, G.M., Stepanyants, A., Bureau, I., Chklovskii, D., and Svoboda, K. (2005). Geometric and functional organization of cortical circuits. *Nat. Neurosci.* **8**, 782–790.

Shepherd, G.M., and Svoboda, K. (2005). Laminar and columnar organization of ascending excitatory projections to layer 2/3 pyramidal neurons in rat barrel cortex. *J. Neurosci.* **25**, 5670–5679.

Shoykhet, M., Land, P.W., and Simons, D.J. (2005). Whisker trimming begun at birth or on postnatal day 12 affects excitatory and inhibitory receptive fields of layer IV barrel neurons. *J. Neurophysiol.* **94**, 3987–3995.

Shu, Y., Hasenstaub, A., and McCormick, D.A. (2003). Turning on and off recurrent balanced cortical activity. *Nature* **423**, 288–293.

Simons, D.J. (1978). Response properties of vibrissa units in rat SI somatosensory neocortex. *J. Neurophysiol* **41**, 798–820.

Simons, D.J., and Land, P.W. (1987). Early experience of tactile stimulation influences organization of somatic sensory cortex. *Nature* **326**, 694–697.

Sjostrom, P.J., Turrigiano, G.G., and Nelson, S.B. (2003). Neocortical LTD via coincident activation of presynaptic NMDA and cannabinoid receptors. *Neuron* **39**, 641–654.

Skibinska, A., Glazewski, S., Fox, K., and Kossut, M. (2000). Age-dependent response of the mouse barrel cortex to sensory deprivation: a 2-deoxyglucose study. *Exp. Brain Res.* **132**, 134–138.

Soltesz, I., and Staley, K. (2006). High times for memory: cannabis disrupts temporal coordination among hippocampal neurons. *Nat. Neurosci.* **9**, 1461–1463.

Somogyi, P., and Klausberger, T. (2005). Defined types of cortical interneurone structure space and spike timing in the hippocampus. *J. Physiol.* **562**, 9–26.

Somogyi, P., Tamas, G., Lujan, R., and Buhl, E.H. (1998). Salient features of synaptic organisation in the cerebral cortex. *Brain Res. Brain Res. Rev.* **26**, 113–135.

Sperk, G. (1994). Kainic acid seizures in the rat. *Prog. Neurobiol.* **42**, 1–32.

Staiger, J.F., Flagmeyer, I., Schubert, D., Zilles, K., Kotter, R., and Luhmann, H.J. (2004). Functional diversity of layer IV spiny neurons in rat somatosensory cortex: quantitative morphology of electrophysiologically characterized and biocytin labeled cells. *Cereb. Cortex.* **14**, 690–701.

Stern, E.A., Maravall, M., and Svoboda, K. (2001). Rapid development and plasticity of layer 2/3 maps in rat barrel cortex *in vivo*. *Neuron* **31**, 305–315.

Sun, Q.Q., Huguenard, J.R., and Prince, D.A. (2006). Barrel cortex microcircuits: thalamocortical feedforward inhibition in spiny stellate cells is mediated by a small number of fast-spiking interneurons. *J. Neurosci.* **26**, 1219–1230.

Szentagothai, J. (1978). The Ferrier Lecture, 1977 The neuron network of the cerebral cortex: a functional interpretation. *Proc. R. Soc. Lond. B. Biol. Sci.* **201**, 219–248.

Tabuchi, K., Blundell, J., Etherton, M.R., Hammer, R.E., Liu, X., Powell, C.M., and Sudhof, T.C. (2007). A neuroligin-3 mutation implicated in autism increases inhibitory synaptic transmission in mice. *Science* **318**, 71–76.

Tamas, G., Buhl, E.H., and Somogyi, P. (1997). Fast IPSPs elicited via multiple synaptic release sites by different types of GABAergic neurone in the cat visual cortex. *J. Physiol.* **500**(Pt 3); 715–738.

Tamas, G., Lorincz, A., Simon, A., and Szabadics, J. (2003). Identified sources and targets of slow inhibition in the neocortex. *Science* **299**, 1902–1905.

Tan, A.Y., Zhang, L.I., Merzenich, M.M., and Schreiner, C.E. (2004). Tone-evoked excitatory and inhibitory synaptic conductances of primary auditory cortex neurons. *J. Neurophysiol* **92**, 630–643.

Thiagarajan, T.C., Piedras-Renteria, E.S., and Tsien, R.W. (2002). alpha- and betaCaMKII Inverse regulation by neuronal activity and opposing effects on synaptic strength. *Neuron* **36**, 1103–1114.

Thompson, S.M., Fortunato, C., McKinney, R.A., Muller, M., and Gahwiler, B.H. (1996). Mechanisms underlying the neuropathological consequences of epileptic activity in the rat hippocampus *in vivo*. *J. Comp. Neurol.* **372**, 515–528.

Thomson, A.M., West, D.C., Hahn, J., and Deuchars, J. (1996). Single axon IPSPs elicited in pyramidal cells by three classes of interneurones in slices of rat neocortex. *J. Physiol.* **496**(Pt 1); 81–102.

Todd, P.K., Malter, J.S., and Mack, K.J. (2003). Whisker stimulation-dependent translation of FMRP in the barrel cortex requires activation of type I metabotropic glutamate receptors. *Brain Res. Mol. Brain Res* **110**, 267–278.

Toyoda, H., Zhao, M.G., and Zhuo, M. (2005). Roles of NMDA receptor NR2A and NR2B subtypes for long-term depression in the anterior cingulate cortex. *Eur. J. Neurosci.* **22**, 485–494.

Turrigiano, G. (2007). Homeostatic signaling: the positive side of negative feedback. *Curr. Opin. Neurobiol* **17**, 318–324.

Turrigiano, G.G., Leslie, K.R., Desai, N.S., Rutherford, L.C., and Nelson, S.B. (1998). Activity-dependent scaling of quantal amplitude in neocortical neurons. *Nature* **391**, 892–896.

Turrigiano, G.G., and Nelson, S.B. (2004). Homeostatic plasticity in the developing nervous system. *Nat. Rev. Neurosci.* **5**, 97–107.

Unnerstall, J.R., Kuhar, M.J., Niehoff, D.L., and Palacios, J.M. (1981). Benzodiazepine receptors are coupled to a subpopulation of gamma-aminobutyric acid (GABA) receptors: evidence from a quantitative autoradiographic study. *J. Pharmacol Exp. Ther.* **218**, 797–804.

Unwin, N. (1989). The structure of ion channels in membranes of excitable cells. *Neuron* **3**, 665–676.

Van der Loos, H., and Woolsey, T.A. (1973). Somatosensory cortex: structural alterations following early injury to sense organs. *Science* **179**, 395–398.

van, V.C., and Sompolinsky, H. (1996). Chaos in neuronal networks with balanced excitatory and inhibitory activity. *Science* **274**, 1724–1726.

Varga, C., Sik, A., Lavallee, P., and Deschenes, M. (2002). Dendroarchitecture of relay cells in thalamic barreloids: a substrate for cross-whisker modulation. *J. Neurosci.* **22**, 6186–6194.

Vicini, S., Wang, J.F., Li, J.H., Zhu, W.J., Wang, Y.H., Luo, J.H., Wolfe, B.B., and Grayson, D.R. (1998). Functional and pharmacological differences between recombinant N-methyl-D-aspartate receptors. *J. Neurophysiol* **79**, 555–566.

Wallace, D.J., and Sakmann, B. (2008). Plasticity of representational maps in somatosensory cortex observed by *in vivo* voltage-sensitive dye imaging. *Cereb. Cortex* **18**, 1361–1373.

Watanabe, M., Inoue, Y., Sakimura, K., and Mishina, M. (1992). Developmental changes in distribution of NMDA receptor channel subunit mRNAs. *Neuroreport* **3**, 1138–1140.

Wehr, M., and Zador, A.M. (2005). Synaptic mechanisms of forward suppression in rat auditory cortex. *Neuron* **47**, 437–445.

Wehr, M., and Zador, A.M. (2003). Balanced inhibition underlies tuning and sharpens spike timing in auditory cortex. *Nature* **426**, 442–446.

Weitlauf, C., Honse, Y., Auberson, Y.P., Mishina, M., Lovinger, D.M., and Winder, D.G. (2005). Activation of NR2A-containing NMDA receptors is not obligatory for NMDA receptor-dependent long-term potentiation. *J. Neurosci.* **25**, 8386–8390.

Welker, C. (1976). Receptive fields of barrels in the somatosensory neocortex of the rat. *J. Comp. Neurol* **166**, 173–189.

Welker, C. (1971). Microelectrode delineation of fine grain somatotopic organization of (SmI) cerebral neocortex in albino rat. *Brain Res.* **26**, 259–275.

White, E.L., and Rock, M.P. (1981). A comparison of thalamocortical and other synaptic inputs to dendrites of two non-spiny neurons in a single barrel of mouse SmI cortex. *J. Comp. Neurol* **195**, 265–277.

Wierenga, C.J., Ibata, K., and Turrigiano, G.G. (2005). Postsynaptic expression of homeostatic plasticity at neocortical synapses. *J. Neurosci.* **25**, 2895–2905.

Wilent, W.B., and Contreras, D. (2004). Synaptic responses to whisker deflections in rat barrel cortex as a function of cortical layer and stimulus intensity. *J. Neurosci.* **24**, 3985–3998.

Wilent, W.B., and Contreras, D. (2005). Stimulus-dependent changes in spike threshold enhance feature selectivity in rat barrel cortex neurons. *J. Neurosci.* **25**, 2983–2991.

Wilson, N.R., Ty, M.T., Ingber, D.E., Sur, M., and Liu, G. (2007). Synaptic reorganization in scaled networks of controlled size. *J. Neurosci.* **27**, 13581–13589.

Wisden, W., Laurie, D.J., Monyer, H., and Seeburg, P.H. (1992). The distribution of 13 GABAA receptor subunit mRNAs in the rat brain I. Telencephalon, diencephalon, mesencephalon. *J. Neurosci.* **12**, 1040–1062.

Wisden, W., and Seeburg, P.H. (1992). GABAA receptor channels: from subunits to functional entities. *Curr. Opin. Neurobiol* **2**, 263–269.

Wong, R.O., and Ghosh, A. (2002). Activity-dependent regulation of dendritic growth and patterning. *Nat. Rev. Neurosci.* **3**, 803–812.

Woolsey, T.A., and Van der Loos, H. (1970). The structural organization of layer IV in the somatosensory region (SI) of mouse cerebral cortex The description of a cortical field composed of discrete cytoarchitectonic units. *Brain Res.* **17**, 205–242.

Woolsey, T.A., and Wann, J.R. (1976). Areal changes in mouse cortical barrels following vibrissal damage at different postnatal ages. *J. Comp. Neurol* **170**, 53–66.

Woolsey, T.A., Welker, C., and Schwartz, R.H. (1975). Comparative anatomical studies of the SmL face cortex with special reference to the occurrence of "barrels" in layer IV. *J. Comp. Neurol* **164**, 79–94.

Yamahachi, H., Marik, S.A., McManus, J.N., Denk, W., and Gilbert, C.D. (2009). Rapid axonal sprouting and pruning accompany functional reorganization in primary visual cortex. *Neuron* **64**, 719–729.

Young III, W.S., Niehoff, D., Kuhar, M.J., Beer, B., and Lippa, A.S. (1981). Multiple benzodiazepine receptor localization by light microscopic radiohistochemistry. *J. Pharmacol Exp. Ther.* **216**, 425–430.

Yuste, R., and Katz, L.C. (1991). Control of postsynaptic Ca2+ influx in developing neocortex by excitatory and inhibitory neurotransmitters. *Neuron* **6**, 333–344.

Zhang, L.I., Tan, A.Y., Schreiner, C.E., and Merzenich, M.M. (2003). Topography and synaptic shaping of direction selectivity in primary auditory cortex. *Nature* **424**, 201–205.

Zhang, Z., and Bodznick, D. (2010). The importance of N-methyl-D-aspartate (NMDA) receptors in subtraction of electrosensory reafference in the dorsal nucleus of skates. *J. Exp. Biol.* **213**, 2700–2709.

Zhang, Z., and Sun, Q.Q. (2011). Development of NMDA NR2 subunits and their roles in critical period maturation of neocortical gabaergic interneurons. *Dev. Neurobiol.* **71**(3); 221–245.

Zhang, Z., Jiao, Y.Y., and Sun, Q.Q. (2011). Developmental maturation of excitation and inhibition balance in principal neurons across four layers of somatosensory cortex. *Neuroscience* **174**, 10–25.

Zhu, J.J., and Connors, B.W. (1999). Intrinsic firing patterns and whisker-evoked synaptic responses of neurons in the rat barrel cortex. *J. Neurophysiol* **81**, 1171–1183.

Subject Index

D

E

O

Q

R

CONTENTS OF RECENT VOLUMES

Volume 39

Volume 40

Volume 41

Volume 42

Volume 43

Volume 44

Volume 45

Volume 46

Volume 47

Volume 48

Volume 49

Volume 50

Volume 51

Volume 52

Volume 53

Volume 54

Volume 55

Volume 60

Volume 61

Volume 62

Volume 63

Volume 64

Volume 65

Volume 66

Volume 67

Volume 68

Volume 69

Volume 70

Volume 71

Volume 72

Volume 73

Volume 74

Volume 75

Volume 76

Volume 77

Volume 78

Volume 79

Volume 80

Volume 81

Volume 82

Volume 83

Volume 84

Volume 85

Volume 86

Volume 87

Volume 88

Volume 89

Volume 90

Volume 91

Volume 92

Volume 93

Volume 94

Volume 95

Volume 96

FSC
www.fsc.org
MIX
Papier | Fördert
gute Waldnutzung
FSC® C083411

Kolibri 360 GmbH
Ferdinand-Jühlke-Straße 7
99095 Erfurt, Deutschland
produktsicherheit@kolibri360.de